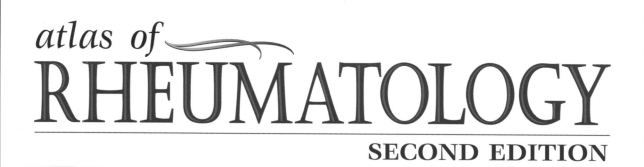

# atlas of RHEUMATOLOGY

## SECOND EDITION

*editor*

## Gene G. Hunder, MD

Professor of Medicine
Mayo Medical School
Mayo Clinic
Rochester, Minnesota

**With 12 contributors**

Developed by Current Medicine, Inc., Philadelphia

## Current Medicine, Inc.

400 Market Street
Suite 700
Philadelphia, PA 19106

Director, Product Development . . . . . *Charles Field*
Editorial Supervisor. . . . . . . . . . . . . . *Fran Klass*
Development Editor . . . . . . . . . . . . . *Bill Edelman*
Editorial Assistant. . . . . . . . . . . . . . . *AnnMarie D'Ortona*
Art and Illustrator Director . . . . . . . . *Wendy Vetter*
Design and Layout . . . . . . . . . . . . . . *Jennifer Knight*
Illustrators . . . . . . . . . . . . . . . . . . . . . *Ann Saydlowski, Larry Ward, Anne Rains*
Production Director . . . . . . . . . . . . . . *Lori Holland*
Assistant Production Manager . . . . . *Simon Dickey*
Indexer. . . . . . . . . . . . . . . . . . . . . . . . *Dorothy Hoffman*

Atlas of rheumatology / edited by Gene G. Hunder ; with 12
   contributors.
      p.  cm.
  Includes bibliographical references and index.
  ISBN 1-57340-171-4  (alk. paper)
   1. Rheumatism—Atlases.   2. Arthritis—Atlases 3. Connective
tissues—Diseases—Atlases.    I. Hunder, Gene G.
   [DNLM: 1. Rheumatic Diseases—atlases.    WE 17 A88063343 1998]
RC927.A856    2000
616.7'23—dc21
DNLM/DLC                                    01-43307
for Library of Congress                     CIP

ISBN: 1-57340-171-4

Printed in Italy by Offset Print Veneta S.r.l.
10 9 8 7 6 5 4 3 2 1

Arthritis and its related musculoskeletal disorders constitute the most common chronic illnesses in the United States. These conditions adversely affect the quality of life of those who are struck by them, require increased use of health care resources, and, because they are the leading cause of disability in the United States, have a significant impact on the national economy. Physicians and other health care workers in many disciplines have been involved in the care and study of patients with these diseases. As a result, our understanding of and ability to treat these diseases have improved continuously.

This *Atlas of Rheumatology* is designed to help clinicians learn about this group of diseases and develop an understanding of their possible causes, clinical features, laboratory findings, and treatments, using an attractive pictorial format. Because more than 100 separate types of arthritis have been described, unfortunately all could not be included. The illustrations shown in the *Atlas* have been carefully selected by recognized experts, who served as authors of the eight chapters, to provide the reader with the essential information needed to get a clear picture of these important diseases. For their successful efforts I am deeply grateful. I am also indebted to editorial workers who have maintained high standards to create a clear, attractive final product.

**Gene G. Hunder, MD**
*Rochester, Minnesota*

CHAPTER 1
_____

## Rheumatoid Arthritis, Juvenile Rheumatoid Arthritis, and Related Conditions
Eric L. Matteson

CHAPTER 2
_____

## Osteoarthritis and Crystal–Associated Synovitis
Stephen L. Myers

CHAPTER 3
_____

## Systemic Lupus Erythematosus, Antiphospholid Syndrome, Scleroderma, and Inflammatory Myopathies
Graham R.V. Hughes and Munther A. Khamashta

CHAPTER 4
_____

## Vasculitides
Loïc Guillevin

**Kenneth T. Calamia, MD**
Assistant Professor of Medicine
Mayo Medical School
Mayo Clinic Jacksonville
Jacksonville, Florida

**Marc D. Cohen, MD**
Associate Professor of Medicine
Mayo Medical School
Mayo Clinic Jacksonville
Jacksonville, Florida

**Loïc Guillevin, MD**
Professor
Internal Medicine
University of Paris, North
Bobigny, France

**Graham R.V. Hughes, MD**
Head of Lupus Research Unit
St. Thomas' Hospital
London, England

**Munther A. Khamashta, MD**
Senior Lecturer
Guy's and St. Thomas' Medical and
  Dental School
London, England

**Muhammed Asim Khan, MD**
Professor
Department of Medicine
Division of Rheumatology
MetroHealth Medical Center
Cleveland, Ohio

**Marcia Ko, MD**
Resident
University of Arizona
Tucson, Arizona

**Michael J. Maricic, MD**
Associate Professor
Department of Medicine
University of Arizona
Tucson, Arizona

**Eric L. Matteson, MD**
Associate Professor
Department of Internal Medicine
Division of Rheumatology
Mayo Medical School
Rochester, Minnesota

**David M. Menke, MD**
Assistant Professor of Pathology
Mayo Medical School
Mayo Clinic Jacksonville
Jacksonville, Florida

**Stephen L. Myers, MD**
Professor
Department of Medicine
Indiana University
Indianapolis, Indiana

**Leonard Sigal, MD**
Associate Professor
Departments of Medicine and Pediatrics
Robert Wood Johnson Medical School
New Brunswick, New Jersey

# 1

# Rheumatoid Arthritis, Juvenile Rheumatoid Arthritis, and Related Conditions

Rheumatoid arthritis is a chronic systemic inflammatory disease characterized by joint destruction. It is the most common inflammatory arthritis, affecting approximately 1% of the world's population [1]. The actual incidence varies by race and geographic location, and appears to be somewhat lower in African blacks and among Chinese, and as high as 5% among the Pima Indians of North America.

The cause of rheumatoid arthritis is unknown. There is strong evidence that the disease occurs in genetically predisposed individuals, probably after exposure to an as yet unknown antigen(s). There are probably multiple genetic factors involved. In white populations, this genetic predisposition appears to be associated with major histocompatibility complex antigens of the human lymphocyte antigen (HLA-D) locus. The B lymphocyte alloantigen HLA-DR4 is present in about 70% of patients with rheumatoid arthritis, compared with 28% of controls (relative risk of four- to five-fold) [2]. Gender plays a clear role, as females are affected more often than males in a ratio of about 3:1. Among the numerous agents implicated in the pathoetiology of rheumatoid arthritis are viruses such as Epstein-Barr virus and parvovirus, and bacteria including mycobacteria. These agents may promote either directly, through molecular mimicry, or indirectly through other pathways. Other autoimmune processes have also been implicated in establishing and perpetuating the disease [3].

Over half of patients with rheumatoid arthritis have insidious onset of articular symptoms over a period of several weeks to months. In one third of patients, the onset is rapid, occurring over a few days to weeks [4]. The majority of patients have oligoarthritis (involvement of <6 joints) at the outset, which is often asymmetric; acute monoarticular arthritis is uncommon as the initial disease manifestation. About 10% to 20% of patients may have an initial flare followed by a prolonged remission [5].

The systemic manifestations of rheumatoid arthritis including Felty's syndrome are typically seen in patients who have high titers of rheumatoid factor, rheumatoid nodules, and severe articular disease. Some of the extra-articular manifestations, such as vasculitis, neurologic, cervical spine, and tracheolaryngeal involvement can be life threatening.

The majority of patients with rheumatoid arthritis have a polycyclic articular course. Although the disease expression is variable, most patients eventually develop destructive arthritis which in some patients causes only mild impairment, but in others is severely disabling. In most patients, the extent of disability is determined within the first several years of disease, with slow worsening of functional capacity thereafter. After 12 years of disease, only 17% of patients are without disability, and 16% are completely disabled [6]. Matched-survivorship may be as low as 50% of that of a normal control population [7]. This understanding of the natural history emphasizes the need for early disease recognition. Modern therapeutic interventions can limit joint damage and disability, and improve survival chances.

Sjögren's syndrome is the second most common rheumatic disease after rheumatoid arthritis [8]. Its leading clinical manifestations are keratoconjunctivitis sicca and xerostomia; about 50% of patients with primary Sjögren's syndrome develop systemic manifestations including arthritis. Raynaud's phenomenon, lymphadenopathy, and lung involvement, among others [8]. Adult Still's disease is a form of polyarthritis with systemic manifestations seen in systemic juvenile rheumatoid arthritis. It is relatively rare, as is remitting seronegative symmetric synovitis with pitting edema (so-called RS3PE syndrome), another form of adult-onset polyarthritis which can occur in isolation or associated with polymyalgia rheumatica, hematopoietic malignancies, or even rheumatoid arthritis.

Juvenile rheumatoid arthritis also widely known as juvenile chronic arthritis, is a term denoting several chronic arthritic conditions of childhood, the cause(s) of which is unknown. There is no clear genetic predisposition, except in patients with pauciarticuar disease or spondyloarthropathies, which may be associated with HLA-B27 [9]. Subtypes of juvenile rheumatoid arthritis include systemic-onset disease (10%), with typical-fever pattern and rash, but also lymphadenopathy, hepatosplenomegaly, and pericardial or pleural effusion; polyarticular onset (40%); and pauciarticular onset (50%), often associated with iridocyclitis.

## Diagnostic Criteria

### AMERICAN RHEUMATISM ASSOCIATION REVISED CRITERIA FOR THE DIAGNOSIS OF RHEUMATOID ARTHRITIS

| | |
|---|---|
| 1. Morning stiffness | Morning stiffness in and around the joints, lasting at least 1 h before maximal improvement |
| 2. Arthritis of 3 or more joint areas | At least 3 joint areas (out of 14 possible areas; right or left proximal interphalangeal, metacarpophalangeal, wrist, elbow, ankle, metatarsophalangeal joints); simultaneously have had soft tissue swelling or fluid (not bony overgrowth alone) as observed by a physician |
| 3. Arthritis of hand joints | At least 1 area swollen (as defined above) in a wrist, metacarpophalangeal, or proximal interphalangeal joint |
| 4. Symmetric arthritis | Simultaneous involvement of the same joint areas (as defined in criterion 2) on both sides of the body (bilateral involvement of proximal interphalangeals, metacarpophalangeals, or metatarsophalangeals, without absolute symmetry is acceptable) |
| 5. Rheumatoid nodules | Subcutaneous nodules over bony prominences or extensor surfaces, or in juxta-articular regions as observed by a physician |
| 6. Serum rheumatoid factor | Demonstration of abnormal amounts of serum rheumatoid factor by any method for which the result has been positive in less than 5% of normal control subjects |
| 7. Radiographic changes | Radiographic changes typical of rheumatoid arthritis on posteroanterior hand and wrist radiographs, which must include erosions or unequivocal bony decalcification localized in, or most marked adjacent to, the involved joints (osteoarthritis changes alone do not qualify) |

**FIGURE 1-1.** The 1987 American Rheumatism Association Revised Criteria for the Classification of Rheumatoid Arthritis. Patients having at least four of these seven criteria (1 to 4 for at least 6 weeks) can be classified as having rheumatoid arthritis. These criteria distinguish rheumatoid arthritis from other forms of arthritis with a specificity of 89% and a sensitivity of about 94%. (*From* Arnett *et al.* [10]; with permission.)

### THE DIFFERENTIAL DIAGNOSIS OF POLYARTHRITIS

**Spondyloarthropathies**

Ankylosing spondylitis
Reiter's syndrome
Inflammatory bowel disease
Behçet's syndrome
Enteric infections, especially *Yersinia,*
 *Salmonella, Shigella, Campylobacter jejuni*
Whipple's disease
Psoriatic arthritis

**Infectious**

Bacterial endocarditis
HIV infection
Bacterial sepsis
Viral syndromes, especially hepatitis B,
 parvovirus, rubella, Epstein-Barr, others
Acute rheumatic fever
Lyme disease
Gonococcal arthritis

**Metabolic and Endocrine Disorders**

Gout
Pseudogout (Calcium pyrophosphate dihydrate deposition disease)
Hemochromatosis
Hemoglobinopathies
Hyper- and hypothyroidism
Hyperlipoproteinemia
Hypertrophic osteoarthropathy

**Connective Tissue Syndromes**

Systemic lupus erythematosus
Dermatomyositis/polymyositis
Mixed connective tissue disease
Scleroderma

**Other**

Still's disease
Relapsing polychondritis
Familial Mediterranean fever
Intermittent hydrarthrosis
Hypereosinophilic syndrome
Malignancy
Osteoarthritis
Sarcoidosis
Multicentric reticulohistiocytosis
Vasculitis
Polymyalgia rheumatica and giant cell arteritis
Heritable polyarthropathies

**FIGURE 1-2.** Differential diagnosis of polyarthritis. The differential diagnosis of polyarthritis, arthritis of six or more joints, is extensive. A careful history, persistence of symmetric joint swelling, and the typical laboratory and radiographic features aid in establishing an accurate diagnosis of rheumatoid arthritis. HIV—human immunodeficiency virus.

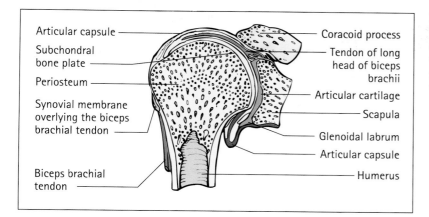

**FIGURE 1-3.** Diagram of a diarthrodial joint—the glenohumeral articulation. Diarthrodial joints have articular surfaces of cartilage that are surrounded by a fibrous capsule. The articular capsule is adjoined to tendons, periosteum, ligaments, and fascia. The synovium covers the internal aspect of the capsule and the intercapsular periosteum, but not the articular surface itself.

Articular capsule
Subchondral bone plate
Periosteum
Synovial membrane overlying the biceps brachial tendon
Biceps brachial tendon
Coracoid process
Tendon of long head of biceps brachii
Articular cartilage
Scapula
Glenoidal labrum
Articular capsule
Humerus

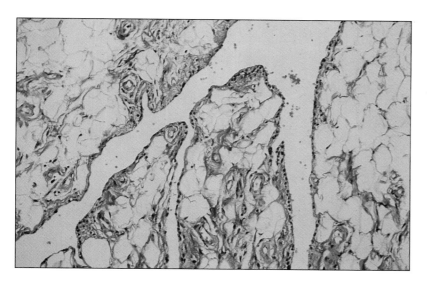

**FIGURE 1-4.** Histology of normal articular synovium. The normal synovial membrane is composed of a flat layer, usually one or two cells thick, overlying the subsynovial stroma. Unlike other membranes, the cells of the synovial lining do not contain true epithelial tissue or basement membranes. Synovial blood vessels course throughout the stroma. There are two major types of synoviocytes: type A is macrophage-like, and type B is fibroblast-like (hematoxylin and eosin, medium power) [3]. (*Courtesy of* Thomas A. Gaffey, MD.)

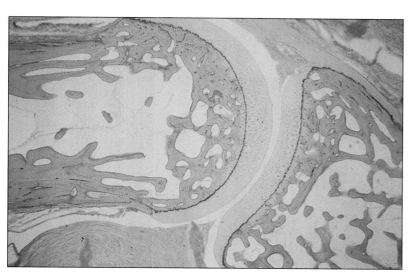

**FIGURE 1-5.** Histology of a normal diarthrodial joint. Sagital section through a normal proximal interphalangeal joint. The bone structure is intact, as is the articular cartilage and joint capsule. A thin layer of synovium is visible in the internal aspect of the capsule (hematoxylin and eosin, low power) [11]. (*Courtesy of* Thomas A. Gaffey, MD.)

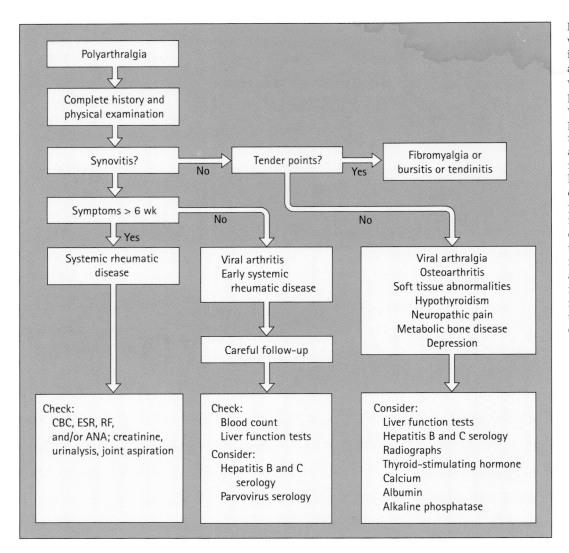

FIGURE 1-6. Initial evaluation of the patient with polyarthritis. A careful history and physical examination are essential. Disease features and time course help to guide the initial workup and management. Polyarthritis persisting for more than 6 weeks is consistent with rheumatoid arthritis; viral syndromes with polyarthritis are usually self-limited. Arthralgias may be accompanied by muscle pain. In the absence of true joint swelling, proximal weakness and elevated creatine phosphokinase levels suggest myositis. Patients over 50 years of age with arthralgias and myalgias may have polymyalgia rheumatica. Initial laboratory tests include a complete blood count (CBC), erythrocyte sedimentation rate (WEST), and rheumatoid factor (RF) among others. A joint aspiration may be helpful to demonstrate inflammation and rule out infection and crystalline diseases in the appropriate clinical setting. ANA—antinuclear antibodies; ESR—erythrocyte sedimentation rate. (*Adapted from* Ad Hoc Committee on Clinical Guidelines [11]; with permission.)

---

## *Epidemiology*

### EPIDEMIOLOGY OF RHEUMATOID ARTHRITIS

| | |
|---|---|
| Gender | Female–male ratio is 3:1 |
| Incidence | Annually 25–30 new cases /100,000 population |
| Prevalence | Occurs in 1% of the adult population of North America and Europe |
| | The prevalence in males over 65 years of age is about 1.9%, and for females about 5.0% |
| Genetics | Greatest risk in persons who are HLA-DR4 and HLA-DR1 positive |
| Pattern age of onset | Usually polyarticular, affecting the wrist, metacarpophalangeal and proximal interphalangeal joints. At onset 20% of patients have monoarticular disease, whereas 80% have multiple (2 or more) joints involved. |
| Peak age of onset | Between about 20–50 years of age |

FIGURE 1-7. Epidemiology of rheumatoid arthritis. Rheumatoid arthritis affects approximately 1% to 2% of the adult population worldwide. The incidence of rheumatoid arthritis is approximately 30 cases per 100,000 person years for women between the ages of 18 and 64. Genetic factors play a role; monozygotic twins have an 11-fold increase in risk compared with dizygotic twins, although penetrance is low (34% in monozygotic, 3% in dizygotic twins) [12]. There are probably several genetic loci predisposing to the development of rheumatoid arthritis, including the class II major histocompatibility complex alleles DR4. These alleles likely regulate the immune response to a putative environmental agent important in the etiology of the disease.

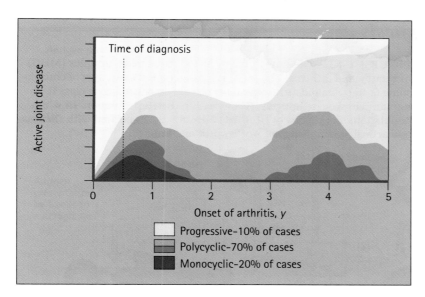

**FIGURE 1-8.** Clinical course of joint disease in rheumatoid arthritis. The articular disease of rheumatoid arthritis is usually polycyclic and progressive. However, in about 20% it is monocyclic, with remission for at least 1 year after the onset. In a minority of patients it is relentlessly active with an ever-increasing number of joints involved and severity of joint involvement with the passing years. Predictors of aggressive, erosive disease include positive rheumatoid factor, persistent polyarticular disease, presence of rheumatoid nodules and other extraarticular disease manifestations, being a young woman, positive p-ANCA, HLA-DR4. (*Adapted from* Masi AT and coworkers [13]; with permission.)

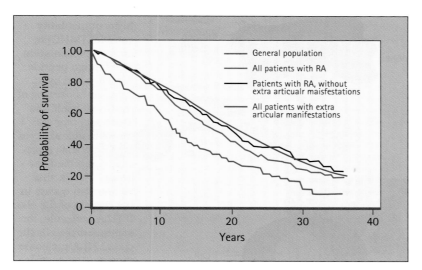

**FIGURE 1-9.** Mortality in rheumatoid arthritis is related to disease severity and comorbid factors. The median age at death is about 4 years younger than in control populations, as seen in Figure 1-9 [14]. Predictors of outcome include gender and age of onset (younger patients are at higher risk of poor outcome), systemic disease (patients with extraarticular disease, particularly vasculitis, have a shortened life expectancy, compared with those who do not), radiographic evidence of erosions, rheumatoid factor seropositivity, presence of rheumatoid nodules, disease duration of greater than 5 years before treatment, functional disability within 1 year of onset, presence of several comorbidities, and socioeconomic status, especially poor educational achievement [15].

---

### STEINBROCKER FUNCTIONAL CLASSIFICATION OF RHEUMATOID ARTHRITIS

| | |
|---|---|
| Class I | No limitations |
| Class II | Function is adequate for normal activities despite joint discomfort or limitation of motion |
| Class III | Function is inadequate for most self care and vocational activities |
| Class IV | Patient is largely or wholly unable to manage self-care and may be restricted to a wheelchair or bed |

**FIGURE 1-10.** Steinbrocker functional classification of rheumatoid arthritis. Most patients with active rheumatoid arthritis fall into class II or III of the Steinbrocker classification. Functional classification is an important indicator of the impact of the disease on the patient's sense of well being and is useful in planning for future health needs, including joint surgery. (*From* Steinbrocker and coworkers [16].)

### CRITERIA FOR REMISSION OF RHEUMATOID ARTHRITIS

For a patient to be considered to be in clinical remission, at least five of the following must be present for at least 2 consecutive months:

1. Morning stiffness of not more than 15 min
2. No fatigue
3. No joint pain
4. No joint tenderness or pain on motion
5. No soft tissue swelling in joints or tendon sheaths
6. Westergren erythrocyte sedimentation rate of less than 30 mm/h (females) or 10 mm/h (males)

**FIGURE 1-11.** The American College of Rheumatology criteria for remission of rheumatoid arthritis. Long-term remission is rare, and probably occurs in less than 5% of patients with disease of 5 or more years' duration. Intermittent remission is seen in 10% to 20% of patients who have periods of clinically quiescent disease that are longer than periods of active disease. Most patients (about 75%) have a progressive, erosive, disabling disease course. (*From* Pinals and coworkers [5]; with permission.)

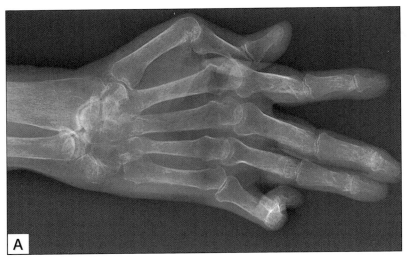

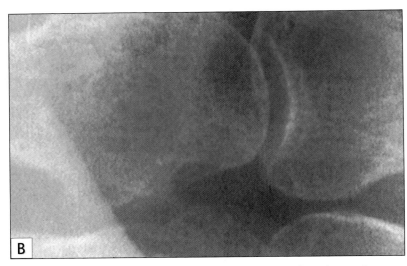

**FIGURE 1-30.** Marginal erosions. Marginal erosions are typical of rheumatoid arthritis, and are evident in this radiograph, especially in the metacarpophalangeal joints (**A**). Extensive erosions affect a number of the proximal interphalangeal joints as well. There is also advanced erosive disease of the carpal bones. Closeup of the marginal erosion from the radial aspect of the second metacarpophalangeal joint (**B**).

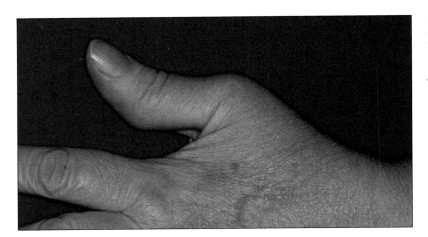

**FIGURE 1-31.** Thumb deformity in rheumatoid arthritis. The typical thumb deformity in rheumatoid arthritis is flexion at the metacarpophalangeal and hyperextension at the proximal interphalangeal joint. Prehension becomes markedly limited, and the proximal interphalangeal joint becomes the pressure-bearing surface. Rheumatoid nodules frequently develop over the volar aspect of the thumb proximal interphalangeal joint. (*Courtesy of* Alan T. Bishop, MD.)

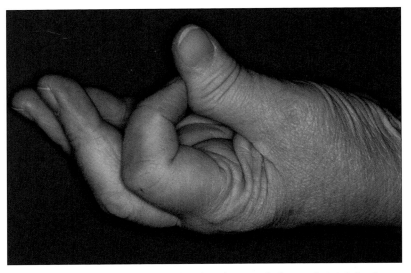

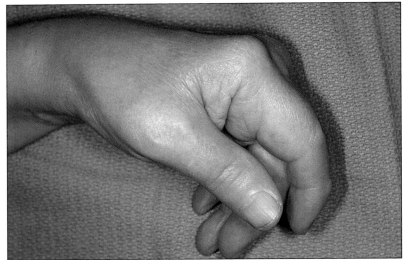

**FIGURE 1-32.** Instability of the thumb interphalangeal (IP) joint in rheumatoid arthritis. Instability of the thumb IP joint is demonstrated by forced lateral deviation by the index finger. The thumb IP joint is flail, and unstable for prehension. (*Courtesy of* Alan T. Bishop, MD.)

**FIGURE 1-33.** Volar subluxation of the metacarpophalangeal joint in rheumatoid arthritis. Subluxation of the index finger is evident. The subluxation initially may be reducible; later it may become fixed and is often associated with ulnar deviation, resulting in a dysfunctional grip. (*Courtesy of* Alan T. Bishop, MD.)

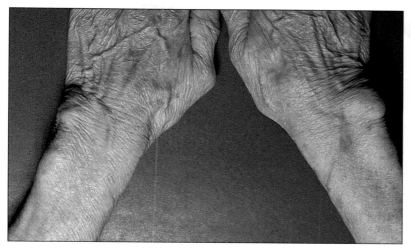

**FIGURE 1-34.** Ulnar styloid prominence in rheumatoid arthritis. Chronic synovitis in the wrists has resulted in carpal ligament laxity, leading to prominence of the ulnar styloid processes. There is profound interosseous muscle wasting, and tenosynovitis of the extensor carpi ulnaris of the left hand.

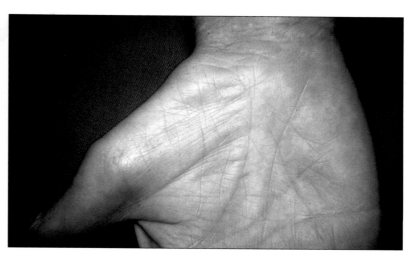

**FIGURE 1-35.** Carpal tunnel syndrome. Synovitis in the wrist can lead to median nerve compression resulting in thenar atrophy, dysesthesias, and weak grip.

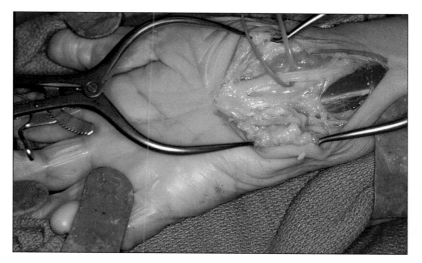

**FIGURE 1-36.** Carpal tunnel release. At carpal tunnel release, the median nerve is looped, the transverse carpal ligament resected, and the hypertrophic synovium excised. (*Courtesy of* Alan T. Bishop, MD.)

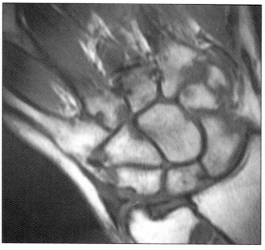

**FIGURE 1-37.** Wrist synovitis—magnetic resonance imaging (MRI). MRI permits detailed study of soft tissue and bones, and can demonstrate the extent of proliferative and erosive disease at an earlier stage and in more detail than conventional radiographic techniques. The T1-weighted image shows multiple erosions in the carpus and distal ulna as well as defined areas of decreased signal. Synovial proliferation is present, especially at the distal carpal row and proximal metacarpophalangeal joint. (*Courtesy of* Richard P. Polisson, MD.)

**FIGURE 1-38.** Nodular tenosynovitis. Several rheumatoid nodules are visible on the exposed hand extensor tendons. There is abundant synovitis, with proliferation and hypervascularity. The nodules may erode into the tendons, leading to their rupture. (*Courtesy of* Thomas A. Gaffey, MD.)

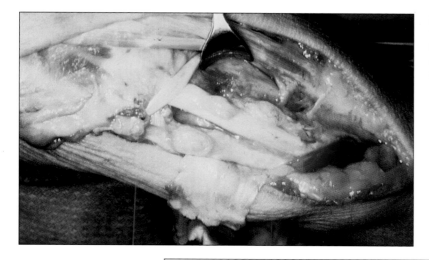

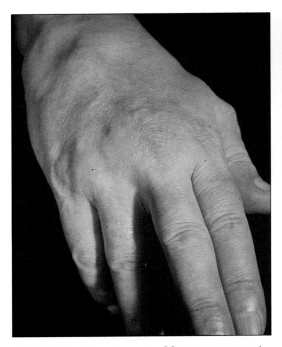

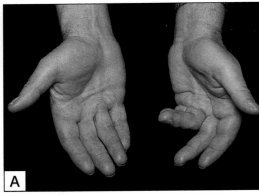

A

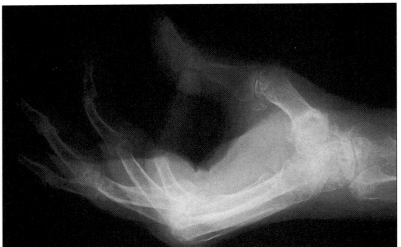

B

**FIGURE 1-39.** Rupture of finger extensors in rheumatoid arthritis. Rupture of the extensors of the fourth and fifth digits is caused by active synovitis, and invasive synovial proliferation. Wrist instability with prominence of the eroded ulnar styloid process can also shear the ulnar tendons.

**FIGURE 1-40.** Stenosing tenosynovitis (trigger finger). **A,** Synovitis of the tendon sheaths can lead to swelling, limitation of motion, and tendon rupture. Stenosing tenosynovitis can lead to "trigger finger," evident in the fourth finger of the left hand. Triggering occurs when the inflamed tenosynovial tissue cannot move through the tendon sheath. Stenosis of the A-1 pulley can be palpated in the palm just proximal to the affected metacarpophalangeal joint. **B,** Stenosing tenosynovitis. Tenosynovitis of the flexor tendon can lead to the trigger finger syndrome. With tenosynovitis, the digit is blocked in the flexed position (*arrow with vertical bar*), making extension difficult or even impossible. If the affected tendon is able to pass through the fibrous tendon sheath, a palpable "pop" may be detected. The action may be painful. The tendon may also be blocked in the extended position (*arrow*). Swelling of the tenosynovium proximal to the stenosed annular ligaments may be palpable in the palm as swelling. (*Courtesy of* Alan T. Bishop, MD.)

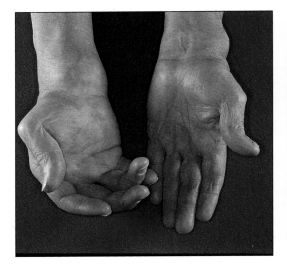

**FIGURE 1-41.** Acute tenosynovitis in rheumatoid arthritis. Massive wrist synovitis and tenosynovitis of the flexor tendons are evident in active disease. Flexion contractures have developed in the left hand, which improved with therapy. Swelling of flexor synovial sheaths is apparent in the right hand proximal to the swollen carpus, especially the flexor carpi radialis.

**FIGURE 1-42.** Metacarpophalangeal arthroplasty. Function and cosmetic appearance resulting from metacarpophalangeal subluxation may be improved by arthroplasty. (*Courtesy of* Alan T. Bishop, MD.)

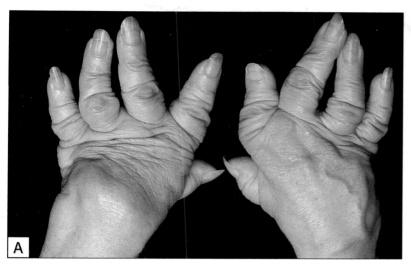

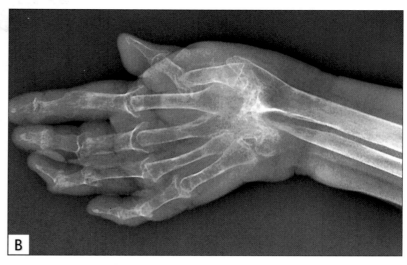

**FIGURE 1-43.** Arthritis mutilans. **A,** Severe long standing rheumatoid arthritis can lead to joint and bony erosion and resorption, with shrinkage of the hand (operetta glass hand). The metacarpophalangeals, carpal bones, proximal interphalangeals, and capsules are destroyed, resulting in extreme joint instability and loss of function. **B,** Radiograph—arthritis mutilans. There is total destruction of the distal radius, ulna and carpal bones, with ankylosis of some of the carpus bones. Resorption of multiple bones of the wrist and phalanges is evident, as is profound osteopenia.

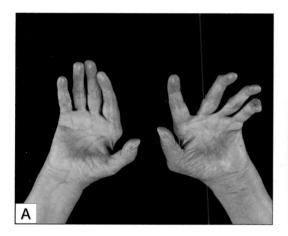

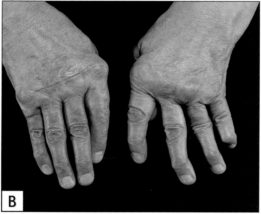

**FIGURE 1-44.** Advanced rheumatoid arthritis of the hands—metacarpophalangeal replacement. Chronic synovitis of the wrists and finger joints in long-standing rheumatoid arthritis is seen. Volar subluxation and ulnar deviation at the metacarpophalangeals led to considerable hand dysfunction especially in the more affected dominant right hand, in which metacarpophalangeal joint replacement has been undertaken. Swan neck deformities are present in multiple digits, especially the third to fifth digits of the left hand. The palmar view (**A**) dramatically demonstrates global muscle wasting from long-standing disease. Dorsal view (**B**).

## Elbow and Shoulder

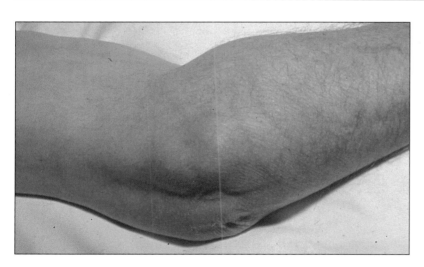

**FIGURE 1-45.** Elbow synovitis in rheumatoid arthritis. Massive swelling of the elbow is easily seen below the radial head. When the joint proper is swollen, the patient is unable to fully extend or completely flex at the elbow. With long-standing disease, a flexion contracture may be the result. Olecranon bursitis is also present, with ulceration. Skin breakdown over the olecranon bursa or olecranon nodules may lead to septic arthritis or septic bursitis.

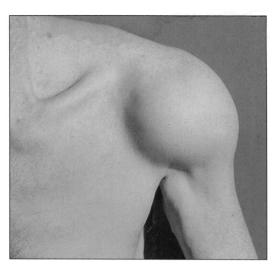

**FIGURE 1-46.**
Rheumatoid arthritis of the shoulder. Radiograph shows massive chronic swelling of the left shoulder. Such swelling usually occurs in advanced disease, and often appears in patients with rotator cuff arthropathies. In addition, there is swelling of the sternoclavicular joint, which may also become eroded.

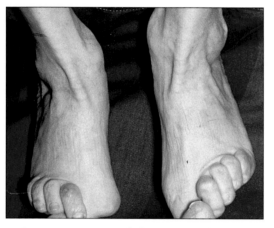

**FIGURE 1-47.**
Subluxation of the shoulder. Extensive erosive changes of the humeral head, erosion of the glenohumeral articulation, marginal erosions, and medial bone resorption have led to loss of articular integrity with superior subluxation of the humerus. Profound osteopenia is present, common in long standing rheumatoid arthritis. (*Courtesy of* Robert H. Cofield, MD.)

## Foot, Knee, Hip, Neck, and Spine

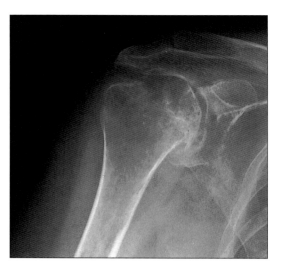

**FIGURE 1-48.** Symmetric synovitis of the feet in early rheumatoid arthritis. Swelling of the right second and third toes and the second toe of the left foot in a 26-year-old patient with rheumatoid arthritis of 6 months' duration. There is also swelling of the first to third metatarsophalangeal joints of the right foot, and the first to fourth metatarsophalangeals of the left foot. This swelling may be apparent on visual inspection, but digital palpation by the examiner confirms the synovitis. The skin proximal to the affected metatarsophalangeals often appears swollen, as it is in this patient.

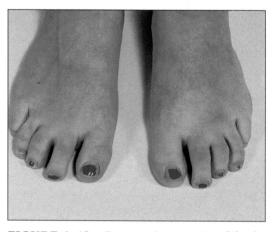

**FIGURE 1-49.** Toe deformities of rheumatoid arthritis. Overlapping of the second and third toes over the first toe of the right foot with marked hallux valgus is seen. Hammer toe deformities (hyperextension of the distal metatarsophalangeal, flexion of the proximal interphalangeal, and extension of the distal interphalangeal joints) are present. Claw toe (extension of the distal metatarsophalangeal and flexion of the proximal interphalangeal with flexion or neutral position of the distal interphalangeal) deformities are also frequently present. Calluses are often present over the protruding proximal interphalangeals, caused by shoes that are too tight to accommodate the deformed foot. Inflammation of the bursa overlying the first distal metatarsophalangeal seen here on the right foot is frequent in hallux valgus. There is almost complete dorsal subluxation at the interphalangeal joint of the left great toe as well.

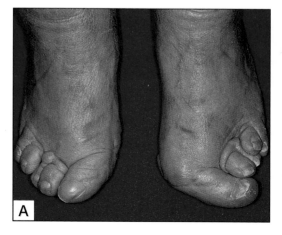

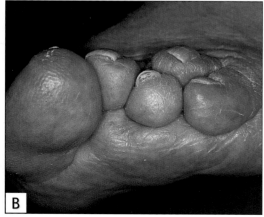

**FIGURE 1-50.** Metatarsal resection. Subluxation at the distal metatarsophalangeal joint may cause severe metatarsalgia, which in some patients is unimproved with custom shoes and inserts. Metatarsal resection can provide significant symptomatic relief, although synovitis may persist. There is marked hallux valgus of the left great toe following metatarsal resection. **A,** The toes are flail; synovitis was persistent and is evident in the inset. The minor toes are flail and some overlap. **B,** None approximate the standing surface, the result of the resections and persistent synovitis.

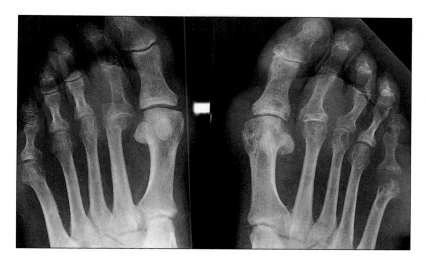

**FIGURE 1-51.** Radiograph of erosive arthritis of the feet. Extensive symmetric erosive changes are evident especially in the metatarsophalangeals and proximal interphalangeals of multiple joints, with advanced destruction of many of the distal metatarsophalangeal heads. Subchondral sclerosis and subchondral cysts are present. Rheumatoid nodules have developed on the left and right fifth distal metatarsophalangeal heads and the distal right first metatarsophalangeal head. Extensive soft tissue swelling is evident around many of the toes.

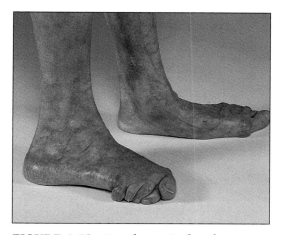

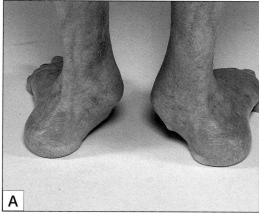

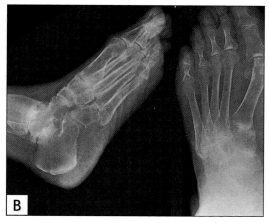

**FIGURE 1-52.** Pes planus. Profound pes planus in a 70-year-old women with rheumatoid arthritis of more than 25 years' duration (same patient as in Fig. 1-54). Malrotation of the toes, especially of the right foot, is evident. The patient was able to walk with supportive shoewear, and declined orthopedic intervention. Also evident is livido reticularis, seen in many patients with vasculopathies. This patient had suffered repeated lower extremity ulcerations; the medial aspect of the left lower extremities demonstrates hyperpigmentation and skin atrophy at the site of one such ulceration.

**FIGURE 1-53.** Hindfoot deformity (same patient as 1-52). **A,** Profound valgus of the tibiotalar joint. Valgus deformity is more common than varus malpositioning, although both may be seen in rheumatoid arthritis. These deformities are often associated with pes planus. Patients with these and other rheumatoid foot deformities are usually not able to walk comfortably barefooted. **B,** Midfoot and hindfoot deformities. Radiograph demonstrates advanced rheumatoid arthritis of the foot, affecting especially the talar joints, mid as well as forefoot. There is marked joint space narrowing of the ankles with loss of bony integrity, sclerosis, subchondral cyst formation at multiple sites including the mortis and the talonavicular, and navicular-cuneiform articulations, and erosive metatarsophalangeal disease. Surgical defects are present on the head of the first metatarsophalangeal joint. The gait became increasingly antalgic with progressive hindfoot instability, requiring splinting, orthotics, and eventually ankle fusion.

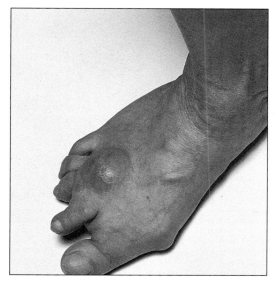

**FIGURE 1-54.** Splayfoot and reactive bursitis in rheumatoid arthritis. Synovitis of the forefoot has compromised the integrity of the capsuloligamentous structures, causing loss of the transverse arch with resultant splaying of the forefoot. The heads of the distal second and third metatarsophalangeal joints are dislocated plantarly, so that the toes cannot make contact with the ground. Improper shoewear has led to formation of a reactive bursa over the third metatarsophalangeal. Adequate shoewear is adapted to the individual foot anatomy. In this patient, the shoe was neither wide enough nor was the toe box of adequate size, leading to the reactive bursitis. Pressure ulcerations may result, which can become infected and are often very difficult to treat. Corrective surgery is often required to improve function and lessen pain.

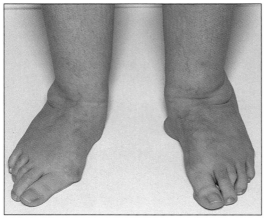

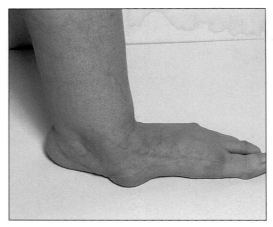

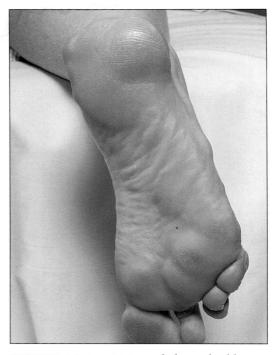

**FIGURE 1-55.** Rheumatoid foot deformities. Chronic synovitis has led to hallux valgus of the right great toe and fibular deviation, especially of the first three toes. An inflamed bursa has formed on the medial aspect of the right first metatarsalphalangeal joint. Profound flatfoot has developed caused by chronic distention and instability of the joint capsules and supporting ligaments of the midfoot and hindfoot. The medial malleoli, tali, and navicular bones of both feet are medially and plantarly rotated, projecting over the medial margin of the foot.

**FIGURE 1-56.** Pes planus. Medial aspect of the left foot shown in Figure 1-55. There is marked pes planus, and a large bursa has formed over the dislocated tarsal bones.

**FIGURE 1-57.** Metatarsophalangeal subluxation and rheumatoid nodules. Metatarsophalangeal subluxation is often accompanied by callous formation, apparent over the distal first and fourth metatarsophalangeal heads. The toes are superiorly subluxed, the third toe to such an extent that it is not visible on this view. Rheumatoid nodules often develop at pressure points; three can be seen around the heel.

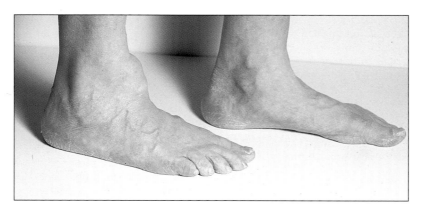

**FIGURE 1-58.** Tenosynovitis of the foot. A large tenosynovial cyst is present on the left anterior tibial tendon in this 60-year old man with a 5-year history of rheumatoid arthritis. Rupture of this tendon results in loss of the longitudinal foot arch and pes planus. Peroneus tenosynovitis affects the right foot.

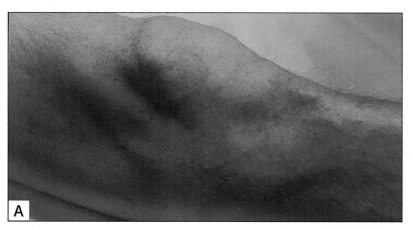

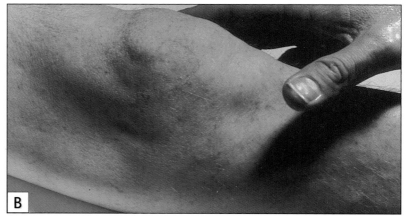

**FIGURE 1-59.** Demonstration of the "bulge sign." **A,** Although massive swelling is obvious, the presence of lesser knee swelling can be demonstrated using the "bulge sign." **B,** To elicit this sign, the examiner compresses the intra-articular fluid from the medial aspect of the knee and then strokes the lateral aspect, forcing the fluid to appear at the medial aspect, or visa versa.

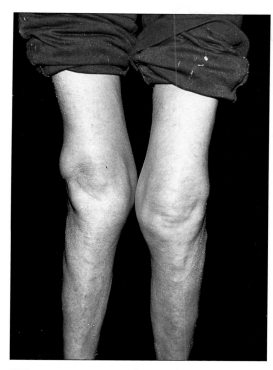

FIGURE 1-60.  Muscle atrophy in chronic arthritis. Chronic synovitis of the knees and profound muscle wasting of the leg muscles are seen in a patient with long standing rheumatoid arthritis. The knees are in varus, and there is a leg length discrepancy which followed total hip arthroplasty.

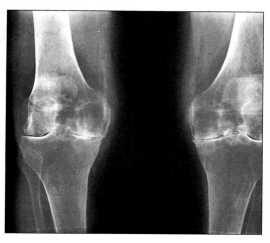

FIGURE 1-61.  Rheumatoid arthritis of the knee. This radiograph of the knees is from a patient with rheumatoid arthritis of 15 years' duration. The disease is symmetric involving both knees, as well as within each joint, affecting both the medial and lateral compartments. Periarticular osteoporosis, marginal erosions, subchondral sclerosis, and a relative lack of secondary hypertrophic changes can be seen. (*Courtesy of* Ronald G. Swee, MD.)

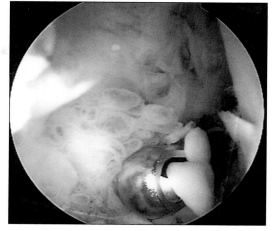

FIGURE 1-62.  Arthroscopy of knee synovitis. Arthroscopy of the posterior medial compartment of the knee demonstrates chronically inflamed synovium in a patient with rheumatoid arthritis. The length and thickness of the synovial villi are increased. The villi are engorged and erythematous. The medial condyle appears as the white structure oriented vertically at the far right of the picture; the shaver is located posteromedially. There is modest degeneration of the articular cartilage of the femoral condyle. In early rheumatoid arthritis, arthroscopy demonstrates synovial changes only, with hypertrophic highly vascularized villi. Later, pannus develops as joint destruction occurs. Degenerative changes similar to those seen in osteoarthritis may be seen in patients with well-controlled disease. (*Courtesy of* Michael E. Torchia, MD.)

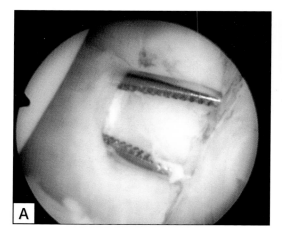

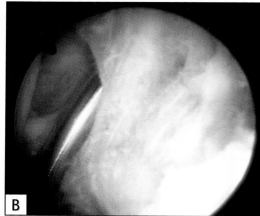

FIGURE 1-63.  Chronic synovitis of the knee. This 25-year-old patient with rheumatoid arthritis for 18 months had been treated with second-line antirheumatic drugs and experienced remission of clinically active synovitis, but had a persistently swollen, boggy left knee joint. **A**, At arthroscopy, minimal inflammation with increased vascularity is demonstrated. The medial condyle of the femur is at the left margin in this view of the knee posterior medial capsule. **B**, The fibrotic proliferated synovium appearing as a dense whitish membrane. The patient underwent arthroscopic synovectomy with good result. (*Courtesy of* Michael E. Torchia, MD.)

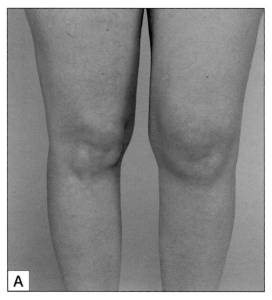 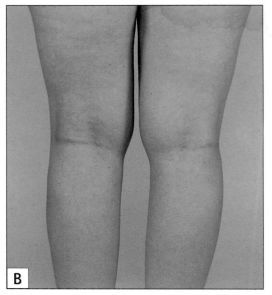 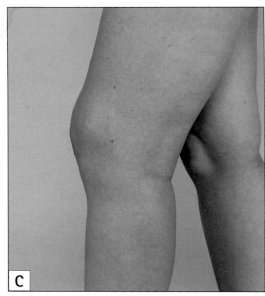

**FIGURE 1-64.** Baker's cyst in rheumatoid arthritis. Posterior herniation of the left knee joint capsule into the popliteal space is seen in a patient with early rheumatoid arthritis. These cysts may reach large size, but are usually more subtle, as in this patient. **A**, **B**, and **C**, The popliteal space appears full, and the normal calf contour is changed. Often, as in this 24-year-old patient, intra-articular swelling is present. The cyst may rupture and dissect into the calf muscles, causing further pain, swelling, erythema, and even a positive Homans' sign, simulating a deep venous thrombosis. The presence of a Baker's cyst can be verified by arthrography, ultrasonography, or magnetic resonance imaging.

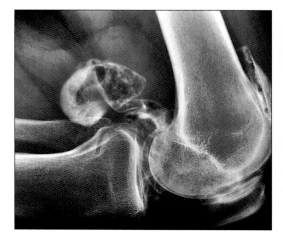 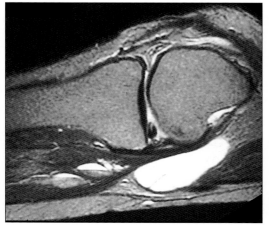 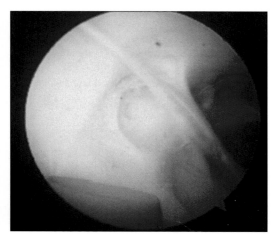

**FIGURE 1-65.** Baker's cyst—arthrogram. Conventional arthrography of a small popliteal cyst. Synovial hypertrophy led to the development of an inflammatory polyp, which appears radiolucent in the superior portion of the cyst. (*Courtesy of* Ronald G. Swee, MD.)

**FIGURE 1-66.** Baker's cyst—magnetic resonance image (MRI). MRI demonstrates a Baker's cyst in a patient with well-controlled, early rheumatoid arthritis and previous knee trauma. There is an extensive horizontal tear involving the body and posterior horn of the medial meniscus associated with degeneration of the meniscus and some loss of articular cartilage. There is a minimal amount of fluid in the knee joint. A 4 ( 2 cm Baker's cyst is seen posteromedially. A couple of smaller cysts are seen inferiorly. Fluid levels are likely related to debris. (*Courtesy of* Michael E. Torchia, MD.)

**FIGURE 1-67.** Arthroscopy of a Baker's cyst. Arthroscopic view of the interior of a Baker's cyst in a patient with well-controlled rheumatoid arthritis. The cyst is approached through the posterior medial portal, and the blue cannula at the bottom of the picture is in the posterior portion. Several plicae are visible. The synovium was not inflamed. Management options for Baker's cysts include observation, glucocorticoid injection, arthroscopic decompression, and open surgical removal, especially for large or symptomatic cysts. (*Courtesy of* Michael E. Torchia, MD.)

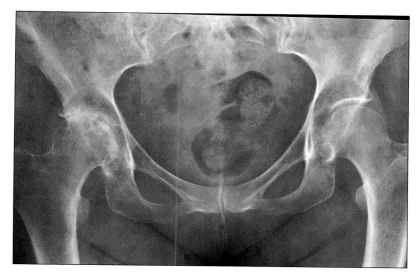

**FIGURE 1-68.** Hip disease in rheumatoid arthritis. The entire joint surface is involved in rheumatoid arthritis from the outset, unlike osteoarthritis, which in weight-bearing joints initially affects the weight bearing surfaces. The joint disease is symmetric, although as seen in this patient's radiograph, one joint may be more affected than the other. Subchondral cyst formation, reactive sclerosis, and joint space narrowing are more advanced in the right hip joint of this patient. Secondary changes of osteoarthritis are often present in longstanding rheumatoid joint disease. (*Courtesy of* Ronald G. Swee, MD.)

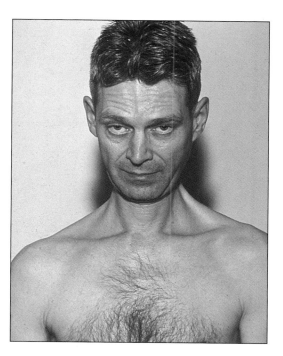

**FIGURE 1-69.** Subluxation of C1–2. This patient has had rheumatoid arthritis for 15 years. His head is held in a fixed flexed posture, and he must gaze upward in order to see ahead.

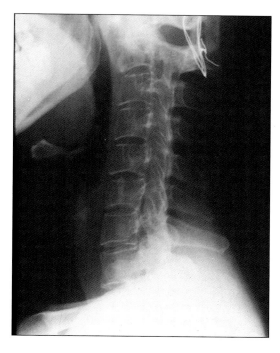

**FIGURE 1-70.** Radiograph of C1–2 fusion. A posterior fusion of C1–2 has been performed on the patient seen Figure 1-69 by cement and wire fixation. The patient is pain-free and able to view normally following the procedure.

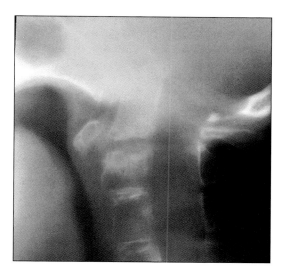

**FIGURE 1-71.** Atlantoaxial subluxation with basilar invagination. In some patients, synovitis leads to erosion of the odontoid process with cervical instability, which can cause pain, limitation of cervical motion, and compromise of the spinal cord, including death. The tomogram shows settling of the skull onto the odontoid process, which protrudes above Chamberlain's line extending from the hard palate to the foramen magnum. Basilar invagination is less common than atlantoaxial instability, which can be measured as the distance in from the posterior aspect of the arch of the atlas to the anterior aspect of the odontoid process, a distance of about 3 mm in normal adults, and may be evident in the neutral position or on extension of the cervical spine. (*Courtesy of* Miguel E. Cabanela, MD.)

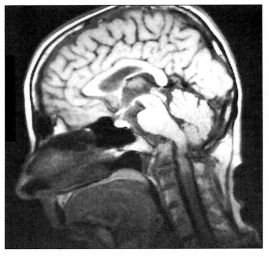

**FIGURE 1-72.** Magnetic resonance image of basilar invagination. The T1-weighted sagittal view from the same patient as in Figure 1-71 demonstrates impingement of the brain stem with protrusion of the eroded odontoid process into the foramen magnum. (*Courtesy of* Miguel E. Cabenela, MD.)

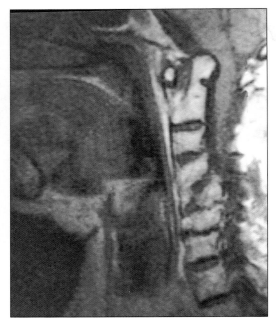

**FIGURE 1-73.** Cervical spine involvement in rheumatoid arthritis. Features of cervical spine involvement in rheumatoid arthritis include odontoid erosion, vertebral collapse, and subluxation of vertebral bodies. These changes may lead to cervical myelopathy, seen on this T-1 weighted magnetic resonance image (MRI). The MRI appearance of proliferated synovium is especially apparent where it is eroding into the anterior aspect of the odontoid process.

## Clinical Features—Extra-articular

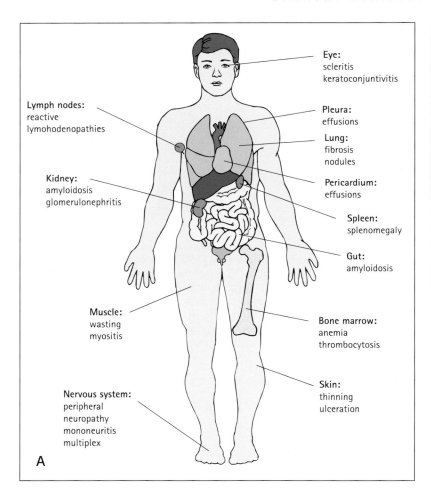

Eye:
scleritis
keratoconjuntivitis

Lymph nodes:
reactive
lymohodenopathies

Pleura:
effusions

Lung:
fibrosis
nodules

Kidney:
amyloidosis
glomerulonephritis

Pericardium:
effusions

Spleen:
splenomegaly

Gut:
amyloidosis

Muscle:
wasting
myositis

Bone marrow:
anemia
thrombocytosis

Skin:
thinning
ulceration

Nervous system:
peripheral
neuropathy
mononeuritis
multiplex

A

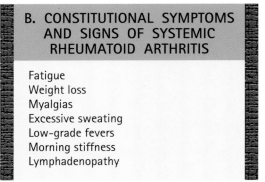

**B. CONSTITUTIONAL SYMPTOMS AND SIGNS OF SYSTEMIC RHEUMATOID ARTHRITIS**

Fatigue
Weight loss
Myalgias
Excessive sweating
Low-grade fevers
Morning stiffness
Lymphadenopathy

**FIGURE 1-74.** Systemic rheumatoid arthritis. **A,** Extraarticular disease manifestations affect about 42% of patients with rheumatoid arthritis and can include multiple organ systems. [15]. **B,** Constitutional symptoms and signs. Constitutional symptoms and signs can vary with disease activity. Most patients with active arthritis experience more than one hour of morning stiffness.

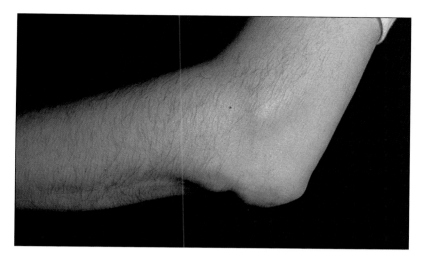

**FIGURE 1-75.** Bursitis and nodulosis. Subcutaneous rheumatoid nodules commonly form over pressure points such as the olecranon (arm rest), feet (shoewear and plantar surfaces), fingers (gripping), and scapula, occiput, ischium, and sacrum from sitting and lying. The nodules are firm, and may be mobile or, when adherent to the periosteum, fixed. As in this patient with nodules and olecranon bursitis, the nodules may be within subcutaneous tissue overlying the bursae. Only about 20% of patients with rheumatoid arthritis develop rheumatoid nodules, and most patients with rheumatoid nodules are positive for rheumatoid factor. Although nodules usually regress with improvement of disease activity, in some patients methotrexate treatment promotes nodule formation.

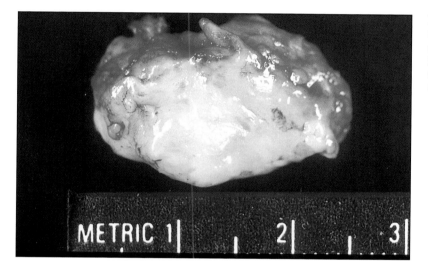

**FIGURE 1-76.** Rheumatoid nodule—gross appearance. This subcutaneous nodule was removed from the olecranon of a patient with longstanding rheumatoid arthritis. The nodule is about 3 cm in diameter, and is covered by a fibrous capsule. The yellow tissue is from fibrinoid necrosis; the fleshy tissue is the fibrous nodule. (*Courtesy of* Thomas A. Gaffey, MD.)

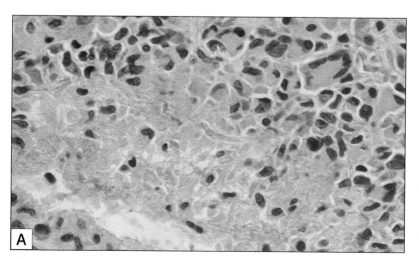

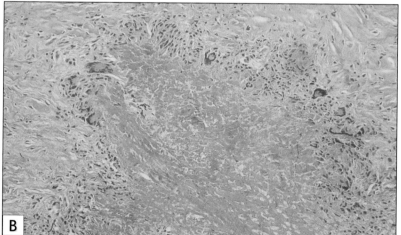

**FIGURE 1-77.** Rheumatoid nodule—histology. **A**, In the active inflammatory nodule, there is fibrinoid necrosis, with surrounding mononuclear inflammatory cells, palisading histiocytes, and multinucleated giant cells that have formed from aggregating histiocytes. Small vessel vasculitis is likely important in the pathoetiology of the rheumatoid nodule (hematoxylin and eosin, medium power).

**B**, Granulomatous transformation of a rheumatoid nodule is evident. There is prominent central fibrinoid necrosis, surrounding palisading histiocytes, and an outer layer of chronic fibrosing connective tissue with inflammatory cells including plasma cells, lymphocytes and fibroblasts (hematoxylin and eosin, low power). (Parts **A** and **B**, *Courtesy of* Thomas A. Gaffey, MD.)

*Rheumatoid Arthritis, Juvenile Rheumatoid Arthritis, and Related Conditions*

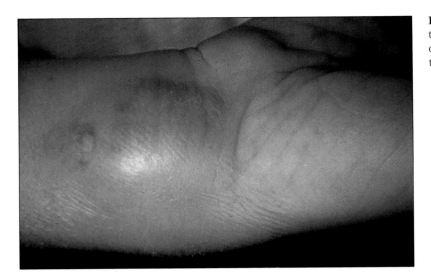

**FIGURE 1-78.** Synovial cyst. A large synovial cyst has developed over the distal volar-radial aspect of the wrist. These cysts develop as a result of synovial hypertrophy and herniation of inflamed synovial tissue through the overlying fascia.

## Ocular Involvement in Active RA

### MAJOR FORMS OF OCULAR INVOLVEMENT IN RHEUMATOID ARTHRITIS

- Keratoconjunctivitis sicca
- Scleritis
- Episcleritis
- Uveitis
- Episcleral nodules
- Brown's syndrome (diplopia on upward gaze caused by tenosynovitis of the superior oblique muscle tendon sheath)

**FIGURE 1-79.** Major forms of ocular involvement in rheumatoid arthritis. Keratoconjuntivitis sicca (secondary Sjögren's syndrome) is the most common ophthalmic complication of rheumatoid arthritis. Episcleritis and scleritis occur independent of the joint activity, and usually can be treated topically. Severe nodular scleritis requires systemic treatment, and may progress to scleromalacia perforans, leading to blindness. Episcleral nodules and Brown's syndrome are rare. Ocular complications of drug treatment for rheumatoid arthritis include cataracts and glaucoma from glucocorticoid treatment (common), and antimalarial associated retinopathy (rare).

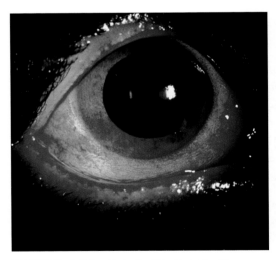 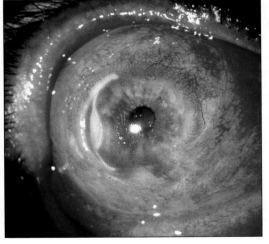 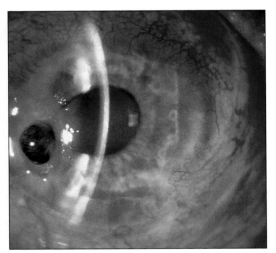

**FIGURE 1-80.** Episcleritis. Episcleritis generally occurs in the setting of active rheumatoid arthritis. The onset is often sudden, with redness of the eye and eye pain. Visual acuity is usually not affected. Another condition, keratoconjuntivitis sicca, is the most common ocular manifestation of rheumatoid arthritis (see section on Sjögren's syndrome further on.).

**FIGURE 1-81.** Scleritis. Scleritis is a serious complication of rheumatoid arthritis which can lead to permanent loss of vision if left untreated. Symptoms include pain and loss of visual acuity. Scleritis often occurs in patients with long standing rheumatoid arthritis, and as in this case may be nodular. Many patients with scleritis have had vasculitis and other systemic disease manifestations. It is often much more resistant to treatment than episcleritis.

**FIGURE 1-82.** Scleromalacia perforans (same patient as Fig. 1-81). Scleritis may lead to destruction of the sclera with herniation of intraocular contents ("scleral melt"). Visual loss is permanent.

### PULMONARY INVOLVEMENT IN RHEUMATOID ARTHRITIS

Interstitial pneumonitis and fibrosis
Pulmonary (rheumatoid) nodules
Pleuritis and pleurisy
Bronchiolitis obliterans
Obstructive lung disease
Pneumoconiosis (Caplan's syndrome)
Isolated pulmonary arteritis

**FIGURE 1-83.** Pulmonary involvement in rheumatoid arthritis. Pulmonary fibrosis and mild obstructive changes are the most common forms of lung disease in rheumatoid arthritis. Pleural effusions are usually asymptomatic until they become large enough to impair respiration. The fluid is exudative, and the pleural glucose is characteristically low. The nodules are typically pleural based, and may cavitate. Caplan's syndrome is an unusual syndrome of pneumoconiosis in patients with rheumatoid arthritis exposed to mineral dusts. Acute interstitial pneumonitis is rare, as is isolated pulmonary arteritis. Interstitial lung disease complicates some treatments, including gold and d-penicillamine. (*From* Walker and Wright [22]; with permission.)

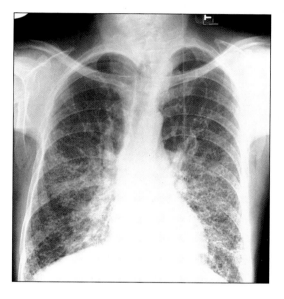

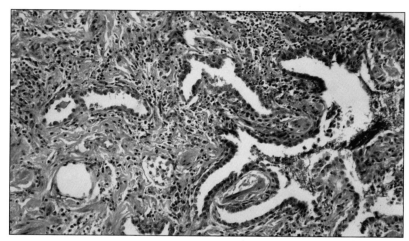

**FIGURE 1-84.** Pulmonary fibrosis. Pulmonary fibrosis occurs in up to 25% of patients with rheumatoid arthritis [23]. Interstitial changes are highly correlated with smoking. The chest radiograph shows a diffuse interstitial infiltrate, which initially usually occurs in the lower lung fields, with a reticular-nodular pattern and pleural involvement. A restrictive pattern is seen on pulmonary function testing.

**FIGURE 1-85.** Interstitial pneumonitis in rheumatoid arthritis. Diffuse interstitial pneumonitis with sclerosing alveolitis. Inflammatory cells including lymphocytes are prominent (hematoxylin and eosin, medium power).

### PLEURAL FLUID IN RHEUMATOID ARTHRITIS

| | |
|---|---|
| Color | Yellow to slightly turbid |
| Cells | Mononuclear cell predominates; usually <5000 cells μL |
| Protein | >4 gm/dL |
| Glucose | 10–50 mg/dL |
| Complement | Low |
| Lipids | High |

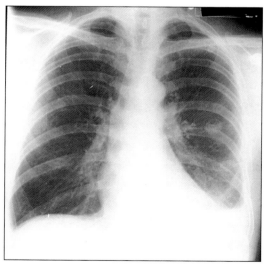

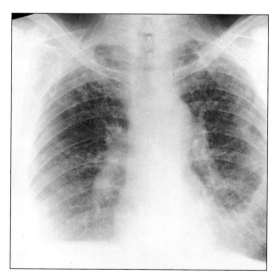

**FIGURE 1-86.** Pleural fluid in rheumatoid arthritis. The pleural fluid in rheumatoid arthritis is classified as an exudate. Pleural fluid glucose is low because of impaired transport of glucose into the pleural space. The most important differential diagnosis based on low-glucose level is pleural-based infection. Pleural biopsy may show nonspecific inflammation and fibrosis.

**FIGURE 1-87.** Pulmonary nodule and pleural effusion—radiograph. Pulmonary nodules may occur singly or in clusters. Single lesions have the appearance of a coin lesion. They are pleural-based, and may cavitate, as has the nodule in the left midlung field of this patient. A bronchopleural fistula may then form. A rheumatoid pleural effusion is present at the left lung base.

**FIGURE 1-88.** Caplan's syndrome. Pneumoconiosis in rheumatoid arthritis promotes the fibroblastic response and the formation of pulmonary nodules. Termed Caplan's syndrome, this complication is rare and is classically seen in the setting of coal dust exposure. In this radiograph nodules are seen throughout the peripheral lung fields, with hazy modeled densities extending from the perihilar areas superiorly, and extensive pulmonary fibrosis. The nodules have the histologic appearance of rheumatoid nodules, with central necrosis that can contain coal dust.

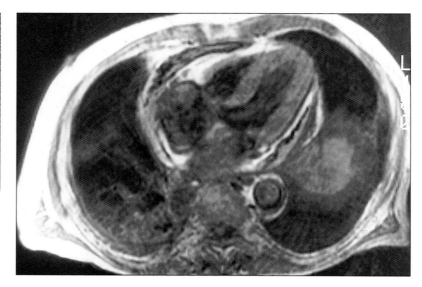

**FIGURE 1-89.** Cardiac involvement in rheumatoid arthritis. Pericarditis is common in rheumatoid arthritis, and can be demonstrated by echocardiography or at autopsy in 50% of patients. Myocarditis is rare, and may be associated with rheumatoid nodular infiltrates of the myocardium. Coronary vasculitis usually occurs in the setting of systemic vasculitis. (*From* Bonfiglio and Atwater [24]; with permission.)

**FIGURE 1-90.** Pericarditis in rheumatoid arthritis. Pericarditis typically occurs in seropositive patients with nodular disease, and is the most common cardiac manifestation of rheumatoid arthritis. It is usually asymptomatic, but can lead to pericardial effusion and fibrosis with cardiac tamponade. This magnetic resonance image demonstrates constrictive pericarditis. The white structure around the pericardium is the pericardial fat, the gray is the pericardial wall. The dense white infiltrate between the pericardium and gray myocardium is pericardial fluid.

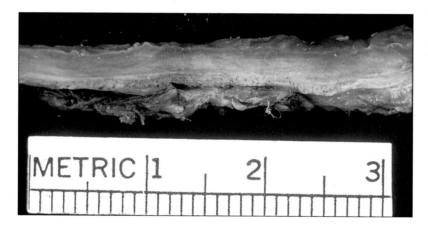

**FIGURE 1-91.** Pericarditis. Gross anatomic specimen of a patient with constrictive rheumatoid pericarditis. At the top is the outer layer of the pericardium overlaid with fat; the fibrotic, thickened pericardium is beneath.

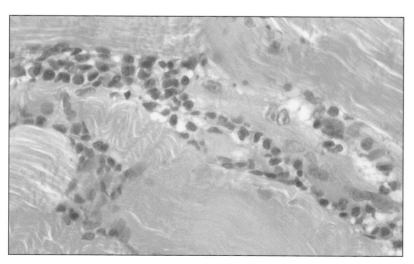

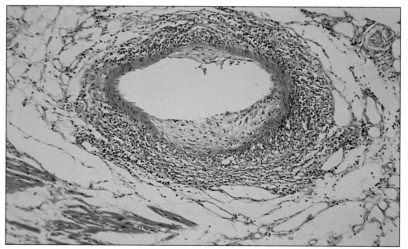

**FIGURE 1-92.** Myositis in rheumatoid arthritis. Myositis is rare in rheumatoid arthritis, and may affect the cardiac and skeletal musculature. The muscle is cut longitudinally in this photomicrograph. There is lymphoplasmacytic infiltrate, round cell infiltrate in the muscle interstitium, and degeneration of the sarcolemmal nuclei (hematoxylin and eosin, high power).

**FIGURE 1-93.** Rheumatoid vasculitis. Systemic vasculitis in rheumatoid arthritis involves small and medium-size arteries, including the coronary arteries. It is uncommon, usually occurring in patients who have had their disease for 10 years or more. In this photomicrograph, necrotizing arteritis with adventitial inflammation and medial destruction is seen. These changes are indistinguishable from those of polyarteritis nodosa. (hematoxylin and eosin, low power.)

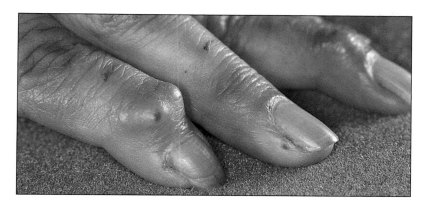

**FIGURE 1-94.** Rheumatoid vasculopathy. Rheumatoid vasculopathy is a rather unusual manifestation of small vessel arteritis. This condition manifests as small, well-localized infarctions which may occur over rheumatoid nodules (nodules on the third and fifth distal interphalangeal joints of this patient), or present as nail-fold infarctions (ulnar aspect of the fourth and fifth digits). When they occur in isolation or with leg ulcers only, without evidence of other systemic inflammation, gangrene or a sensorimotor neuropathy, they usually do not require specific treatment, especially increased immunosuppression or higher doses of corticosteroids.

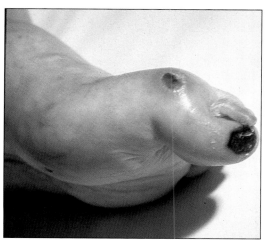

**FIGURE 1-95.** Digital ulcerations in rheumatoid vasculitis. There are two ulcers on the great toe of this patient with rheumatoid arthritis. The ulcers are like those seen in some other forms of vasculitis, including polyarteritis nodosa. Unlike patients with isolated nail-fold infarction, this patient had diffuse vasculitis and required high doses of glucocorticoids for management of the inflammatory disease.

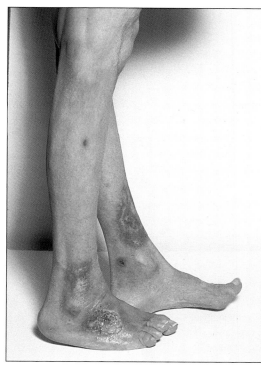

**FIGURE 1-96.** Extensive rheumatoid vasculitis. Extensive ulcerations of the lower extremities of this patient are from rheumatoid vasculitis. There is profound muscle and skin atrophy, thinning of the skin, and hyperpigmentation. A partially healed, weeping ulcer is present on the lateral aspect of the left foot.

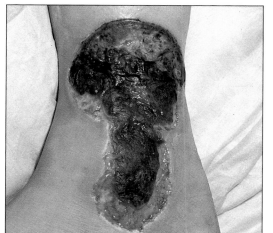

**FIGURE 1-97.** Large ulceration in rheumatoid vasculitis. Large ulceration on the medial aspect of the right lower extremity in a patient with long-standing rheumatoid arthritis. The ulcers are characteristically well demarcated, and have the appearance of having been cut out by a cookie cutter. They are often difficult to heal. Vasculitis may occur in patients in the early stages of the disease, but is more typical of patients with disease of 10 years or longer. Confirmation of vaculitis may be obtained by biopsy; frequently there is evidence of neural involvement. Skin, nerve or muscle biopsy may be required to confirm the diagnosis.

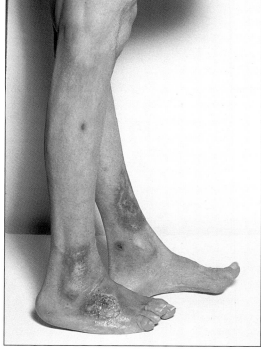

**FIGURE 1-98.** Vasculitis and mononeuritis multiplex. Cutaneous infarctions in a patient with long-standing rheumatoid arthritis. Vasculitis of the arteries supplying the peripheral nerves has led to multiple peripheral neuropathies (mononeuritis multiplex), with bilateral footdrop. The resultant ulcerations often heal poorly. These manifestations frequently portend a poor prognosis.

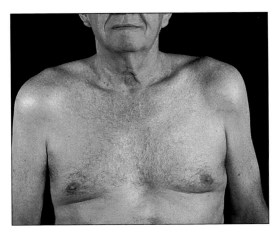

**FIGURE 1-99.** "Shoulder pad" sign in rheumatoid arthritis and secondary amyloidosis. Bilateral shoulder swelling (shoulder pad sign) is seen in a patient with long-standing rheumatoid arthritis and secondary amyloidosis. This patient also has sternoclavicular arthritis on the left side. Patients with primary amyloidosis may also develop this sign, along with subcutaneous nodules, which may be confused with rheumatoid nodules.

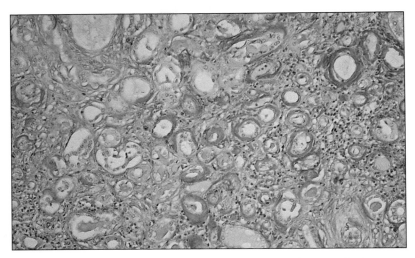

**FIGURE 1-100.** Seondary amyloidosis. The secondary amyloidosis of rheumatoid arthritis is rare, and occurs in patients with long standing disease. Amyloidosis may affect almost any organ, including the skin, kidney, liver, spleen, and heart. In this renal tissue polarized photomicrograph, amyloid deposits appear green (Congo red, low power).

## *Laboratory Features and Synovial Histology*

### LABORATORY FEATURES OF RHEUMATOID ARTHRITIS

Hematologic
  Anemia
  Eosinophilia
  Thrombocytosis
  Large granular lymphocytes (especially in Felty's syndrome)
Hepatic
  Increased levels of alkaline phosphatase, aspartate amino-
    transferase, and γ glutamyltransferase
  Decreased albumin and prealbumin
Acute-phase reactants
  Elevated erythrocyte sedimentation rate
  Elevated C-reactive protein

**FIGURE 1-101.** Laboratory features of rheumatoid arthritis. These laboratory features are nonspecific and reflect both acute and chronic inflammation, although they do not always directly correlate with disease activity. In the patient with rheumatoid arthritis and abnormal laboratory findings, other causes must always be considered, for example, drug toxicity in patients with anemia or elevated liver enzymes.

### DIFFERENTIAL DIAGNOSIS OF DISEASES ASSOCIATED WITH RHEUMATOID FACTOR

| Disease | Prevalence, % | Other Diseases |
|---|---|---|
| Rheumatic Diseases | | Scleroderma |
| Rheumatoid arthritis | 80 | Intersitial fibrosis |
| Juvenile rheumatoid arthritis | 20 | Chronic bronchitis |
| Systemic lupus erythematosus | 40 | Chronic liver disease |
| Sjögren's syndrome | 90 | Silicosis |
| Cryoglobulinemia | 90 | Sarcoidosis |
| Infections | | Malignancies, especially hematopoietic |
| Subacute bacterial endocarditis | 40 | Parasitic infections |
| Viral hepatitis | 25 | Kala-azar, malraia, schistosomiasis, |
| Leprosy | 25 | filariasis, trypanosomiasis |
| Tuberculosis | 10 | Other chronic infections |
| | | Syphilis, brucellosis, salmonellosis |
| | | Acute viral infections; HIV |

**FIGURE 1-102.** Differential diagnosis of diseases associated with rheumatoid factor. Many conditions are associated with the presence of rheumatoid factor. In some of these, especially infectious diseases, rheumatoid factor is only transiently present. In rheumatoid arthritis, the rheumatoid factor titer is not a useful indicator of disease activity. (*From* Tighe and Carson [25]; with permission.)

## CLASSIFICATION OF SYNOVIAL EFFUSIONS

| Fluid | Appearance | Leukocyte count/mm3 |
|---|---|---|
| Normal | Clear, colorless | <200, with <25% PMNs |
| Noninflammatory | Clear, yellow | 200–2000 with <25% PMNs |
| Inflammatory | Cloudy, yellow | 2000–100,000 with >50% PMNs |
| Septic | Purulent | >80,000 with >75% PMNs |

**FIGURE 1-103.** Classification of synovial effusions. Normal and noninflammatory synovial fluid (such as may be seen in osteoarthritis) is viscous with low cellularity. In inflammation, the fluid becomes turbid, and viscosity decreases. In patients taking glucocorticosteroids, antimetabolites and immunosuppressive agents, the cell count is an unreliable indicator of the possibility of infection, because cell counts in these patients may not be dramatically increased, and are indistinguishable from patients with active synovitis but uninfected joints. PMN—polymorphonuclear neutrophil leukocytes. (*From* Schumacher and Reginato [26]; with permission.)

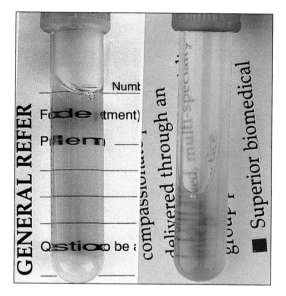

**FIGURE 1-104.** Examination of synovial fluid. Examination of the synovial fluid gives a valuable clue to the etiology of an inflammatory arthritis. While the appearance is nonspecific, the synovial fluid in active rheumatoid arthritis (*tube on the right*) is usually somewhat cloudy, with reduced viscosity, and contains greater than 2000 leukocytes /mm$^3$. Normal joint fluid (*tube on the left*) is clear or yellow tinged, with less than 200 leukocytes/mm$^3$. Depending on the clinical scenario, the synovial fluid may be evaluated by cultures and Gram stain to aid in detection of infectious causes. Crystalline disease is diagnosed by the presence of urate, calcium pyrophosphate, hydroxyapatite and other crystals under microscopy.

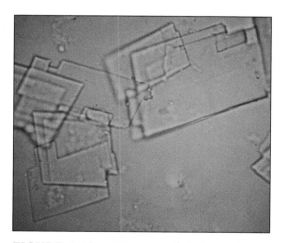

**FIGURE 1-105.** Presence of cholesterol crystals in synovial fluid. Cholesterol crystals may occasionally be seen in the synovial fluid of patients with rheumatoid arthritis, or, as in this case, in the fluid aspirated from an inflamed olecranon bursa. The presence of cholesterol crystals is nonspecific, and their diagnostic significance is uncertain. The cholesterol crystals seen here under normal light microscopy are flat, rectangular in shape, and often have notched corners.

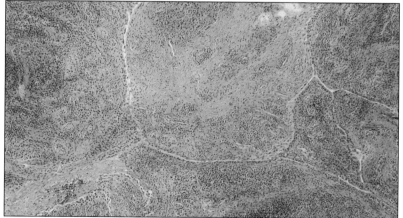

**FIGURE 1-106.** Synovial hypertrophy. Photomicrograph shows section through the synovium from the knee of a patient with rheumatoid arthritis. There is an intense cellular infiltrate forming lymphoid follicules. Each lobule represents a synovial frond (hematoxylin and eosin, low power). (*Courtesy of* Thomas A. Gaffey, MD.)

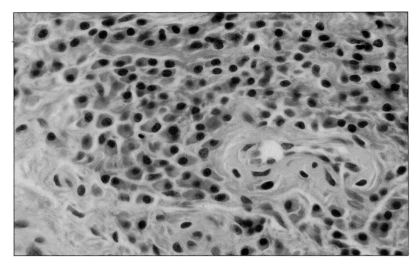

**FIGURE 1-107.** Synovitis in rheumatoid arthritis. Synovial biopsy is rarely performed as a diagnostic procedure to confirm the diagnosis of rheumatoid arthritis. The histopathologic changes are characteristic but not specific for rheumatoid arthritis. Features of the inflamed synovium include synovial hyperplasia, angiogenesis, subsynovial fibrosis, perivascular infiltrates, and the presence of plasma cells. Macrophages, mast cells, histiocytes, and multinucleated giant cells may also be seen. These features are present throughout the disease course. As in this photomicrograph, there are marked perivascular lymphoplasmacytic infiltrates, a hallmark of active disease (hematoxylin and eosin, high power). (*Courtesy of* Thomas A. Gaffey, MD.)

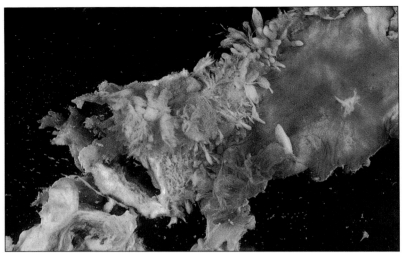

**FIGURE 1-108.** Synovial hypertrophy and pannus formation. Gross anatomic appearance of hypertrophied synovium and invasive pannus recovered from a patient with rheumatoid arthritis at the time of joint arthroplasty. Many of the hypertrophied synovial fronds appear relatively avascular, characteristic of long-standing or nearly "burned out" disease. Mature pannus is aggressively invasive and contributes, together with interarticular inflammatory processes such as the release of inflammatory mediators and enzymatic action, to the characteristic joint destruction. The synovium does not proliferate like a tumor in the capsule, but rather the villus fronds proliferate like branches of ferns from a common stalk [3]. The villi may infarct and be aspirated as debris or "rice bodies." (*Courtesy of* Thomas A. Gaffey, MD.)

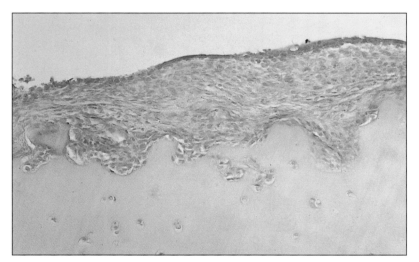

**FIGURE 1-109.** Invasive pannus—histopathology. Invasion of tumor-like proliferation formation and destruction of the articular cartilage of an interphalangeal joint from a 19-year-old woman with chronic rheumatoid arthritis. In this photomicrograph compact avascular masses of synovial origin (*top*) are seen invading into the articular surface, with unmasking of collagen at the cartilage border. (hematoxylin and eosin, high power). (*Courtesy of* Hans-Georg Fassbender, MD.)

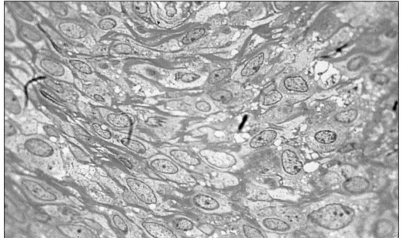

**FIGURE 1-110** Tumor-like proliferation of synovium. High-power photomicrograph of undifferentiated compact synovial cell formation (tumorlike proliferation). The tissue is avascular and contains no inflammatory cells. Normal synovial stromal cells are oval to spindle shaped, with an elongated to oval shaped nucleus. With proliferation, as in this example, the cells become rounded to polyhedral and some are multinuclear; the nuclei are vesicular and contain up to two nucleoli [27]. (methylene blue). (*Courtesy of* Hans-Georg Fassbender, MD.)

## TREATMENT OF RHEUMATOID ARTHRITIS: GENERAL PRINCIPLES

Disease and general education

Rest periods, including daytime rest

Enhancement of self-esteem

Support from family, friends, coworkers, support groups

Pain relief: medications, physical modalities (heat, cold, TENS, splints)

Occupational therapy and physical therapy for joint protection and functional enhancement

Splints, orthotics, adaptive and adequate shoewear, adaptive devices

Range-of-motion exercises (for affected joints)

Appropriate stretching, strengthening, and conditioning exercises

Handicap stickers, home modifications

Counseling: disease, occupational, and coping skills

Surgery: joint replacement and stabilization; tendon repair; removal of cysts, bursae, and nodules; relief of entrapment neuropathies

**FIGURE 1-111.** Treatment of rheumatoid arthritis—general principles. The importance of early therapeutic intervention and the role of nonmedicinal therapies for rheumatoid arthritis cannot be overstated. A carefully considered treatment approach helps the patient cope with the emotional, physical, social, and financial consequences of the disease. Occupational and physical therapy are important to enhance joint function while protecting joints from overuse. Home modifications may include lowering the height of counters, widening doorways and hallways, and installing railings, especially in the bathroom. The principal goals of joint replacement surgery are pain relief and improvement of function. TENS—transcutaneous electrical nerve stimulation.

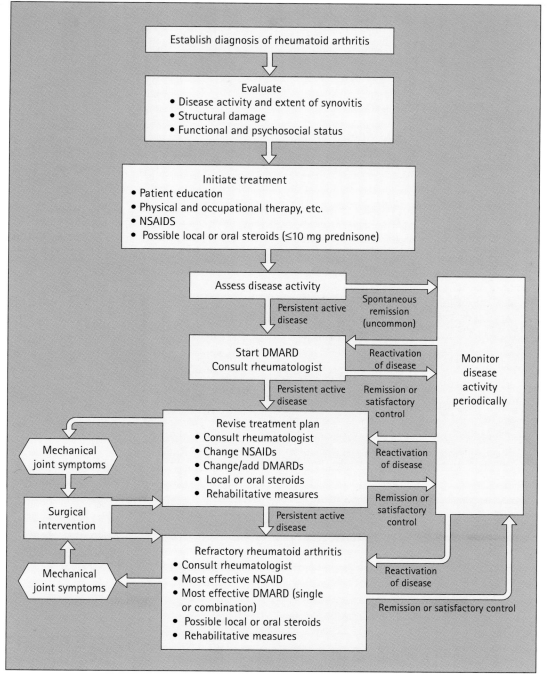

**FIGURE 1-112.** Management of rheumatoid arthritis. This algorithm outlines the management of rheumatoid arthritis. After the diagnosis has been established, early therapeutic intervention is important to control disease, preserve function, and improve disease outcome. Initial interventions to control symptoms include the use of nonsteroidal anti–inflammatory drugs (NSAIDs) and sometimes glucocorticosteroids. For patients in whom the diagnosis is established, slower-acting second-line drugs should be initiated early in the disease course. The disease process is dynamic, and frequent reevaluation is necessary to good disease management. Consultation with a rheumatologist helps to guide diagnostic and therapeutic decision making. DMARDs—disease modifying antirheumatic drugs. (*From* Ad Hoc Subcommittee on Clinical Guidelines [28]; with permission.)

## PHARMACOTHERAPEUTIC TREATMENT FOR RHEUMATOID ARTHRITIS

Analgesics and anti-inflammatory drugs
  NSAIDs, including aspirin
Second-line or "disease modifying" antirheumatic drugs
  Hydroxychloroquine
  Methotrexate
  Sulfasalazine
  Azathioprine
  Gold
  Cyclosporine
  Leflunomide
  TNF-α antagonists
    Etanercept
    Infliximab
Others: experimental; D-penicillamine, immuoabsorption column, minocycline; other antimetabolic and chemotherapeutic agents, including cyclophosphamide and chlorabmucil
Glucocorticoids

**FIGURE 1-113.** Pharmacotherapeutic treatment for rheumatoid arthritis. The goals of modern therapy are to relieve pain and swelling, and ultimately to prevent functional impairment and joint damage. Nonsteroidal anti-inflammatory drugs (NSAIDs) include aspirin, ibuprofen, naproxen, indomethacin, celecoxib, rofecoxib, and a host of others. These medications are used to relieve the pain, swelling, and stiffness caused by rheumatoid arthritis. Simple analgesics, such as acetaminophen, are not antiphlogistic, but may be needed for patients who cannot tolerate NSAIDs. Second-line agents are employed to modify the underlying disease process and improve disease control. They should be initiated as soon as the diagnosis of rheumatoid arthritis is established. These drugs are used to slow the progression of joint damage and control systemic disease manifestations. The mechanisms of action of these agents are variable. Some, especially biological response modifiers, such as the tumor necrosis factor-alpha (TNF-α antagonists, inhibit specific inflammatory processes [28a–28d]. Glucocorticoids are frequently used to gain control of a disease flare, and as treatment for organ-threatening systemic manifestations, such as vasculitis and nodular scleritis. Because of drug intolerances or poor disease control on NSAIDs and second-line therapy, many patients still require long-term, low-dose glucocorticoids (usually less than 15 mg/day) for management of the inflammatory disease.

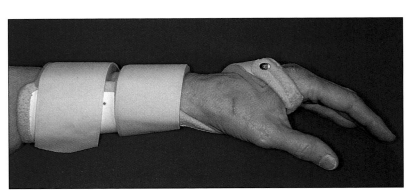

**FIGURE 1-114.** Wrist splint. Splinting contributes greatly to pain relief and stabilization of the affected joint. Both active and resting splinting are used. This is an example of a splint used to immobilize the wrist of a patient with active rheumatoid arthritis. This splint permits the use of the fingers, and can be worn during activity and at rest. Splints and orthotics, including shoe inserts, do not prevent joint deformities in this disease.

# Juvenile Rheumatoid Arthritis

## Criteria and Types

### JRA—DEFINITION

Age of onset <16 y of age
Exclusion of other causes of childhood arthritis
Continuous presence of arthritis for at least 6 wk
Arthritis is defined as:
  Joint swelling or effusion, or
  Two of the following: joint tenderness, decreased ROM, pain on ROM, or joint warmth

**FIGURE 1-115** Criteria for the diagnosis of juvenile rheumatoid arthritis (JRA). In 1977 the American Rheumatism Association defined criteria for the diagnosis of JRA. ROM—range of motion. (*From* Brewer and coworkers [29]; with permission.)

### JRA—CLASSIFICATION

**Based on the predominant clinical features during the first 6 mo of disease:**

Systemic onset: Daily intermittent fevers which are typically manifest in the afternoons or evenings, often associated with rash and arthritis (either polyarticular or pauciarticular)
Polyarticular: Arthritis involving of ≥ 5 joints, without systemic features
Pauciarticular: Arthritis involving ≤ 4 joints, without systemic features

**FIGURE 1-116.** Classification of juvenile rheumatoid arthritis (JRA). JRA, also know as juvenile chronic arthritis, is a term for several forms of childhood arthritis. Clinical classification of the type of JRA is based on the presence or absence of systemic features, and the number of diarthrodial joints involved. (*From* Brewer and coworkers [29]; with permission.)

## JRA–DIFFERENTIAL DIAGNOSIS

### Seronegative Spondyloarthropathies

Ankylosing spondylitis
Reiter's disease
Arthritis associated with psoriasis
Arthritis associated with inflammatory
 bowel disease

### Systemic Connective Tissue Diseases

Systemic lupus erythematosus
Scleroderma and related conditions
Overlap syndromes (MCTD, *etc.*)
Sj\#154>gren's syndrome

### Idiopathic Inflammatory Myopathies

### Systemic Vasculitides

Large-sized vessel (Takayasu's, *etc.*)
Medium-sized vessel (Wegener's, *etc.*)
Small-sized vessel (Henöch-Schonlein purpura, *etc.*)
Other (Beçhet's, *etc.*)

### Infectious

Septic arthritis
Osteomyelitis

### Postinfectious

Rheumatic fever
Lyme disease

### Other Systemic Illness

Chronic active hepatitis
Familial Mediterranean fever
Sarcoidosis
Pigmented villonodular synovitis

### Periaticular Pain: Metabolic

Bone marrow expansion leukemia, sickle cell, *etc.*
Metastatic disease (*eg*, neuroblastoma)
Primary bone/cartilage tumors
Hypertrophic osteoarthropathy

### Periarticular Pain: Nonmetabolic

Overuse syndromes
"Growing pains"
Fibromyalgia
Somatization

### Trauma

**FIGURE 1-117.** Differential diagnosis of juvenile rheumatoid arthritis (JRA). The differential diagnosis for JRA is quite broad. Many of these diagnoses have clinical features that differentiate them from the various types of JRA. At the outset, it may be difficult to distinguish these various conditions. MCTD—mixed connective tissue disease.

## Epidemiology

## JRA–EPIDEMIOLOGY

Systemic JRA: 10% to 15% of new cases
Polyarticular JRA: 15% to 20% of
 new cases
Pauciarticular JRA: 65% to 75% of
 new cases

**FIGURE 1-118.** Epidemiology of juvenile rheumatoid arthritis (JRA). Data are from a population-based study in Rochester, Minnesota. Compared with other nonpopulation-based studies, a higher proportion of pauciarticular JRA was observed in this study. (*From* Peterson *et al.* [30]; with permission.)

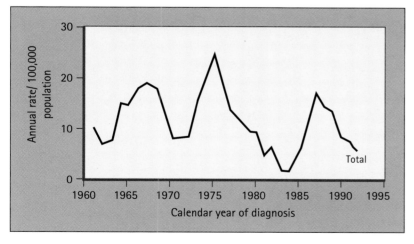

**FIGURE 1-119.** Annual incidence of JRA. Three year moving average of the incidence of JRA in Rochester, Minnesota. The significance of this variation in incidence rate for JRA is unclear.
For this study:
 Incidence: 11.7 (8.7%, 14.8%) cases/100,000 year, age-adjusted
 Prevalence: 86.1 (36.9%, 135.3%) per 100,000.
(*From* Peterson *et al.* [30]; with permission.)

*Rheumatoid Arthritis, Juvenile Rheumatoid Arthritis, and Related Conditions*

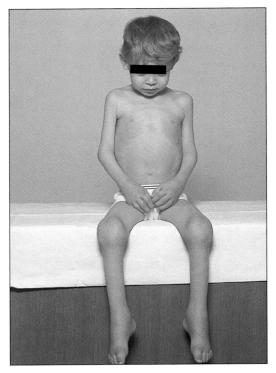

**FIGURE 1-120.** Juvenile rheumatoid arthritis (JRA)—polyarticular disease. This child has florid polyarticular JRA. There are large effusions in the knees, ankles, hands, and wrists. The limited extension of the neck is indicative of cervical spine involvement. Prominent muscular atrophy of the extremities is secondary to persistent arthritis disease. Disease-related growth retardation is evident.

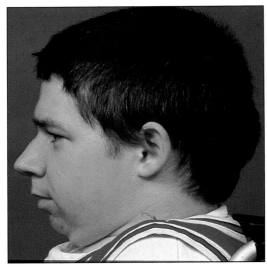

**FIGURE 1-121.** Micrognathia in juvenile rheumatoid arthritis (JRA). This child has impressive micrognathia as a sequelae of JRA, evident on this lateral photograph. (*Courtesy of* Suzanne L. Bowyer, MD.)

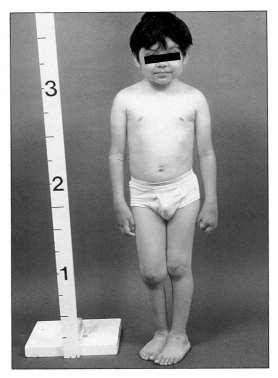

**FIGURE 1-122.** Knee involvement in juvenile rheumatoid arthritis (JRA). Toddlers and preschoolers who present with pauciarticular JRA frequently have knee involvement. Shown here is a toddler with a moderate-sized knee effusion. Knee effusions from pauciarticular JRA are frequently not very painful in this age group. (*Courtesy of* Donald A. Person, MD.)

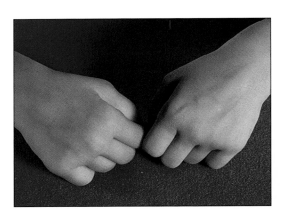

**FIGURE 1-123.** Polyarticular juvenile rheumatoid arthritis (JRA)—synovitis. Tenosynovitis and synovitis of the hands and wrists are frequent in children with the polyarticular form of JRA. There is marked swelling of the extensor tendons of the wrists and metacarpophalangeal joints.

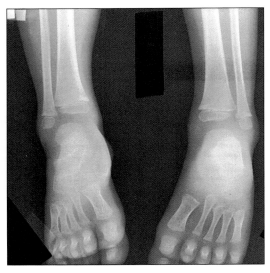

**FIGURE 1-124.** Radiograph of soft tissue swelling in juvenile rheumatoid arthritis (JRA). Early in the course of JRA, soft tissue swelling may be the only radiographic finding. This 2-year-old boy with systemic-onset JRA had a polyarticular course including ankle effusions. There is radiodense soft tissue swelling over the medial malleoli.

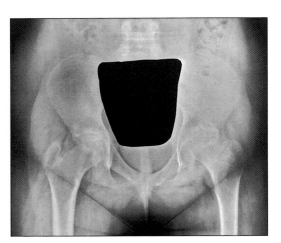

**FIGURE 1-125.** Hip involvement in juvenile rheumatoid arthritis (JRA). Hip involvement in JRA may be associated with a worse overall outcome. This is due to the limited blood supply to the growing femoral epiphysis and because of its critical nature in weight bearing and ambulation. In spite of very aggressive medical management, destructive changes as seen on this radiograph may occur. There are changes on both the femoral and acetabular sides of the hip.

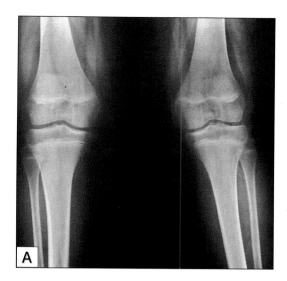
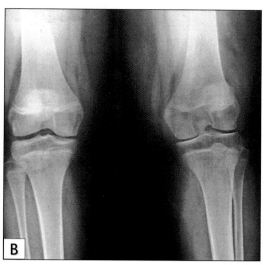

**FIGURE 1-126.** Radiographic progression of knee involvement in juvenile rheumatoid arthritis (JRA). Shown are radiographs (**A** and **B**) of standing knee films on an 11-year-old girl with JRA taken 16 months apart. There is significant loss of the medial joint space of the left knee with bony overgrowth of the medial femoral condyle. Some degree of widening of the femoral condyles of the right knee also can be appreciated.

## Extra-articular Sites

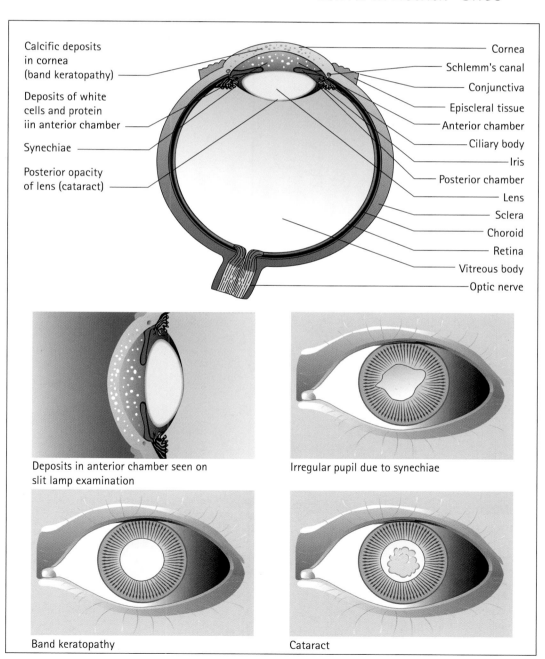

Calcific deposits in cornea (band keratopathy)

Deposits of white cells and protein iin anterior chamber

Synechiae

Posterior opacity of lens (cataract)

Cornea
Schlemm's canal
Conjunctiva
Episcleral tissue
Anterior chamber
Ciliary body
Iris
Posterior chamber
Lens
Sclera
Choroid
Retina
Vitreous body
Optic nerve

Deposits in anterior chamber seen on slit lamp examination

Irregular pupil due to synechiae

Band keratopathy

Cataract

**FIGURE 1-127.** Ocular involvement in juvenile rheumatoid arthritis (JRA). The spectrum of eye involvement in JRA is broad. Almost always, it is initially asymptomatic. Young children with pauciarticular JRA are at greatest risk for eye involvement, especially if they have positive antinuclear antibody serology. (*Adapted from* Netter [31].)

*Rheumatoid Arthritis, Juvenile Rheumatoid Arthritis, and Related Conditions*

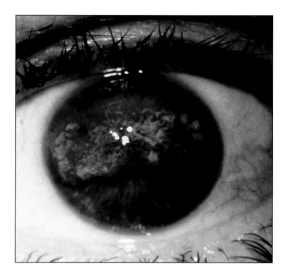

**FIGURE 1-128.** Band keratopathy in juvenile rheumatoid arthritis (JRA). After prolonged uveal inflammation in children with JRA, dense bands may form in the anterior chamber, which may severely compromise vision.

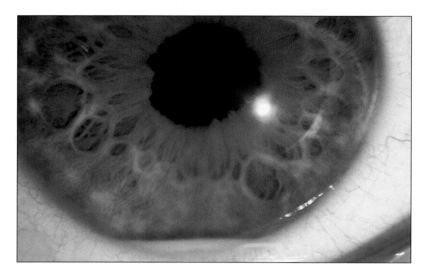

**FIGURE 1-129.** Hypopyon in juvenile rheumatoid arthritis (JRA). This 6-year-old girl with antinuclear antibody–negative pauciarticular JRA has an accumulation of pus in the inferior aspect of the anterior chamber of the left eye. She also has some irregularity of the shape of the pupil secondary to synechia. Hypopyon is an uncommon manifestation of uveitis in children with JRA.

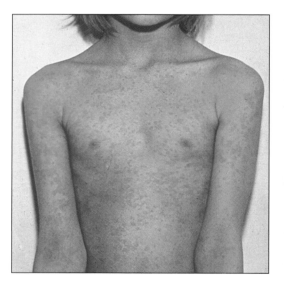

**FIGURE 1-130.** Rash in systemic-onset juvenile rheumatoid arthritis (JRA). This girl with systemic-onset JRA has a florid, diffuse, nonvesicular rash, which is most prominent during an afternoon fever spike.

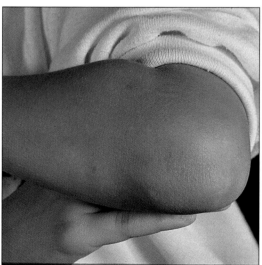

**FIGURE 1-131.** Rheumatoid nodules in juvenile rheumatoid arthritis (JRA). Rheumatoid nodules are seen on the olecranon surface of the left elbow of this girl with polyarticular JRA. While less frequently seen in children, nodules are a marker of more aggressive disease, as they are in adults with rheumatoid arthritis.

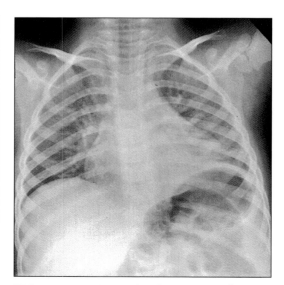

**FIGURE 1-132.** Pericarditis in juvenile rheumatoid arthritis (JRA). Pericarditis is occasionally seen in children with systemic onset JRA. This child had a small pericardial effusion on echocardiography. The cardiac silhouette is mildly enlarged. Pleural effusions may also be seen in children with systemic-onset JRA.

# Laboratory Features

## JRA—LABORATORY STUDIES

Rule out other causes for joint symptoms
   (infection, *etc.*)
Assess acuity of disease (systemic onset)
   Acute-phase reactants
   Anemia
   Serositis
Assess prognosis
   RF: Less than 10%; worse prognosis
   ANA: Usually pauciarticular; increases relative risk of uveitis
   Radiographs: Radiographic changes are associated with worse
      prognosis

**FIGURE 1-133.** Laboratory studies in juvenile rheumatoid arthritis (JRA). Laboratory studies in JRA are often neither specific or sensitive for the diagnosis. They can provide prognostic information including increased risk for worse outcome with positive rheumatoid factor (RF). Children with pauciarticular JRA who are antinuclear antibody (ANA) positive are at increased risk for uveitis. Levels of acute-phase reactants, degree of anemia, and evidence of serositis on radiographs are studies frequently used in the management of children with systemic-onset JRA.

# Treatment

## JRA—NONDRUG TREATMENTS

Meeting basic needs: family, socioeconomic, financial issues
Education: patient, family, school
Balance of rest and appropriate physical activity
Physical and occupational therapy
Splinting of actively involved joints
Good general pediatric care

**FIGURE 1-134.** Nondrug treatment for juvenile rheumatoid arthritis (JRA). The impact of JRA may be profound in many areas of the child's daily activities including family, school, and peers/relational issues. As with other children with chronic illness, good primary medical care is very important. Rehabilitative interventions such as occupational and physical therapy, and splinting, can beneficially impact the course of JRA.

## JRA—NSAIDS MOST COMMONLY USED

Aspirin: 60–100 mg/kg/d divided tid
Ibuprofen*: 30–40 mg/kg/d divided tid
Naproxen sodium*: 15–20 mg/kg/d divided bid
Tolmetin sodium: 20–30 mg/kg/d divided tid
Diclofenac: 2–3 mg/kg/d divided bid or tid

*Liquid preparations are available in the United States*

**FIGURE 1-135.** Commonly used nonsteroidal anti-inflammatory drugs (NSAIDs) in juvenile rheumatoid arthritis (JRA). Dosage ranges for commonly used NSAIDs in children with JRA are shown. Suggested baseline laboratory studies for the use of NSAIDs in adults with rheumatoid arthritis include complete blood count with differential, creatinine, alanine aminotransferase, and aspartate aminotransferase Newer cyclooxygenase-2 inhibitors are increasingly being used in children. (*From* ACR Clinical Guidelines Committee [32]; with permission.)

## JRA—FREQUENTLY USED DMARDS

Hydroxychloroquine: 5–27 mg/kg/d qd or divided bid
Sulfasalazine: target dose of 40–60 mg/kg/d divided bid or tid
IM gold: target dose of 1 mg/kg/wk, up to 50 mg/wk; typically 20
   weekly injections, then dose adjusted to clinical response
Methotrexate, 10 mg/M$^2$, given once per week, usually orally
Etanercept, 25 mg subcutaneously, twice weekly

**FIGURE 1-136.** Frequently used disease-modifying antirheumatic drugs (DMARDs) in juvenile rheumatoid arthritis (JRA). Dosage ranges for commonly used DMARDs in children with aggressive or JRA are shown. Methotrexate is frequently used to treat children with aggressive or recalcitrant disease; tumor necrosis factor-alpha (TNF-α antagonists have been demonstrated to be effective in children as well as adults.

## JRA—BASELINE LABORATORY STUDIES FOR MONITORING DMARDS

Hydroxychloroquine: Retinal examination every 6 mo
Sulfasalazine: CBC with differential, AST/ALT; consider G6PD screen
IM gold: CBC with differential, creatinine, urinalysis
Methotrexate: CBC with differential, AST/ALT, albumin, alkaline
   phosphatase, creatinine; consider hepatitis B and C serology

**FIGURE 1-137.** Baseline laboratory studies for the use of disease-modifying antirheumatic drugs (DMARDs). Suggested baseline laboratory studies for the use of DMARDs in adults with rheumatoid arthritis. ALT—alanine aminotransferase; AST—aspartate transaminase; CBC—complete blood count; G6PD—glucose-6-phosphate dehydrogenase; IM—intramuscular. (*From* ACR Clinical Guidelines Committee [32]; with permission.)

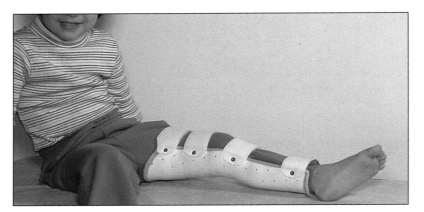

**FIGURE 1-138.** Splinting in juvenile rheumatoid arthritis (JRA). This child has been fitted with a knee splint which will be used at night time to allow the knee to be in a more extended position when the child sleeps. Splinting is often used to facilitate the maintenance of a more appropriate alignment of clinically involved joint in children with JRA.

## Outcome

### JRA—PROGNOSIS

Poorer prognosis is associated with
  Systemic-onset disease
  Polyarticular disease
  (+) Rheumatoid factor
  Need for treatment with systemic
    corticosteroids
  Younger age at onset of disease
  Female gender

**FIGURE 1-139.** Prognosis in juvenile rheumatoid arthritis (JRA). The higher the number of poor prognostic indicators, the greater the need to be aggressive in the initial management of JRA. Good controlled long-term prospective studies of JRA are lacking. Most of the information regarding prognosis in JRA is from case series.

## Related Conditions

### FELTY'S SYNDROME

### FELTY'S SYNDROME—CRITERIA

Chronic (rheumatoid) arthritis
Splenomegaly
Leukopenia

**FIGURE 1-140.** Felty's syndrome—criteria. The original criteria for Felty's syndrome were first described in 1924. (*From* Felty [33].)

## Clinical Features

### FELTY'S SYNDROME—CLINICAL FEATURES

Rheumatoid arthritis, usually seropositive, nodular
Two-thirds are female
Increased frequency of Drw4
Splenomegaly
Granulocytopenia
Leg ulcers
Recurrent infections
Other extra-articular features
  Sjögren's syndrome
  Episcleritis

**FIGURE 1-141.** Felty's syndrome—clinical features. This syndrome usually occurs in patients with long-standing, nodular rheumatoid arthritis, although one third may not have active synovitis at the time of diagnosis.

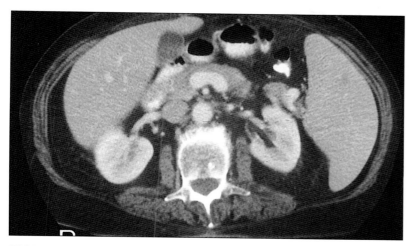

**FIGURE 1-142.** Marked splenomegaly. Marked splenomegaly is seen on this computed tomography scan in a patient with Felty's syndrome. The spleen may be mildly enlarged to massively increased in size in rheumatoid arthritis. Splenomegaly is not uncommon in patients without neutropenia, and is thought to be related to the systemic lymphoid hyperplasia common in rheumatoid arthritis. About one third of patients with neutropenia and rheumatoid arthritis do not have splenomegaly. (*Courtesy of* Timothy J. Welch, MD.)

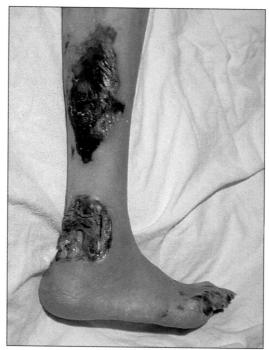

**FIGURE 1-143.** Leg ulcers in Felty's syndrome. Leg ulcers are frequently seen in patients with Felty's syndrome. They tend to be over the anterior aspect of the tibia, and are often very difficult to manage. In this patient, the ulcers were associated with rheumatoid vasculitis, including involvement of the toes. (*Courtesy of* Robert M. Valente, MD.)

## Laboratory Features

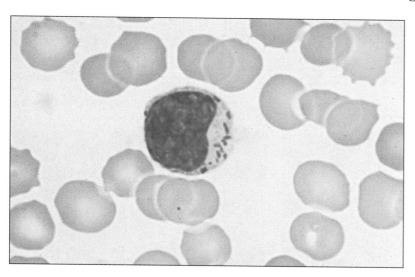

**FIGURE 1-144.** Felty's syndrome—large granular lymphocytes (LGL). This photomicrograph shows the large granular lymphocytes that are frequently seen in patients with Felty's syndrome. These cell populations are often polyclonal, but may be a single cell line. The significance of LGL is unclear. They may also be present in patients with rheumatoid arthritis who do not have Felty's syndrome.

## Treatment

**FELTY'S SYNDROME—TREATMENT**

Evaluate for infection
Splenectomy
Gold injections, possibly other DMARDs,
  including methotrexate
Stimulate production of granulocytes
  Testosterone
  Lithium
  Colony stimulating factor

**FIGURE 1-145.** Treatment of Felty's syndrome. Treatment of patients has been difficult. Many of these patients are using immunosuppressive medications for their rheumatoid arthritis and have granulocytopenia, predisposing to recurrent infections. While splenectomy can improve the features of hypersplenism, including anemia, leukopenia, and thrombocytopenia, it is not clear that the frequency of infections after splenectomy is decreased. A number of agents have been tried to increase the number of circulating granulocytes, with variable success. DMARDs—disease modifying antirheumatic drugs.

## SJÖGREN'S SYNDROME— CLINICAL FEATURES

Sicca symptoms (especially keratocon-
  junctivitis and xerostomia)
Parotid enlargement
Arthralgia/arthritis
Renal tubular acidosis
Raynaud's phenomenon
Palpable purpura/vasculitis
Central/periperal nervous system
Interstitial lung disease
Autoantibodies
Evidence of reticuloendothelial activation
Increased relative risk of lymphoma

**FIGURE 1-146.** Sjögren's syndrome—
clinical features. Sjögren's syndrome is a
systemic autoimmune illness with many clinical and laboratory features. Significant dry
eyes and dry mouth along with other mucosal
surfaces (sicca) are very common features.
The eye dryness is associated with filamentary
keratitis. Parotid gland enlargement is
frequently bilateral. Musculoskeletal manifestations and autoantibodies are also common
features.

## SJGREN'S SYNDROME— DIAGNOSTIC TESTS

Ophthalmologic
  Schirmer's test
  Rose-Bengal staining
Minor salivary gland biopsy
Elevated levels of acute-phase reactants
Evidence of B-cell activation
  Hypergammaglobulinemia
  Autoantibodies
    Rheumatoid factors
    Cryoglobulins
    Antinuclear antibodies, including
      SSA (Ro), SSB (La)

**FIGURE 1-147.** Sjögren's syndrome—diagnostic tests. Eye dryness can be quantitated by
a Schirmer's test, and evidence of filamentary
keratitis can be detected by Rose-Bengal
staining. A biopsy of a minor salivary gland of
the lower lip can detect lymphoid aggregates
consistent with Sjögren's syndrome. Autoantibodies are frequently found in patients with
Sjögren's syndrome, but antibodies to SSA (Ro)
or SSB (La) are more specific for Sjögren's
syndrome. SSA—Sjögren's antigen A;
SSB—Sjögren's antigen B.

## SJÖGREN'S SYNDROME— ASSOCIATED DISEASES

Primary Sjögren's
Secondary Sjögren's
  Rheumatoid arthritis
  Systemic lupus erythematosus
  Scleroderma
  Inflammatory myopathies
  Other connective tissue diseases
Lymphoproliferative disorders

**FIGURE 1-148.** Associated diseases in
Sjögren's syndrome. Sjögren's syndrome
frequently occurs with or after the onset of
another connective tissue disease such as
rheumatoid arthritis or scleroderma (secondary
Sjögren's). It may also occur without another
connective tissue disease (primary Sjögren's).
The relative risk of lymphoproliferative disorders, especially lymphoma, is increased in
patients with Sjögren's syndrome.

## Clinical Features

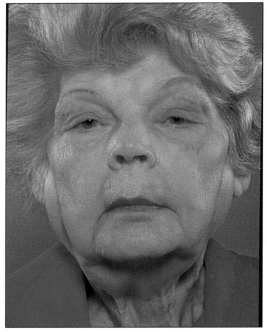

**FIGURE 1-149.** Parotid enlargement in
Sjögren's syndrome. There is marked bilateral
enlargement of the parotid glands in this
patient with Sjögren's syndrome.

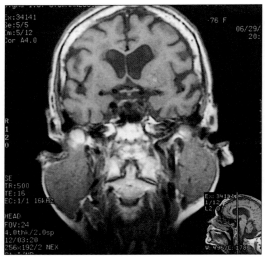

**FIGURE 1-150.** Bilateral parotid enlargement—magnetic resonance imaging (MRI).
This coronal view MRI of the head demonstrates the massive bilateral parotid enlargement of the patient seen in Figure 1-149.

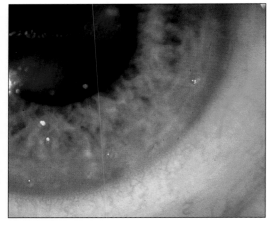

**FIGURE 1-151.** Keratitis in Sjögren's
syndrome—Rose-Bengal stain. Positive Rose-
Bengal staining is seen in this patient with
Sjögren's syndrome. The area of punctate
staining (light pink) around the inferior
periphery of the cornea is due to corneal
damage (keratitis).

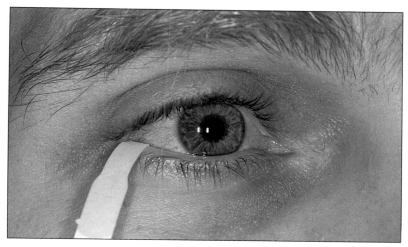

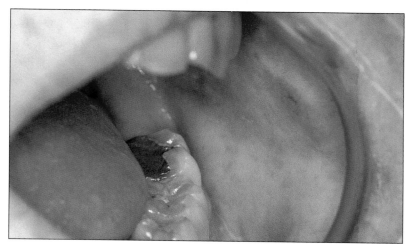

**FIGURE 1-152.** Schirmer's test. Schirmer's test is used to assess eye dryness. Less than 5 mm of wetness on the paper at 5 minutes is significant but not very sensitive or specific for Sjögren's syndrome. This patient had a normal Schirmer's test. (*Courtesy of* Keith H. Baratz, MD.)

**FIGURE 1-153.** Xerostomia (dry mouth) in Sjögren's syndrome. This woman has secondary Sjögren's syndrome associated with scleroderma. The parched appearance, mucosal atrophy, and evidence of mechanical irritation to the buccal mucosa are due to the profound dryness.

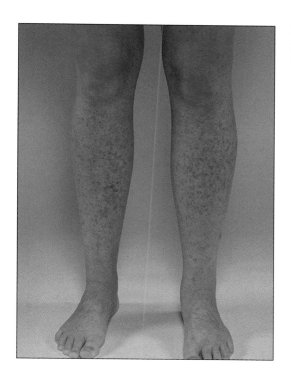

**FIGURE 1-154.** Sjögren's syndrome—palpable purpura. Palpable purpura is not uncommon in patients with Sjögren's syndrome. It is secondary to immune complex deposition and subsequent small vessel vasculitis. (*Courtesy of* Audrey M. Nelson, MD.)

## Laboratory Features

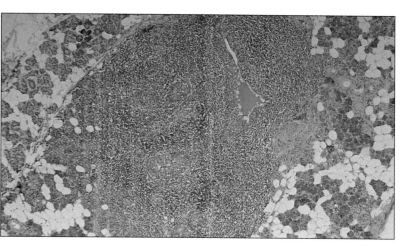

**FIGURE 1-155.** Salivary gland histology in Sjögren's syndrome. Low-power photomicrograph of a minor salivary gland biopsy from the patient seen in Figure 1-149. Note the dense, diffuse lymphocytic infiltrate. In patients with Sjögren's syndrome, most of the lymphocytes are CD4 positive. (Hematoxylin and eosin, medium power.)

## SJÖGREN'S SYNDROME— TREATMENT OPTIONS

Sicca
  Adequate oral fluids with nonsweetened liquids
  Frequent dental visits
  Moisture (artificial tears, ophthalmologic care)
  Avoid drying agents (anticholinergic drugs)
Musculoskeletal
  NSAIDs, antimalarials, low-dose systemic corticosteroids
Vasculitic
  Systemic corticosteroids, cytotoxic agents
Vigilance for osteoporosis, lymphoproliferative malignancies
Treatment of associated disease in secondary Sjögren's

**FIGURE 1-156.** Treatment options in Sjögren's syndrome. Treatment of Sjögren's syndrome, as with other systemic connective tissue diseases, depends on the severity of the various organ systems involved. For organ-threatening disease, aggressive immunosuppressive therapy, including high-dose systemic corticosteroids or cytotoxic agents may be required. The increased relative risk of lymphoproliferative disease suggests the need for surveillance for these conditions in patients with Sjögren's syndrome.

## ADULT STILL'S DISEASE

### ADULT-ONSET STILL'S DISEASE— CLINICAL FEATURES

Arthralgia or arthritis
High fever (>39°C), especially in afternoon and evening
Fleeting, salmon-pink maculopapular rash, most prominent with fever
Anemia and elevated acute-phase reactants
Evidence of reticuloendothelial activation
Serositis

**FIGURE 1-157.** Adult-onset Still's disease—clinical features. The clinical manifestations of adult-onset Still's disease are very similar to systemic-onset juvenile rheumatoid arthritis. (*From* Bywaters [34]; with permission.)

### ADULT-ONSET STILL'S DISEASE— DIAGNOSTIC CRITERIA

**Major Criteria**

Fever of >39°C lasting >1 wk
Arthralgias or arthritis lasting >2 wk
Typical rash
WBC >10,000/mm$^3$ with >80% polymorphonuclear cells

**Minor Criteria**

Sore throat
Lymphadenopathy and/or splenomegaly
Transaminase elevation not secondary to other causes
RF and ANA negative

**FIGURE 1-158.** Diagnostic criteria for adult-onset Still's disease. These are the preliminary criteria for the diagnosis of adult-onset Still's disease (AOSD). The presence of five or more criteria, of which at least two are "major criteria," has a 96% sensitivity and a 92% specificity for the diagnosis of AOSD. ANA—antinuclear antibodies; RF—rheumatoid factor; WBC—white blood cell count. (*From* Yamaguichi *et al.* [35]; with permission.)

**FIGURE 1-159.** Differential diagnosis of adult-onset Still's disease (AOSD). The differential diagnosis of AOSD is quite broad. Frequently, the diagnosis is made after an extensive workup to exclude all other causes of the patient's symptoms.

### ADULT-ONSET STILL'S DISEASE— DIFFERENTIAL DIAGNOSIS

Differential diagnosis of AOSD is very similar to that of a fever of unclear origin

| Infectious | Malignant | Other Connective Tissue Diseases |
|---|---|---|
| Viral | Lymphoma | Vasculitis |
| Bacterial | Leukemia | Rheumatoid arthritis |
| Parasitic | | Systemic lupus erythematosus |
| Other | | Reactive arthropathies (*eg*, serum sickness, postinfectious processes) |

### ADULT-ONSET STILL'S DISEASE—JOINT INVOLVEMENT

May be oligoarthritis or polyarthritis
Frequently destructive
Involvement of "root joints" carries a worse prognosis
Wrist commonly involved
The degree of articular involvement is more indicative of prognosis than extra-articular involvement

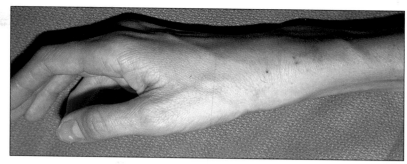

**FIGURE 1-160.** Joint involvement in adult-onset Still's disease (AOSD). The articular involvement of AOSD differs from rheumatoid arthritis. Often the wrist is involved, but the small joints of the fingers may be spared. The symmetry of articular disease typically seen in rheumatoid arthritis may be absent in patients with AOSD. In both, the arthritis can be destructive and deforming. Root joint (especially shoulders, hips, and knees) involvement is a marker of poor prognosis.

**FIGURE 1-161.** Wrist involvement in adult-onset Still's disease (AOSD). Wrist synovitis is seen in a patient with AOSD. Large joint involvement is characteristic of this illness; however, small joint involvement is not uncommon.

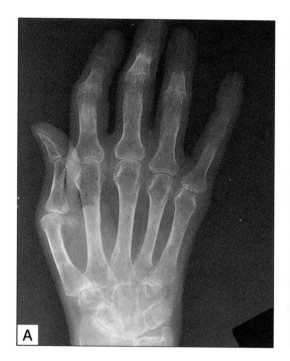

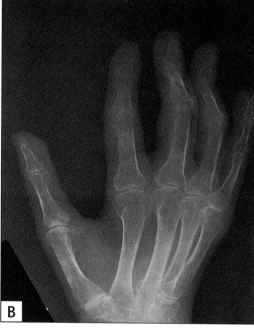

**FIGURE 1-162.** Radiographic changes in adult-onset Still's disease (AOSD). **A** and **B**, Radiograph of hand and wrist of a patient with destructive polyarthritis of AOSD. Periarticular osteopenia and loss of joint space are pervasive. Note the destructive changes at the proximal interphalangeal joints.

## *Clinical Features—Extra-articular*

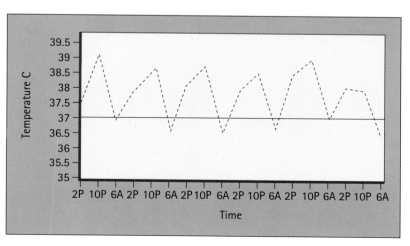

**FIGURE 1-163.** Fever pattern in patients with adult-onset Still's disease (AOSD). The fever pattern in AOSD is characteristically quotidian. During the mornings, the body temperature may be (sub)normal, but in the afternoon or evenings, it may exceed 40°C.

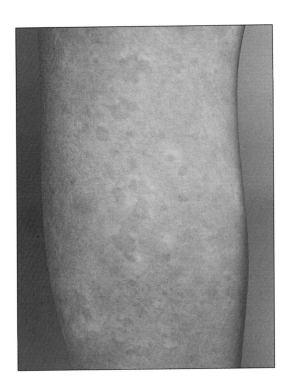

**FIGURE 1-164.** Rash in adult-onset Still's disease (AOSD). The rash of AOSD is usually truncal, nonpruritic, and nonvesicular. Dermatographism may be present, but this finding is nonspecific. The rash is evanescent, often seen only during the time of the fever spikes.

## Laboratory Features

### ADULT-ONSET STILL'S DISEASE—LARBORATORY STUDIES

Acute-phase reactants
  Increased ESR, CRP, thrombocytosis, ferritin
Hypergammaglobulinemia
  Autoantibodies not present
Articular disease
  Erosive disease
Evidence of serositis
Evidence of reticuloendothelial activation
  Lymphadenopathy
  Hepatosplenomegaly

**FIGURE 1-165.** Adult-onset Still's disease (AOSD)—laboratory studies. The laboratory evaluation of patients with AOSD consists of an assessment of acute-phase reactants, extra-articular organ involvement, and articular involvement. Evidence of anemia, serositis, and hepatomegaly are common extra-articular features along with the fever and rash. The joint involvement can range from mild oligoarthritis to a destructive, erosive polyarthritis. CRP—C-reactive protein; ESR—erythrocyte sedimentation rate.

## Treatment

### ADULT-ONSET STILL'S DISEASE—TREATMENT

Establish the correct diagnosis
Extra-articular features
  Fevers: aspirin, NSAIDs, systemic glucocorticoids
  Anemia: exclude other causes; attain improved disease control
  Serositis: NSAIDs, systemic glucocorticoids
Articular
  Assess prognosis (number of joints involved, radiographic changes)
  Aspirin, NSAIDs
  Glucocorticoids (systemic and intra-articular)
  Methotrexate
  Other immunosuppressives, possibly TNF-α antagonists

**FIGURE 1-166.** Adult-onset Still's disease (AOSD)—treatment. The treatment of patients with AOSD is based on the evaluation of both the extra-articular and articular features of the disease. Often aspirin and nonsteroidal anti-inflammatory drugs (NSAIDs) are used with systemic glucocorticoids.

# REMITTING SERONEGATIVE SYNOVITIS WITH PITTING EDEMA (RS3PE) SYNDROME

## *Clinical Features*

**RS3PE SYNDROME—CLINICAL FEATURES**

Elderly
Symmetric small joint synovitis
Pitting edema of the hands and feet
Rheumatoid factor negative
Generally favorable outcome

**FIGURE 1-167.** Clinical features of remitting seronegative synovitis with pitting edema (RS3PE) syndrome [36]. There may be clinical overlap with polymyalgia rheumatica. Some patients eventually develop another identifiable rheumatic disease, especially rheumatoid arthritis. RS3PE can occasionally be a paraneoplastic manifestation of an underlying malignancy. Magnetic resonance imaging demonstrates marked tenosynovitis as a major cause of swelling in RS3PE [37].

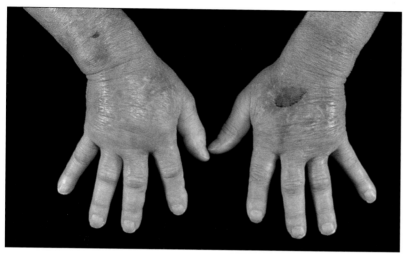

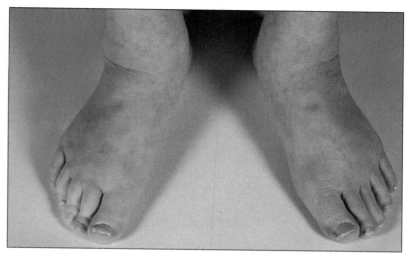

**FIGURE 1-168.** Hand involvement in remitting seronegative synovitis with pitting edema (RS3PE) syndrome. Hand swelling in RS3PE syndrome is characteristically diffuse as in this patient the swelling is due mainly to florid tenosynovitis. In addition to the edema, small joint synovitis is present at the metacarpophalangeal joints and the proximal interphalangeal joints.

**FIGURE 1-169.** Foot involvement in remitting seronegative synovitis with pitting edema (RS3PE) syndrome. As with hand swelling, foot swelling in the RS3PE syndrome is diffuse. This is the same patient seen in Figure 1-168.

## *Treatment*

**RS3PE SYNDROME—TREATMENT**

Establish diagnosis
Careful use of NSAIDs
Low-dose oral prednisone
Antimalarials

**FIGURE 1-170.** Treatment of remitting seronegative synovitis with pitting edema (RS3PE) syndrome. The prognosis is generally favorable, so that aggressive medical treatment is not usually indicated. Antimalarials are favored in recalcitrant disease. Consideration must be given to potential drug-related adverse effects before treating these patients, as they are frequently elderly.

# References

1. Wolfe AM: The epidemiology of rheumatoid arthritis: a review. *Bull Rheum Dis* 1968, 19:518–522.

2. Stastny P:Association of the B-cell alloantigen Drw4 with rheumatoid arthritis. *N Engl J Med* 1978, 298:869–871.

3. Firestein GS: Etiology and pathogenesis of rheumatoid arthritis. In *Textbook of Rheumaology*, edn 5. Edited by Kelley WN, Harris ED, Ruddy S, Sledge CB. Philadelphia: WB Saunders; 1997:851–897.

4. Fleming A, Benn RT, Corbett M, *et al.*: Early rheumatoid disease: Patterns of joint involvement *Ann Rheum Dis* 1976, 35:361–364.

5. Pinals RS, Masi AF, Larsen RA, *et al.*: Preliminary criteria for clinical remission in rheumatoid arthritis. *Bull Rheum Dis* 1982, 32:7–10.

6. Sherrer YS, Block DA, Mitchell DM, *et al.*: The development of disability in rheumatoid arthritis. *Arthritis Rheum* 1986, 29:494–500.

7. Mitchell DM, Spitz PW, Yound DY, *et al.*: Survival, prognosis, and causes of death in rheumatoid arthitis. *Arthritis Rheum* 1986, 29:706–714.

8. Youinou P, Moutsopoulos HM, Pennec YL: Clinical features of Sjögren's syndrome. *Curr Opin Rheumatol* 1991, 3:815–822.

9. Cassidy JT, Petty RE: *Textbook of Pediatric Rheumatology*, edn 3. Philadelphia: WB Saunders; 1995:1–610.

10. Arnett FC, Edworthy SM, Bloch DA, *et al.*: The American Rheumatism Association 1987 Revised Criteria for the Classification of Rheumatoid Arthritis. *Arthritis Rheum* 1988, 31:315–324.

11. Ad Hoc Committee on Clinical Guidelines: Guidelines for the initial evaluation of the adult patient with acute musculoskeletal symptoms. *Arthritis Rheum* 1996, 39:1–8.

12. Mitchell DM: Rheumatoid arthritis. In *Rheumatoid Arthritis: Epidemiology, Etiology, Diagnosis and Treatment*. Edited by Utsinger PO, Zvaifler NJ, Ehrlich GE. Philadelphia: JB Lippincott; 1985:133–150.

13. Masi AT, Feigenbaum SL, Kaplan SB: Articular patterns in the early course of rheumatoid arthritis. *Am J Med* 1983, 75 (Suppl 6A):16–26.

14. Vollertsen RS, Conn DL, Ballard DJ, *et al.*: Rheumatoid vasulitis: survival and associated risk factors. *Medicine* 1986, 65:365–375.

15. Turesson C, O'Fallon WM, Matteson EL, *et al.*: Occurrence of extraarticular disease manifestations is associated with excess mortality in a population-based cohort of patients with rheumatoid arthritis [submitted].

16. Steinbrocker O, Traeger CH, Batterman RC: Therapeutic criteria in rheumatoid arthritis. *JAMA* 1949, 140:659–662.

17. Wordsworth P, Bell J: Polygenic susceptibility in rheumatoid arthritis. *Ann Rheum Dis* 1991, 50:34–36.

18. Gravallese EM, Manning C, Tsay A, *et al.*:Synovial tissue in rheumatoid arthritis is a source of osteoclast differentiation factor. *Arthritis Rheum* 2000, 43:250–258.

18a. Schrieber L:The endothelium in rheumatoid arthritis. In *Rheumatology*. Edited by Klippel JH, Dieppe PA. London: CV Mosby; 1994 3.10–3.10.6.

19. Lane JM, Weiss C: Review of articular cartilage collagen research. *Arthritis Rheum* 1975, 18:553–562.

20. Harris ED Jr: Rheumatoid arthritis: Pathophysiology and implications for therapy. *N Engl J Med* 1990, 322:1277–1289.

21. Pincus T, Callahan LF, Brooks RH, *et al.*: Self-report questionnaire scores in rheumatoid arthritis compared with traditional, physical, radiographic, and laboratory measures. *Ann Intern Med* 1989, 110:259–266.

22. Walker WC, Wright V: Pulmonary lesions and rheumatoid arthritis. *Medicine* 1968, 47:501–520.

23. Walker WC, Wright V: Diffuse interstitial fibrosis and rheumatoid arthritis. *Ann Rheum Dis* 1969, 28:252–259.

24. Bonfiglio T, Atwater EC: Heart disease in patients with seropositive rheumatoid arthritis. *Arch Intern Med* 1969, 124:714–719.

25. Tighe H, Carson DA: Rheumatoid factors. In *Textbook of Rheumatology*, edn 5. Edited by Kelley WN, Harris ED Jr, Ruddy S, Sledge CB. Philadelphia: WB Saunders; 1997, 241–249.

26. Schumacher HR Jr, Reginato AJ: *Atlas of Synovial Fluid Analysis and Crystal Identification*. Philadelphia: Lea & Febiger; 1991.

27. Fassbender H-G: Inflammatory reactions in arthritis. In *Immunopharmacology of Joints and Connective Tissue*. Edited by Davies ME, Dingle JT. London: Harcourt, Brace; 1994:166–198.

28. Ad Hoc Subcommittee on Clinical Guidelines: Guidelines for the management of rheumatoid arthritis. *Arthritis Rheum* 1996, 39:713–722.

28a. Moreland LW, Heck LW Jr, Koopman WJ: Biologic agents for treating rheumatoid arthritis. *Arthritis Rheum* 1997, 40:397–409.

28b. Moreland LW, Baumgartner SW, Schiff MH, *et al.*: Treatment of rheumatoid arthritis with a recombinant human tumor necrosis factor receptor (p75)-Fc fusion protein. *N Engl J Med* 1997, 337:141–147.

28c. Weinblatt ME, Kremer JM, Bankhurst AD, *et al.*: A trial of etanercept, a recombinant tumor necrosis factor receptor:Fc fusion protein, in patients with rheumatoid arthritis receiving methotrexate. *N Engl J Med* 1999, 340:253–259.

28d. Maini R, St Clair EW, Breedveld F, *et al.*: Infliximab (chimeric anti-tumour necrosis factor α monoclonal antibody) versus placebo in rheumatoid arthritis patients receiving concomitant methotrexate: A randomised phase III trial. *Lancet* 1999, 354:1932–1939.

29. Brewer EJ, Bass J, Baum J, *et al.*: JRA Criteria Subcommittee of the Diagnosis and Therapeutic Criteria Committee of the American Rheumatism Association: Current proposed revision of the JRA criteria. *Arthritis Rheum* 1977, 20(Suppl):195–199.

30. Peterson LS, Mason T, Nelson A, *et al.*: Juvenile rheumatoid arthritis in Rochester, Minnesota. Is the epidemiology changing? *Arthritis Rheum* 1996, 39:1385–1390.

31. Netter FH: Rheumatic diseases. In *The Cibe Collection of Medical Illustrations*, vol 8, part II. Summit, NJ: Ciba Giegy, 1990, 176.

32. ACR Clinical Guidelines Committee: Guidelines for monitoring drug therapy in rheumatoid arthritis. *Arthritis Rheum* 1996, 39:723–731.

33. Felty AR: Chronic arthritis in the adult, associated with splenomegaly and leucopenia. *Johns Hopkins Hosp Bull* 1924, 35:16–20.

34. Bywaters EGL: Still's disease in the adult. *Ann Rheum Dis* 1971, 30:121–133.

35. Yamaguichi M, Ohta A, Tsunematsu T: Preliminary criteria for the diagnosis of adult Still's disease. *J Rheumatol* 1992, 19:424–430.

36. McCarthy DJ, O'Duffy JD, Pearson L, *et al.*: Remitting seronegative symmetrical synovitis with pitting edema. *JAMA* 1985, 254:2763–2767.

37. Cantini F, Salvarani C, Olivieri I, *et al.*: Remitting seronegative symmetrical synovitis with pitting oedema (RS3PE) syndrome: a prospective follow up and magnetic resonance imaging study. *Ann Rheum Dis* 1999, 58:230–236.

# 2

# Osteoarthritis and Crystal-Associated Synovitis

## STEPHEN L. MYERS

A successful strategy for the clinical management of the patient with osteoarthritis requires an appreciation of the natural history of the disease, an assessment of the nature and severity of the pathology present in the symptomatic joint, and an understanding of the pros and cons of the available therapies. Osteoarthritis can produce symptoms in nearly any joint, but it is most strongly associated with work disability and has the greatest socioeconomic impact when it affects the hip or knee. Its prevalence increases steadily with age, and by 65 years of age, radiographic evidence of osteoarthritis is present in about 70% of the population.

To the pathologist, osteoarthritis is characterized by structural and mechanical failure of the articular cartilage. Biochemical and metabolic changes occur in the articular cartilage before significant structural damage is visible in the joint, or radiographic signs of the disease appear and considerable capacity of the tissue for repair. Studies of advanced disease show that this reparative effort ultimately fails because mechanical factors and degradative enzymes result in breakdown, fibrillation, and irreversible ulceration of the articular cartilage. Pathologic changes develop in other joint tissues as the disease progresses; osteophytes form at the osteochondral junction, the synovium becomes inflamed and fibrotic, tears and fibrillation damage the menisci, and sclerosis and cystic changes develop in the subchondral bone under the arthritic cartilage.

For the clinician, osteoarthritis is a disease of the whole joint. Joint pain is almost always the principal symptom, but variable degrees of stiffness, muscular weakness, and joint deformity contribute significantly to the patient's reduced functional capacity. It is important to determine what the patient can and cannot do because of their arthritis symptoms and to judge whether comorbid conditions, such as vascular claudication, or neuropathy contribute to the problem. The symptomatic joint and adjacent soft tissue should be inspected for muscle atrophy and swelling and palpated to correctly diagnose symptoms that arise in bursae, ligaments, tendons, or in myofascial tender points. Signs of joint inflammation include local erythema, warmth, swelling, and diffuse tenderness to palpation.

The suspicion of joint inflammation in a patient with osteoarthritis, particularly when a joint effusion or prominent swelling is detected, suggests a coincident crystal-induced arthropathy or even joint sepsis. This should be pursued, without delay, by diagnostic arthrocentesis and analysis of the synovial fluid. Recognition and correct treatment of gouty arthritis is important because chronic, tophaceous gout constitutes a preventable cause of secondary osteoarthritis. One of the clinical manifestations of calcium pyrophosphate dihydrate (CPPD) deposition is acute pseudogout, although many patients with osteoarthritis and evidence of CPPD in their cartilage or synovial fluids do not recall acute attacks of pain and swelling. There is a predilection to deposits of CPPD or basic calcium phosphate (hydroxyapatite) in damaged or osteoarthritic cartilage. Whether synovial fluid crystals of these compounds drive the progression of cartilage destruction in osteoarthritis remains controversial, but they are readily identified in the joint effusions common in advanced disease. The elevated synovial fluid leukocyte count (eg, 1000 to 2000 cells/mm$^3$) and histologic changes of mild synovitis present in many, but not all, patients with osteoarthritis are evidence that chronic inflammation is a sequela of cartilage damage.

Epidemiologic studies often rely on skeletal radiographs of a sample population to detect characteristic changes of osteoarthritis, which include loss of joint space, osteophytes, subchondral cysts, and bony sclerosis. In practice, joint radiographs are not required to initiate treatment; clinical criteria enable a diagnosis of osteoarthritis to be made in patients who are over age 50 and have joint crepitus. Radiographs are useful to evaluate the severity of osteoarthritis in a particular joint and invaluable when evidence of a traumatic injury is present. They may identify conditions that predisposed the patient to develop osteoarthritis or explain the course of the disease. For example, radiographs are required to identify chondrocalcinosis produced by deposition of CPPD or hydroxyapatite in the articular cartilage or adjacent fibrocartilagenous menisci.

No dogmatic approach to the management of symptomatic osteoarthritis is likely to be satisfactory. Simple strategies that provide patient information and psychologic support (*eg*, repeated telephone calls by a skilled nurse) have shown considerable efficacy. Many patients do well with regimens that combine an exercise program, a cane, or an appropriate resting splint with nonnarcotic analgesics. Some show sufficient improvement to wean themselves from medica-

tions entirely. Others respond only to more potent analgesics, anti-inflammatory agents, or intra-articular injections of corticosteroids. Ultimately, some patients require joint arthroplasty. The rationale for treatment that includes anti-inflammatory drugs is strong in patients who have crystal-induced synovitis, but the severity of pre-existing structural damage in the articular cartilage is a critical determinant of therapeutic success.

# Osteoarthritis

## *Symptoms and Examination*

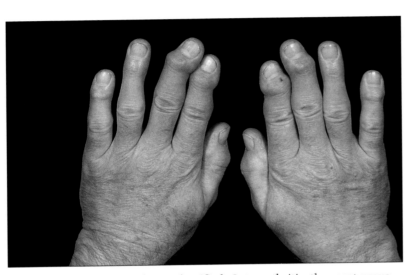

**FIGURE 2-1.** Osteoarthritis classified. Osteoarthritis, the most prevalent form of arthritis in the United States, is characterized by progressive loss of the articular cartilage that comprises the normal weight-bearing surface of the joint and remodeling of the bone beneath and adjacent to that cartilage. The swelling and angular deformities of the distal interphalangeal joints of the second and third fingers seen here are caused by osteoarthritis in these joints.

### PRIMARY OSTEOARTHRITIS

#### Clinical Subsets
Generalized osteoarthritis: affects hands, hips, knees, first CMC and MTP joints, cervical or lumbar spine.
Primary generalized or nodal osteoarthritis: involves DIP and IP joints, females:males 10:1
Erosive osteoarthritis: red, swollen DIP or IP joints; often first CMC, hip, and knee symptoms

**FIGURE 2-2.** Primary osteoarthritis. Several clinical subsets of patients with primary or idiopathic osteoarthritis have been described, although many patients cannot readily be classified into one of these categories on the basis of existing radiographic criteria. To date, useful genetic or immunologic markers that distinguish these subsets of patients have not been identified. Most clinicians will recall patients with *generalized osteoarthritis* that involves three or more joints, who have, for example, symptoms in their spine, knees, hips, in the first carpometacarpophalageal joint (CMC) at the base of the thumb, the distal fingers, and the great toe. The wrists, elbows, and shoulder are typically spared. A second group of patients with generalized osteoarthritis includes women who develop painful swelling of several distal interphalangeal (DIP) or proximal interphalangeal (IP) joints within a year or two of menopause and have a strong family history of osteoarthritis. They have been described as having *nodal osteoarthritis*. Another subset of patients have *erosive osteoarthritis* characterized by the erythema and tenderness that develops in multiple DIP and IP joints and by the development of "erosive" changes and osteophytes at these sites. MTP—metatarsophalangeal.

### WEIGHT-BEARING PAIN

#### Patients with hip or knee osteoarthritis often report pain or difficulty when:
- Walking
- Ascending or descending stairs
- Standing
- Bending, stooping
- Rising from a low chair or the toilet
- Getting in or out of bus, car, or bath
- Adjusting footwear

**FIGURE 2-3.** Weight-bearing pain. Involvement of the weight-bearing joints is the most common cause of disability in osteoarthritis and typically produces pain on walking, using stairs, or eventually, with prolonged standing. Transient stiffness in the involved joint is common after a period of inactivity, but this rarely persists for more than 15 minutes. Although the pain of hip osteoarthritis is usually felt in the groin, in some patients this pain is referred to the thigh or knee. Bending, stooping, or any activity that requires exertion while the hip or knee is flexed tends to produce pain. For example, getting out of a car can be particularly troublesome.

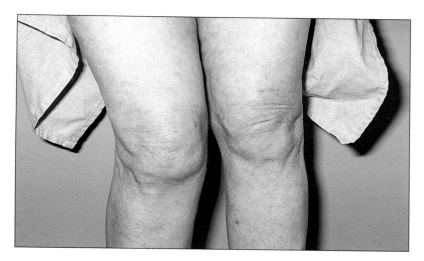

**FIGURE 2-4.** Valgus deformity—knee. This 64-year-old woman has a severe valgus deformity of the right knee and normal alignment of the left knee. Standing radiographs of her right knee showed changes of osteoarthritis in the medial, lateral, and patellofemoral compartments. The bulge seen lateral to the patella in the right knee suggests that a significant synovial effusion is present in the suprapatellar bursa. There is no cutaneous erythema to indicate the presence of acute inflammation in this knee, although more than 50% of specimens of synovial fluid aspirated from osteoarthritic knees contain crystals of either calcium pyrophosphate dihydrate (CPPD) or apatite.

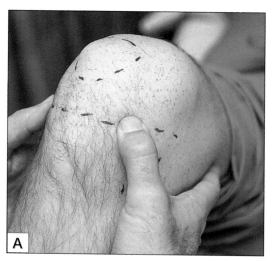
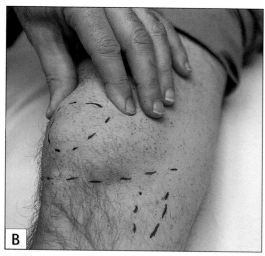

**FIGURE 2-5.** Knee palpation. **A**, Examination of the osteoarthritic knee should include palpation along and proximal to the joint line, indicated by the dashed line beneath the examiner's thumb. Crepitus can be elicited by passive flexion and extension of the joint. Osteophytes that arise at the osteochondral margins of the joint and loose bodies trapped in the gutters along the medial and lateral aspects of femoral condyles or in the suprapatellar bursa can be palpated. Tenderness in these areas suggests underlying synovitis. An estimate of the degree of medial-lateral laxity in the joint can be obtained by applying a valgus and then a varus stress to the joint. The margins of the patella are outlined by a dashed line. **B**, Palpation of the margins of the patella, outlined here by the dashed circle below the examiner's fingers, may reveal osteophytes. The "shrug sign," or knee pain reproduced by pressing above the patella (as illustrated) while the patient contracts the quadriceps muscle, suggests that cartilage pathology is present in the patellofemoral portion of the knee.

**FIGURE 2-6.** Bursa palpation. The examiner's right thumb palpates the anserine bursa. This bursa is below the knee and between the tibia and the pes anserine, a conjoint tendon of the sartorius and gracilis muscles that inserts on the proximal tibia. Pain that arises in the anserine bursa can mimic or exacerbate the pain of knee osteoarthritis and can be reproduced by deep palpation in this area. Local measures, such as hot packs or injection of the bursa with a mixture of bupivacaine and corticosteroids, usually provide effective relief.

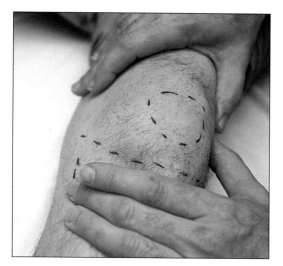

**FIGURE 2-7.** Bulge sign. Most osteoarthritic knees do not contain a substantial joint effusion, and when one is detected synovial fluid should be aspirated for an analysis that includes a cell count and a thorough search for crystals. The technique of eliciting the bulge sign is illustrated. After the examiner compresses the medial aspect of the knee to force synovial fluid into the supralateral portion of the suprapatellar pouch, the thumbs are used to compress that region and force the effusion back to the medial portion of the knee. This produces a readily visible bulge over the medial aspect of the knee proximal to the joint line. This technique may fail when a large knee effusion (> 30 mL) is present or the patient is unable to relax the quadriceps muscle. In such cases, patellar ballotment may be used to confirm the presence of an effusion.

*Osteoarthritis and Crystal-Associated Synovitis*

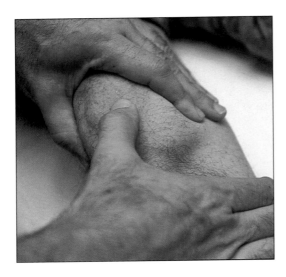

**FIGURE 2-8.** Patellar ballotment. The patella should be balloted to detect large (> 30 mL) knee effusions that distend the suprapatellar bursa enough to make the bulge sign an unreliable test for the presence of an effusion. Here, the left hand has been used to compress the suprapatellar bursa after the patient has relaxed the quadriceps muscle. This maneuver should force the patella away from the femoral trochlea, and depending on the volume and chronicity of the effusion, a gap of several millimeters can be created. Patellar ballotment is then detected by pressing the patella toward the femur with the right thumb.

## Diagnostic Methods

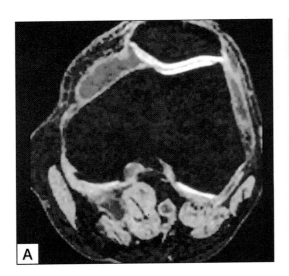
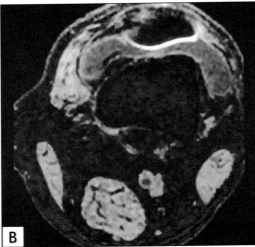

A

B

**FIGURE 2-9.** Magnetic resonance imaging (MRI). **A,** A synovial effusion (*gray area*) is present lateral to the patella in this MRI view of the left knee. This effusion would be readily detected as a bulge sign in the anterolateral aspect of the knee on physical examination of the joint. The smooth contour of apparently normal articular cartilage is visible on the opposed surfaces of the patella and femoral trochlea. **B,** This image of the knee at approximately the superior pole of the patella shows a large synovial effusion (*gray area*) in the suprapatellar bursa. This is an appropriate location for needle aspiration of the joint effusion, using either a medial or lateral approach, because it is proximal to the articular cartilages of the femoral trochlea and the patella.

### INTERPRETATION OF SYNOVIAL FLUID FINDINGS IN JOINTS WITH CLINICAL AND RADIOGRAPHIC EVIDENCE OF OSTEOARTHRITIS

| Example 1 | Example 2 | Example 3 |
|---|---|---|
| Volume < 10 mL | Volume = 10–30 mL | Volume = 10–50 mL |
| Viscosity = Normal | Viscosity = Normal | Viscosity = Reduced |
| WBC < 200 cells/mm$^3$ | WBC 200–2000 cells/mm$^3$ | WBC = 500–50,000 cells/mm$^3$ |
| Birefringent crystals = None | Birefringent crystals = None | Birefringent crystals = Positive |
| Normal synovial fluid: | Possible causes: | Crystal arthropathy: |
|   Hypervolemia |   Apatite crystals |   CPPD |
|   Hypoalbuminemia |   Cartilage factors |   Urate (gout) |
| |   Cartilage debris |   Depo-corticosteroid |

**FIGURE 2-10.** Synovial fluid findings. Normal synovial fluid (Example 1) contains very few leukocytes and no crystals that are birefringent, or visible with the polarizing microscope. Asymptomatic knee effusions seen in patients with congestive heart failure or anasarca typically contain such synovial fluid, as do some osteoarthritic joints. Synovial fluid from most osteoarthritic joints (Example 2) is viscous, and is noninflammatory, or contains fewer than 2000 leukocytes/mm$^3$. Inflammatory factors that may cause such effusions include apatite crystals, which are not birefringent, and both soluble and particulate cartilage debris. Inflammatory synovial fluid, (Example 3) is sometimes obtained from the osteoarthritic joint, and can contain birefringent crystals such as calcium pyrophosphate dihydrate (CPPD) or monosodium urate. Corticosteroid crystals that have been injected into the joint are also birefringent and can cause confusion. WBC—white blood cells.

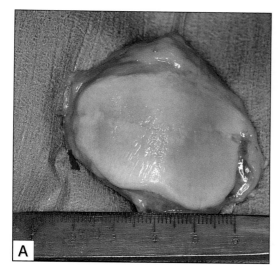

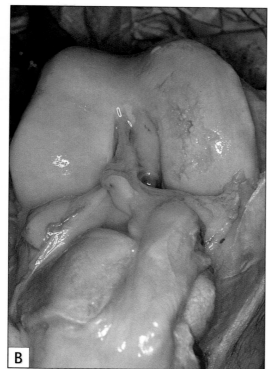

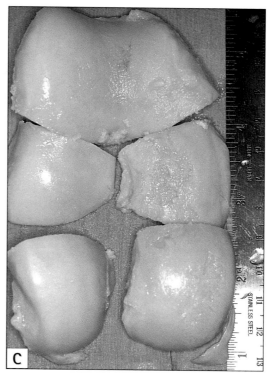

**FIGURE 2-11.** Fibrillated cartilage. **A**, This osteoarthritic patella shows thinned, fibrillated cartilage that has a "crab-meat" appearance. Patients with patellofemoral osteoarthritis often benefit from exercise programs that include isometric strengthening of the quadriceps muscle. **B**, The suprapatellar bursa of this osteoarthritic knee was opened, and the patella was dislocated to expose a large area of eroded cartilage on the medial femoral condyle. Thinning and erosion of the patellar cartilage are also visible. **C**, An osteoarthritic femoral condyle was sawed into sections to display the distribution of roughened, pitted, and fibrillated articular surfaces. The most severe changes in this knee were located on the central and "habitually loaded" area of the medial condyle. In patients with end-stage osteoarthritis who undergo knee arthroplasty, this area often contains no cartilage and the subchondral bone is exposed.

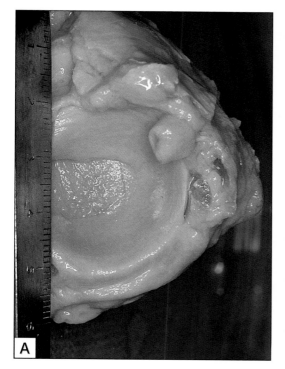

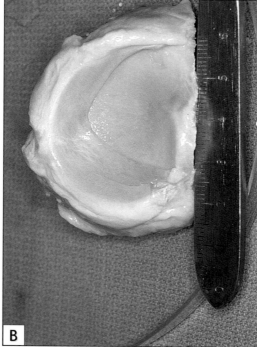

**FIGURE 2-12.** Roughened and pitted articular cartilage. **A**, The lateral tibial plateau is largely covered by the lateral meniscus, a flexible fibrocartilage that plays an important role in load distribution in the knee. This meniscus has a normal appearance. The articular cartilage in the central region of the tibia appears roughened and pitted, which indicates osteoarthritis is present. Changes of more severe osteoarthritis, such as fibrillation or erosion of the cartilage, are not seen. The tibial cartilage beneath the meniscus was grossly normal. Some authorities argue that minor degenerative changes in tibial and patellar cartilage reflect normal aging rather than an early stage of osteoarthritis. **B**, The medial meniscus covers less of the articular surface of the adjacent tibial plateau than the lateral meniscus. The surface of the osteoarthritic articular cartilage on this tibia is pitted, and a small erosion of the articular surface is seen near the thin posterior horn of the meniscus.

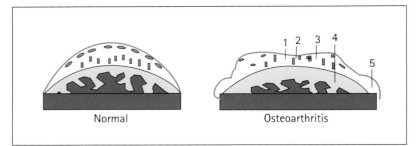

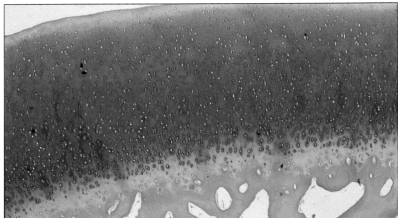

**FIGURE 2-13.** Chondrocytes. The cartilage cells, or chondrocytes, in normal articular cartilage lie parallel to the smooth articular surface near the surface, but in deeper zones of the cartilage they are aligned in columns perpendicular to the surface. Important pathologic changes seen in osteoarthritic cartilage include 1) fissures, or cracks in the cartilage that reflect breakdown of the collagen ``scaffolding'' in the tissue, and its loss of tensile strength; 2) thinning and erosion that can progress to full-thickness defects in the cartilage; 3) focal proliferation (cloning) of chondrocytes and eventual loss of the capacity of the cells to maintain the proteoglycan-rich tissue matrix; 4) thickening and remodeling of the subchondral plate; and 5) endochondral ossification at the joint margins that produces osteophytes.

**FIGURE 2-14.** Normal articular cartilage. In this photomicrograph (10×) of normal articular cartilage, the articular surface (*top*) is smooth, and the bony trabeculae of the subcondral plate comprise the bottom of the frame. The intensity of the red safranin O stain corresponds to the concentration of proteoglycan in the cartilage matrix, which is lowest near the surface of the cartilage. Proteoglycans are very large molecules that rely on complex carbohydrates to hold water in the cartilage matrix and make it resilient.

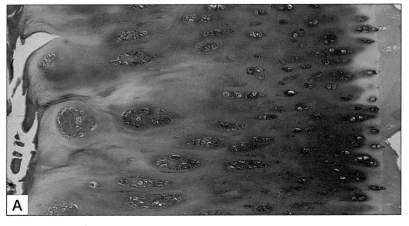

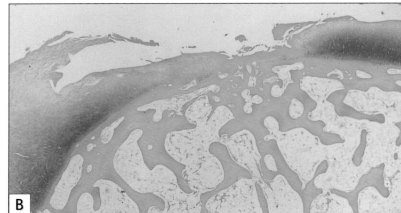

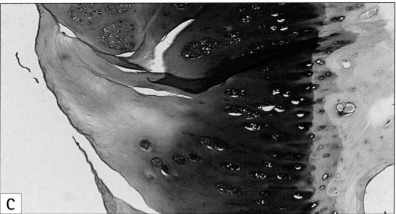

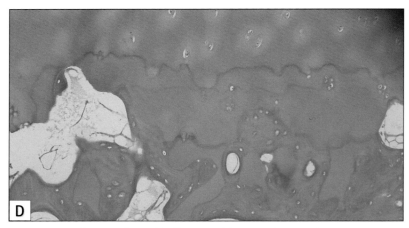

**FIGURE 2-15.** Cartilage defects. **A**, Superficial fibrillation, or cleft formation, is present in the articular cartilage surface on the left in this specimen (25×). Note that the matrix surrounding the proliferating chondrocytes is stained red, indicating continued proteoglycan synthesis by these cells. **B**, Photographed at a low (5×) magnification, this specimen shows a full-thickness defect in the articular cartilage. There is cartilage fibrillation and loss of red safranin staining for proteoglycan at the margins of the ulcerated area. In such advanced lesions, the synovial fluid comes in contact with the subchondral bone which can lead to the formation of bone cysts [1]. **C**, Histologic changes of severe osteoarthritis are seen in this section whose proteoglycans were stained with toluidine

blue (25×). There is deep fibrillation of the cartilage, with prominent chondrocyte clones in some areas and severe cellular depletion and loss of proteoglycan in others. **D**, This photomicrograph (50×) of osteoarthritic articular cartilage taken near the chondro-osseous junction shows several irregular purple lines, or tidemarks. In normal cartilage, a single tidemark separates the articular cartilage matrix, which is not calcified, from a narrow zone of calcified cartilage that lies between cartilage and the cortical surface of the subchondral bone. The multiple tidemarks seen in osteoarthritic cartilage reflect an active, dynamic remodeling of the cartilage–bone interface that can be viewed as an adaptive response to the disease.

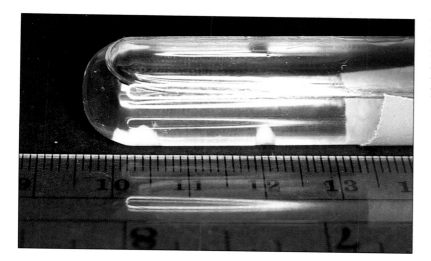

**FIGURE 2-16.** Joint lavage. Several controlled studies have shown symptomatic improvement in patients with knee osteoarthritis who underwent joint lavage with 1 to 3 L saline administered through an arthroscope trochar or a comparable large-bore needle [2]. These 2- to 3-mm tissue fragments recovered during such a lavage proved on histologic examination to be fibrillated cartilage.

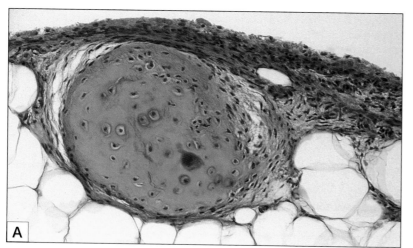

A

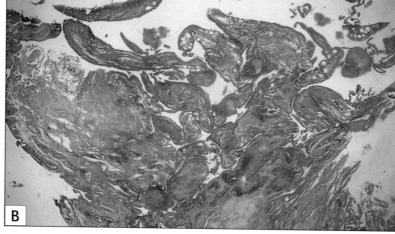

B

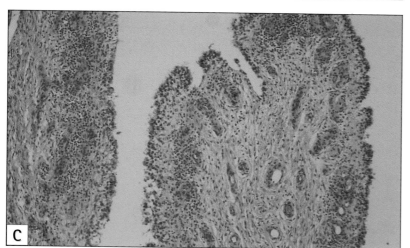

C

**FIGURE 2-17.** Histologic examination of synovium. **A,** Synovium from a patient with advanced osteoarthritis (50×) contains a fragment, or shard, of fibrillated cartilage that has become embedded in the tissue. This fragment has not elicited a local inflammatory response although such debris, or molecules released from the cartilage matrix, may be responsible for the synovial inflammation that eventually develops in most osteoarthritic joints. The loose body seen in a radiograph of the osteoarthritic joint usually represents a calcified fragment of cartilage or bone. **B,** A low-power photomicrograph (10×) of osteoarthritic synovium removed at the time of knee arthroplasty shows marked proliferation of the synovial villi. These minute, finger-like projections of the synovial membrane greatly increase its surface area, and probably facilitate the entrapment and eventual removal of debris from the synovial fluid. The severity of infiltration by chronic inflammatory cells and other inflammatory changes in such specimens often equals that seen in rheumatoid synovium, but osteoarthritic synovium does not form an invasive pannus that damages the joint. **C,** This photomicrograph (50×) of osteoarthritic synovium shows chronic inflammation, with infiltration of the tissue around small synovial blood vessels by mononuclear cells. There is a two- to threefold increase in the thickness of the layer of synovial cells that makes up the lining of the joint cavity. Many of these cells are macrophage-like phagocytes, whereas others produce the hyaluronic acid that imparts viscosity to the synovial fluid. Histologic evidence of acute synovial inflammation, such as fibrin or extravascular neutrophils, is rare in osteoarthritic synovium. None is seen in this specimen.

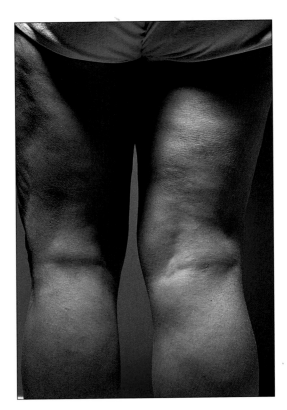

**FIGURE 2-18.** Popliteal cyst. A popliteal, or Baker's cyst is seen in the right knee. These cysts reflect excess synovial fluid production, and although more common in chronic inflammatory arthropathies than in osteoarthritis, they constitute a reversible cause of knee pain. Ultrasound examination of the popliteal fossa is the preferred method of diagnosis, and treatment with intra-articular corticosteroid therapy and rest is usually successful.

### INDICATIONS FOR RADIOGRAPHY OF THE OSTEOARTHRITIC JOINT

Detect narrowing of the joint space that indicates thin, arthritic cartilage

Distinguish involvement of the medial and lateral tibiofemoral and patellofemoral compartments of the knee

Identify linear calcifications (chondrocalcinosis) in cartilage or menisci that suggest CPPD arthropathy

Exclude other arthropathies and skeletal lesions associated with joint pain

**FIGURE 2-19.** Indications for radiography. In the patient with typical symptoms and physical findings of osteoarthritis, radiographs can be used to estimate the severity of cartilage loss in the symptomatic joint. It is important to remember that the radiographic joint space represents the total thickness of the cartilage on both the proximal and distal sides of the joint and may underestimate the severity of cartilage damage. Conversely, technical factors can lead to overestimation of the severity of osteoarthritis. Knee radiographs can be used to evaluate involvement of the patellofemoral joint (skyline views) and the medial and lateral tibiofemoral compartments (weight-bearing, standing, or semiflexed anteroposterior views). Radiographic detection of chondrocalcinosis, or calcification in the articular cartilage or fibrocartilage, suggests the possibility of calcium pyrophosphate dihydrate (CPPD) arthropathy. Radiographs are also required in some situations to exclude uncommon causes of joint pain, such as hypertrophic pulmonary osteoarthropathy or bone tumor.

# Secondary Osteoarthritis

## Causes

### HERITABLE DISORDERS ASSOCIATED WITH SECONDARY OSTEOARTHRITIS

Hemochromatosis
Hemaglobinopathies
Hemophilia
Gaucher's disease
Ochronosis
Wilson's disease
Spondyloepiphyseal, epiphyseal, and other chondro-osseous dysplasia syndromes
Ehler-Danlos and joint hypermobility syndromes

**FIGURE 2-20.** Heritable causes of secondary osteoarthritis. Many heritable diseases can cause secondary osteoarthritis, including hemochromatosis, sickle cell anemia, hemophilia, Gaucher's disease, ochronosis, and Wilson's disease. Conditions that affect joint development, including the spondyloepiphyseal dysplasias, epiphyseal dysplasias, and a variety of chondro-osseous dysplasia syndromes are usually regarded as causes of secondary osteoarthritis. In some families primary osteoarthritis is associated with mild articular dysplasia [3]. Abnormal joint biomechanics are blamed for the occurrence of secondary osteoarthritis in patients with the Ehler-Danlos syndrome, and in those with joint hypermobility or recurrent dislocations.

### ENDOCRINE AND ACQUIRED CAUSES OF SECONDARY OSTEOARTHRITIS

Acromegaly
Hypothyroidism
Hyperparathroidism
Obesity
Frostbite
Paget's disease
Articular fracture
Meniscectomy
Osteonecrosis
Neuropathic arthropathy (Charcot's joints)

**FIGURE 2-21.** Endocrinopathies and other conditions. The endocrine disorders most strongly associated with secondary osteoarthritis are hypothyroidism, hyperparathyroidism, and acromegaly. Obesity is the most common acquired risk factor for osteoarthritis of the knee in women, although this has not proven to be the case for the hip joint, or in men [1]. Articular trauma severe enough to rupture ligaments or fracture cartilage or the subchondral bone is associated with subsequent osteoarthritis, as is repetitive joint injury (*eg*, the ballerina's bunion). Knee meniscectomy is now avoided because it increases the likelihood of osteoarthritis in that joint. Relatively uncommon causes of secondary osteoarthritis include frostbite; Paget's disease; osteonecrosis of the knee, hip, or shoulder; and neuropathic arthropathy.

**FIGURE 2-22.** Inflammatory arthropathies. Erosion or fibrillation of the articular surface of cartilage that has been damaged by the deposition of monosodium urate crystals in gout, or that contains crystals of calcium pyrophosphate dihydrate (CPPD) or apatite, constitutes secondary osteoarthritis. Articular cartilage severely damaged by an inflammatory pannus (eg, in rheumatoid or reactive arthritis) and cartilage whose matrix and cells have been destroyed by joint sepsis may continue to deteriorate and develop typical osteoarthritic changes despite optimal therapy.

## Skeletal Changes

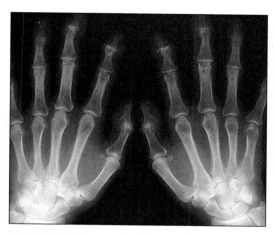

**FIGURE 2-23.** Heberden's and Bouchard's nodes. The radiographic changes that accompany the development of Heberden's and Bouchard's nodes in the distal interphalangeal (DIP) and proximal interphalangeal joints (PIP), respectively, include soft tissue swelling, angular deformities of the distal digits, osteophytes loss of joint space, and subchondral cysts. IP—interphalangeal.

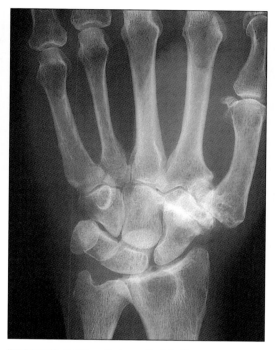

**FIGURE 2-24.** Osteoarthritic first carpometacarpal joint. This severely osteoarthritic first carpometacarpal joint is narrowed and sclerotic, and subluxation of the metacarpal produces "squaring" of the base of the thumb. There is also severe loss of articular cartilage between the trapezium and the scaphoid, and subchondral cysts are present in the scaphoid and distal radius. This man with primary generalized osteoarthritis underwent hip and knee arthroplasties.

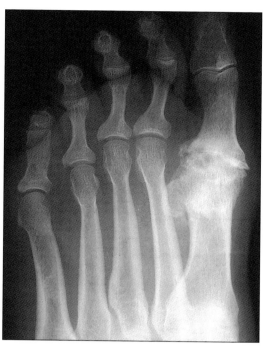

**FIGURE 2-25.** Hallux rigidus. Osteoarthritis of the first metatarsophalangeal joint is referred to as *hallux rigidus* because it results in diminished flexion of the toe and pain [4]. This radiograph shows severe loss of joint space, with osteophyte formation, subchondral sclerosis, and geodes in the metatarsal head. Typically, these osteoarthritic changes involve only the first metatarsophalangeal joint.

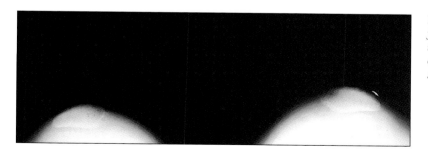

**FIGURE 2-26.** Knee osteoarthritis. Special views of the patellofemoral joint are often required to adequately evaluate knee osteoarthritis. This skyline view shows severe lateral subluxation of both patellae, with small osteophytes on the lateral margins. The patellofemoral joint space appears to be narrowed.

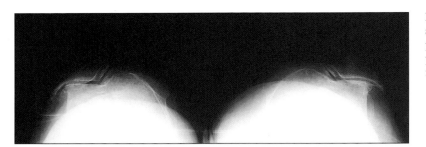

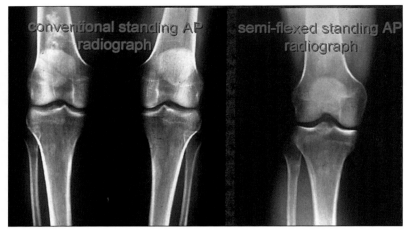

**FIGURE 2-27.** Patellofemoral joint space. The patellofemoral joint space is narrow, and there has been marked remodeling of the joint in this patient with end-stage osteoarthritis that involved the medial, lateral, and patellofemoral compartments. Large osteophytes are present on the medial and lateral aspects of the femoral condyle as well as on the patellae.

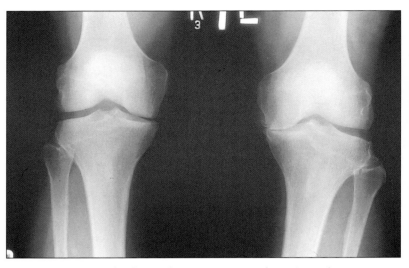

**FIGURE 2-28.** Tibiofemoral joint space, standing view. The tibiofemoral joint space in the medial compartment of the left knee is abnormally narrow, compared to that in the right knee, in this radiograph obtained with the patient standing. Marginal osteophytes are visible. Radiographs that have been obtained with the patient supine cannot be relied on to indicate the severity of joint space narrowing, and thus of cartilage loss, in the osteoarthritic knee.

**FIGURE 2-29.** Joint positioning. Standardized, reproducible positioning of the joint is essential when serial joint radiographs are used to evaluate disease progression. Specialized methods, such as using fluoroscopy to align the x-ray beam with the tibiofemoral joint while the knee is in a standing, semiflexed position, substantially improve the precision and reproducibility of measurements of joint space [5]. AP—anteroposterior.

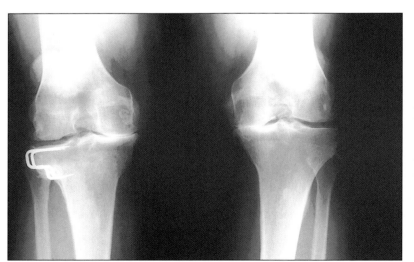

**FIGURE 2-30.** Diminished joint space. This standing knee radiograph shows moderately severe osteoarthritis. The joint space in the medial compartment of both knees is diminished, there is sclerosis of the subcondral bone, and osteophytes have formed. The metallic staple indicates that a tibial osteotomy has been performed in the right knee to temporarily alleviate the patient's knee pain.

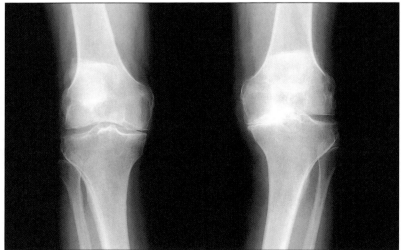

**FIGURE 2-31.** Obliteration of the joint space. There is obliteration of the joint space in the medial compartment of the left but not the right knee. This patient underwent a successful left knee replacement after failing a brief trial of medical management.

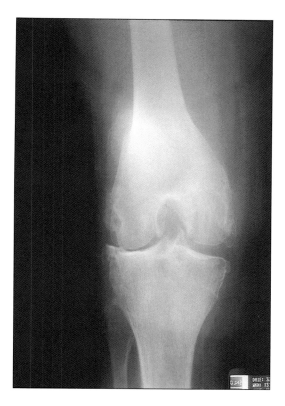

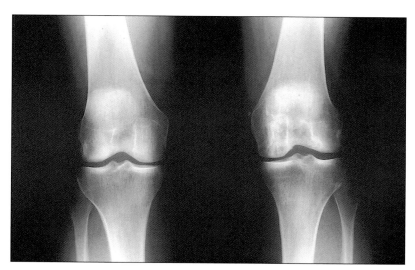

**FIGURE 2-32.**
Lateral tibiofemoral compartment narrowing. When the knee is radiographed in partial flexion, the intercondylar notch is prominent. In this example, the tunnel view radiograph reveals narrowing of the lateral but not the medial tibiofemoral compartment. Large marginal osteophytes are present.

**FIGURE 2-33.** Secondary osteoarthritis. This standing knee radiograph was obtained in a 48-year-old woman with patellofemoral crepitus and 1 to 2 years of knee pain. The slight narrowing of the medial compartment in both knees is consistent with primary osteoarthritis, but the sclerosis and cystic changes of osteonecrosis seen in the femoral condyles of the left knee indicate that she has secondary osteoarthritis. Spontaneous osteonecrosis of the knee typically occurs in older patients and can cause acute knee pain [6].

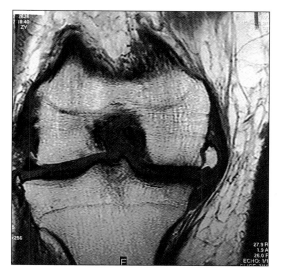

**FIGURE 2-34.** Femoral osteophytes. This coronal magnetic resonance image of the knee is a T1-weighted spin-echo image that shows femoral osteophytes on both the medial and lateral aspects of the joint. The bright signal within the osteophytes is produced by marrow fat.

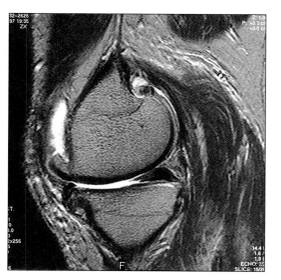

**FIGURE 2-35.** Lack of articular cartilage. In this saggital view magnetic resonance image (MRI) of a knee with advanced osteoarthritis, no articular cartilage remains on the posterior aspect of the femoral condyle to separate the margin of the subchondral cortical bone, which appears black, from the triangular posterior horn at the medial meniscus. The image was displayed as a T2-weighted fast spin-echo image. Studies to test the precision and reliability of MRI techniques that produce three-dimensional "maps" of cartilage thickness in the osteoarthritic knee are underway in several laboratories.

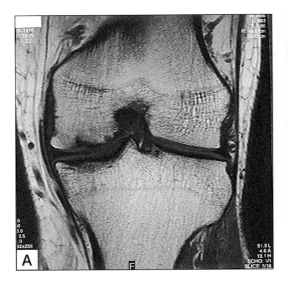

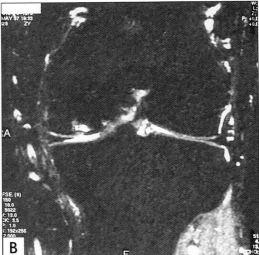

**FIGURE 2-36.** Osteoarthritic cysts. **A**, Osteoarthritic cysts, or geodes, are seen in the subchondral bone of the medial femoral condyle in this coronal T1-weighted spin-echo magnetic resonance image. **B**, In a short tau inversion recovery (STIR) image of this area, synovial fluid (*white hortizontal line within the triangular cartilage*) is visible in the joint space, as well as in the cysts, and in a tear in the medial meniscus.

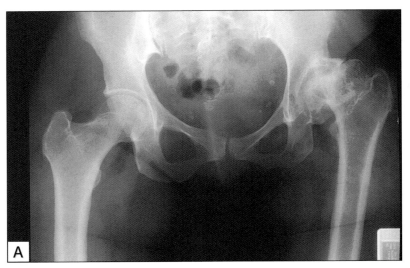

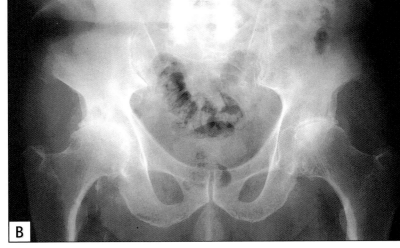

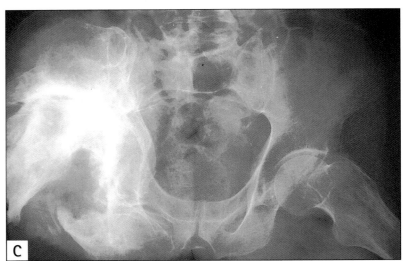

**FIGURE 2-37.** End-stage osteoarthritic changes. Pediatric diseases of the hip, including acetabular dysplasia, slipped capital femoral epiphysis, or Legg-Calve-Perthes disease are believed to be the underlying cause of most adult cases of hip osteoarthritis [7]. **A**, The left hip of this woman with a history of a slipped femoral epiphysis shows end-stage osteoarthritic changes with loss of joint space, subchondral sclerosis and cysts, osteophyte formation, and obvious shortening of the limb. The contralateral hip appears normal. She complained of right knee pain and had radiographic changes of mild osteoarthritis in that joint, which has been described as "long leg arthropathy." **B**, Radiographic changes of bilateral hip osteoarthritis in a man with primary generalized osteoarthritis include the severely narrowed joint space, osteophytes on both the femoral and acetabular aspects of the joint, and subchondral sclerosis. **C**, Severe destruction of the right hip with marked bony sclerosis, osteophytosis, and protrusion of the acetabulum has occurred in this patient with Charcot's arthropathy and neurosyphilis. Neuropathic arthropathy is also complication of syringomyelia and diabetic neuropathy. It has been described as "osteoarthritis with a vengeance."

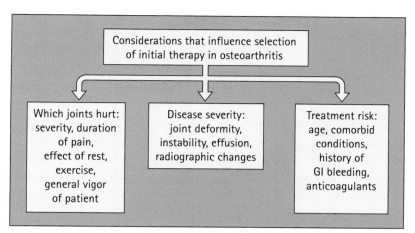

**FIGURE 2-38.** Selection of therapy. Many factors must be considered when the initial therapy for a patient with osteoarthritis is selected. One approach is to inventory the symptomatic joints and evaluate the impact arthritis has had on the patient's daily activities. The musculoskeletal examination and, when appropriate, evaluation of synovial fluid or radiographs are then used to determine the overall severity of cartilage damage, joint deformity, muscular atrophy, and joint inflammation in the affected joints. This evaluation should confirm the diagnosis of osteoarthritis. Finally, the relative risks of the treatment options available for this particular patient are assessed. The elderly are at particular risk for gastrointestinal (GI) bleeding when treated with anti-inflammatory agents and frequently have comorbid conditions that will affect the treatment plan.

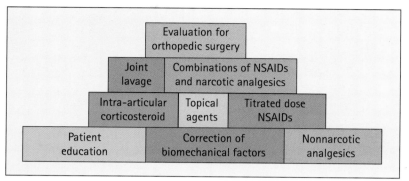

**FIGURE 2-39.** Treatment pyramid. Because osteoarthritis often involves small, large, and spinal joints in the same patient, treatment algorithms that focus on only the hip or knee can be problematic. A stepwise approach, or therapeutic pyramid, first teaches the patient about the condition, and then attempts to improve the patient's biomechanics. A trial of one or more simple analgesics is also often appropriate. Intra-articular injections of corticosteroids and systemic administration of nonsteroidal anti-inflammatory drugs (NSAIDs) have proven efficacious in the treatment of symptomatic osteoarthritis [8]. Topical agents, including capsaicin, provide additional relief in some cases. Patients who fail to obtain sufficient benefit from these steps, or whose symptoms progress over time, may require NSAIDs combined with a nonnarcotic or narcotic analgesic. Viscosupplementation with hyaluronan derivatives can reduce or eliminate pain in up to 85% of patients with osteoarthritis of the knee. These agents are being investigated for their potential efficacy in other joints affected by osteoarthritis [9,10]. Knee pain may also respond to an arthroscopic joint lavage that is performed under local anesthesia, if no surgical intervention (eg, debridement of a torn meniscus) is indicated. This approach reserves consideration of surgical management (ie, joint replacement) for patients who fail medical management and/or viscosupplementation.

## ADJUNCTS TO PHARMACOLOGIC THERAPY IN OSTEOARTHRITIS

Ambulatory assists (*eg*, cane, walker)
Adaptive devices
Splints, wraps, braces
Topical capsaicin or analgesic
Exercise to strengthen muscles
Stretching to maintain or improve joint motion
Joint lavage

**FIGURE 2-40.** Adjuncts to pharmacologic therapy. Alternatives or adjuncts to systemic drug therapy in osteoarthritis include ambulatory assists that reduce pain on ambulation and adaptive devices that reduce the strain placed on a symptomatic joint. A wide variety of splints, wraps, or braces can be used to position, support, or limit the excursion of the arthritic joint, and topical agents can be used to provide local analgesia. Therapeutic exercises strengthen and stabilize joints and can reduce joint pain; stretching and joint range-of-motion exercises help maintain mobility. Joint lavage is practical only in the knee.

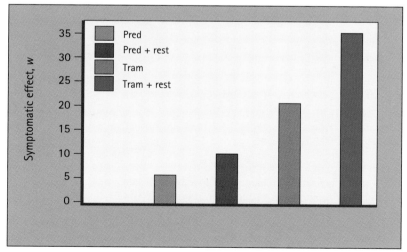

**FIGURE 2-41.** Corticosteroid therapy. Intra-articular corticosteroid therapy is used in the osteoarthritic joint to obtain prompt, albeit temporary, relief of joint swelling and reduce pain. It is routinely combined with analgesics and other treatment modalities. Although systemic absorption of intra-articular methylprednisolone acetate can be demonstrated, and subcutaneous extravasation of glucocorticoid may produce localized hyperpigmentation or lipoatrophy, this therapy is well tolerated. The duration of the symptomatic response to intra-articular corticosteroid can be improved by resting the injected joint for several days [11]. Pred—prednisolone; Tram—triamcinalone.

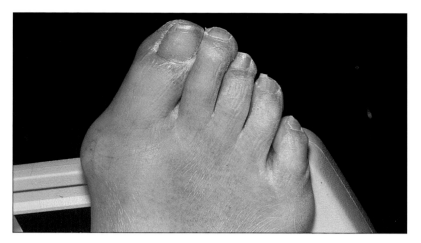

**FIGURE 2-42.** Crystal-induced synovitis. Acute crystal-induced synovitis is caused by the slow deposition in joint tissue of crystals of monosodium urate (gout), calcium pyrophosphate dihydrate (pseudogout), or apatite (*eg*, calcific tendonitis) and their subsequent acute release into the synovial fluid. Phagocytosis of these crystals in the joint stimulates a brisk, neutrophil-mediated inflammatory response. Each of these crystals is also associated with more indolent, chronic synovial inflammation in joints that show evidence of secondary osteoarthritis. Podagra, or acute pain in the first metatarsophalangeal joint that is accompanied by local redness, tenderness, and swelling (as illustrated here), is a common presentation of acute gout.

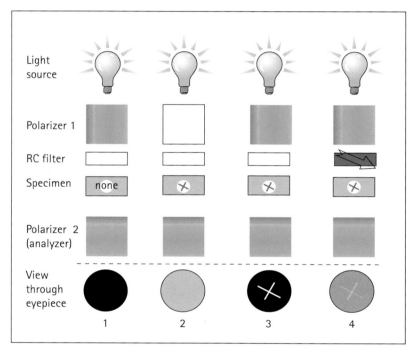

**FIGURE 2-43.** Polarizing microscopy. The unique elements of a polarizing microscope equipped for the identification of birefringent (*ie*, light-bending) crystals, including monosodium urate and calcium pyrophosphate dihydrate (CPPD), are two optical polarizers and a first-order red compensator (RC) filter. In this diagram, 1) no light reaches the eyepiece when the polarizers are correctly adjusted for crystal viewing, and neither the RC filter nor a specimen of crystal is in the optical path; 2) if one polarizer is removed (or rotated 90°), crystals are nearly transparent and can be difficult to identify; 3) urate and CPPD crystals are easily seen when a correct, perpendicular alignment of the polarizers has been obtained; 4) the addition of the RC filter to the optical path changes the background from black to magenta, enabling urate and CPPD crystals to be distinguished by their color and orientation, as well as by their shape. Urate crystals are always *negatively* birefringent, and when the long axis of this crystal parallels the optical axis of the RC filter (*black arrow*), it appears yellow. If the urate crystal is rotated clockwise, or counterclockwise, its color fades, and then changes to blue as its long axis falls perpendicular to the axis of the RC. In contrast, crystals of CPPD are *positively* birefringent and appear blue when their long axis is aligned with the axis of the RC filter. Because they have opposite birefringence, if two parallel crystals of CPPD and urate are viewed with the RC filter in place, one crystal appears blue and the other yellow.

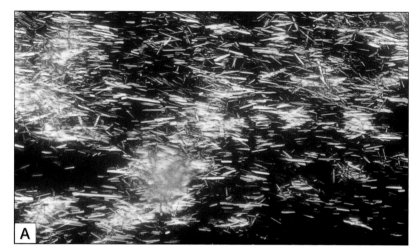

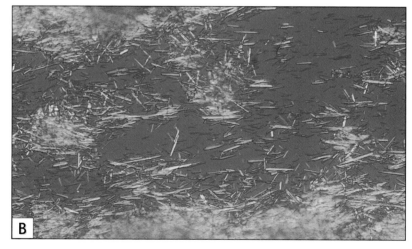

**FIGURE 2-44.** Gouty aspirates. **A,** Aspiration of a tophaceous nodule or chronic gouty bursitis routinely yields a few drops of chalky or bloody fluid that is sufficient to confirm a diagnosis of gout when the specimen is viewed with a polarizing microscope (50×). This suspension of brightly birefringent, needle-shaped urate crystals contained a few erythrocytes but no leukocytes. **B,** This suspension of brightly birefringent, needle-shaped urate crystals aspirated from a gouty tophus was photographed in the polarizing microscope (50×) with a red compensator filter in place. These negatively birefringent crystals appear yellow when they lie parallel to the optical axis of the compensator and blue when perpendicular to it.

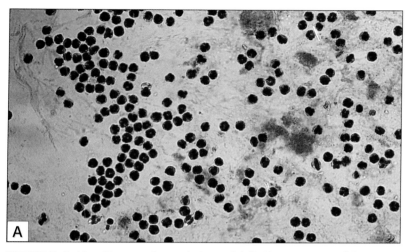

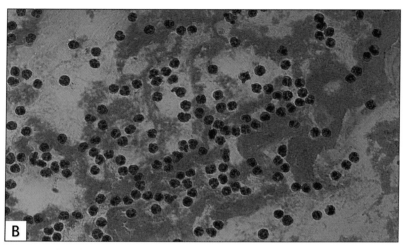

**FIGURE 2-45.** Knee aspirate. **A**, Synovial fluid was aspirated from a painful knee during an acute attack of gout. To obtain a differential leukocyte count, it was fixed in alcohol and stained with a modified Wright's-Geimsa stain. Many mononuclear cells and neutrophils are visible, and when viewed with the polarizing microscope (25×), several cells contain brightly birefringent, needle-shaped crystals. An extracellular crystal is also present. The morphology of these crystals strongly suggests that they are monosodium urate, although crystals of some corticosteroid esters (*eg*, triamcinolone acetate) have a similar appearance. **B**, The stained preparation of gouty synovial fluid from the same patient was examined after adding the first-order red compensator to the optical path to confirm that the crystals were negatively birefringent. Intracellular and extracellular crystals of monosodium urate are visible on the magenta background (25×).

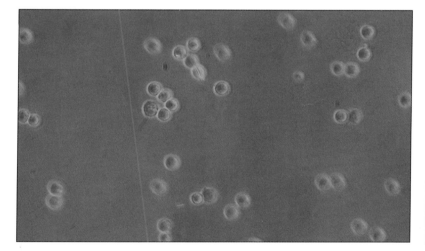

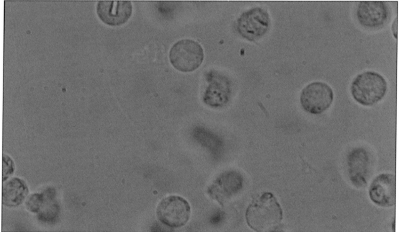

**FIGURE 2-46.** Aspirate under polarizing microscope. Synovial fluid aspirated from a painful knee during an acute attack of gout was photographed with a polarizing microscope (50×) equipped with a first-order red compensator filter. Numerous synovial fluid leukocytes are visible, and several contain acinar (needle-shaped) crystals of monosodium urate. Crystals whose long axis is aligned with the optical axis of the red compensator are yellow; those perpendicular to the axis are blue because they are negatively birefringent.

**FIGURE 2-47.** Synovial fluid leukocytes. Synovial fluid aspirated from a painful knee during an acute attack of arthritis was photographed with a polarizing microscope (10×) equipped with a first-order red compensator filter. Numerous synovial fluid leukocytes are visible, and several contain blunt or rhomboid-shaped crystals of calcium pyrophosphate monohydrate (CPPD). These crystals are positively birefringent, and when their long axis is aligned with the optical axis of the red compensator they appear blue. When they lie perpendicular to this axis, CPPD appears yellow.

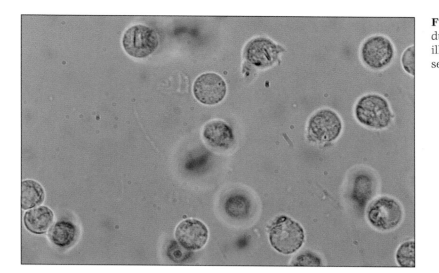

**FIGURE 2-48.** Phase contrast microscopy. Synovial fluid aspirated during an acute attack of pseudogout and viewed with phase contrast illumination shows calcium pyrophosphate dihydrate crystals within several leukocytes (100×).

## Diagnosis

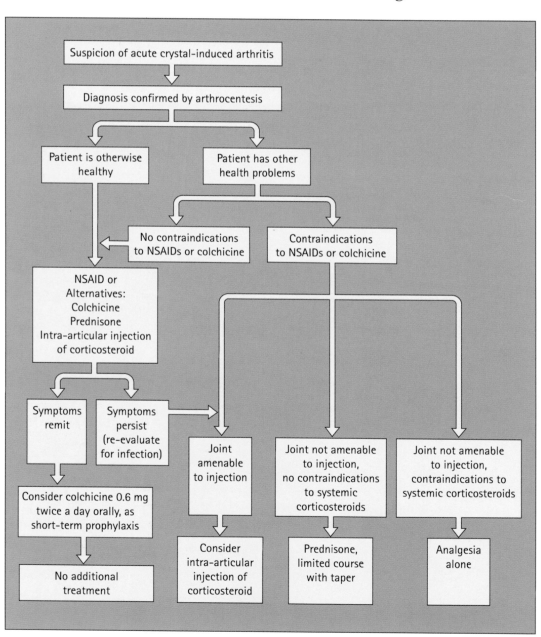

**FIGURE 2-49.** Synovial fluid analysis. The key to accurate diagnosis of crystal-induced synovitis is synovial fluid analysis. This treatment algorithm presents one approach to the management of a typical episode of acute gout, pseudogout, or calcific tendonitis. Joint aspiration itself produces substantial relief in some patients. NSAID—nonsteroidal anti-inflammatory drug. (*Adapted from* George and Mandell [12].)

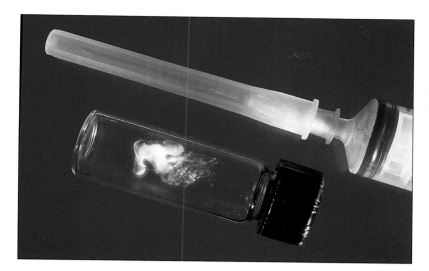

**FIGURE 2-50.** Aspirate from an olecranon bursa. Both acute and chronic olecranon bursitis occur in gout. A fluctuant area in an olecranon bursa that contained numerous pale yellow subcutaneous nodules was aspirated with a syringe to obtain this pasty white material. When viewed with a polarizing microscope, this proved to be a suspension of monosodium urate crystals, confirming that the nodules were gouty tophi. Such chalky white bursal aspirates have been described as urate milk.

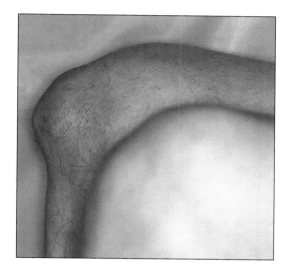

**FIGURE 2-51.** Tophaceous deposits. This man with a long history of tophaceous gout developed prominent tophaceous deposits in the prepatellar bursa of the right knee.

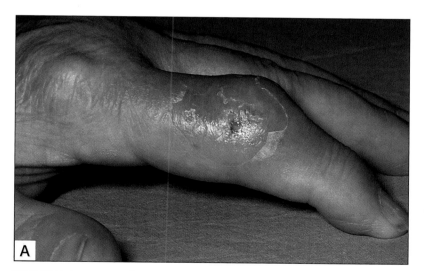
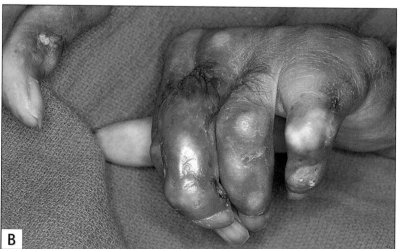

**FIGURE 2-52.** Tophaceous gout. **A,** Tophaceous gout produced chronic swelling and serous drainage in this finger. Examination of a drop of this fluid under the polarizing microscope confirmed the diagnosis. **B,**. The flexion deformities in the hands of this patient with tophaceous gout are associated with destructive erosions of bone and cartilage in multiple joints, and large tophi. Patients with swollen fingers and radiographic evidence of erosive arthritis are sometimes mistakenly assumed to have rheumatoid arthritis until urate crystals are identified by careful examination of synovial fluid or the drop or two of bloody fluid that can be aspirated from a tophaceous ``nodule.''

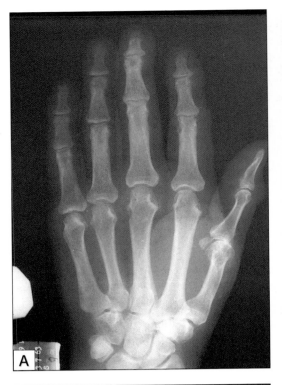

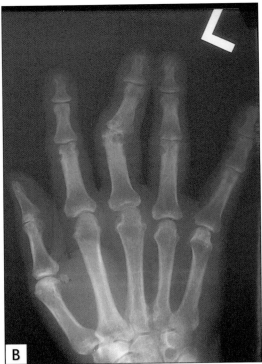

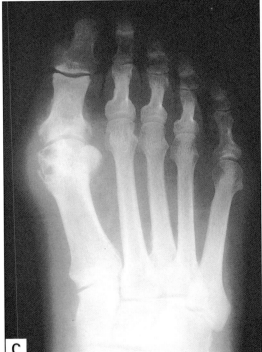

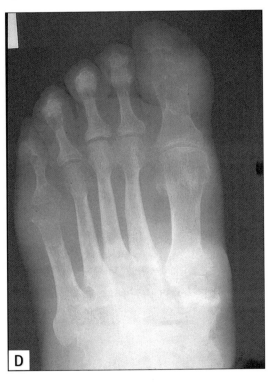

**FIGURE 2-53.** Erosions. **A**, In this radiograph a gouty erosion is present in the second interphalangeal joint. **B**, Severe joint destruction is evident in the gouty third and fourth interphalangeal joints. Reduction of the serum uric acid to < 7 mg/dL allows for gradual dissolution of tophaceous deposits, and such erosions can resolve. **C**, The erosion of the medial aspect of the first metatarsal head in this patient with a 1-year history of gout appears cystic and has an ``overhanging edge'' of cortical bone that helps distinguish it from the erosions seen in other inflammatory arthropathies, as well as from osteoarthritis. Aspiration of this site is likely to yield urate crystals even in the absence of podagra. **D**, The increased soft tissue density over the fifth metatarsal head and first interphalangeal joints is a result of gouty tophi. There is severe erosive destruction of these joints.

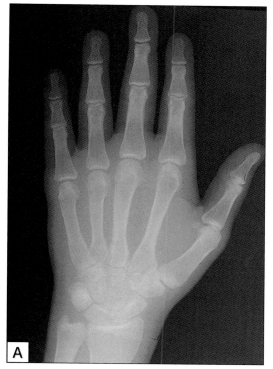

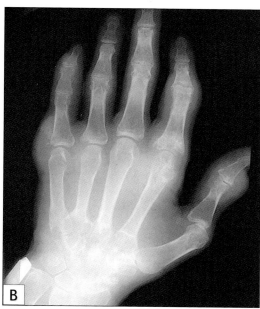

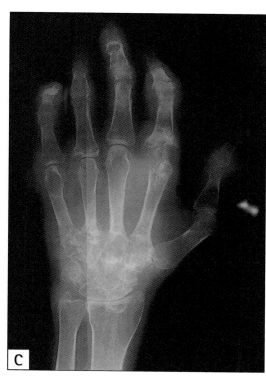

**FIGURE 2-54.** Treatment of hyperuricemia. Physicians differ in their approach to the treatment of hyperuricemia in the patient who has the diagnosis of gout confirmed by crystal analysis, radiographic findings, and clinical data. For example, 30% of the respondents in a recent survey of French rheumatologists never prescribed urate-lowering drugs [13]. This approach is supported by anecdotes that some patients suffer only a single attack of gout, and by the observation that in others, years pass between episodes of acute joint inflammation.

However, the progressive, tophaceous joint destruction that occurs in some patients with gout presents a strong argument to the contrary. **A**, **B**, and **C**, This series of three radiographs documents the peripheral joint destruction and tophi formation (note progression of second metacarpophalangeal joint erosion and loss of joint space) that occurred over 10 years in a patient with gout, persistent hyperuricemia, and alcoholism. His serum uric acid level ranged from 8 to 11 mg/dL during this interval.

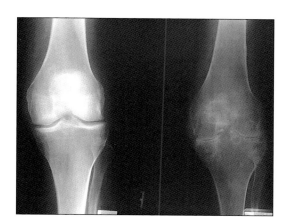

**FIGURE 2-55.** Severe osteopenia in untreated gout. The initial radiograph of the right knee of a 40-year-old man with gout (*left*) appeared normal. When the study was repeated (*right*), after 7 years of hyperuricemia and numerous episodes of acute gout, severe osteopenia was present, there was loss of joint space in both the medial and lateral tibiofemoral compartments, and an erosion was present on the lateral aspect of the femoral condyle.

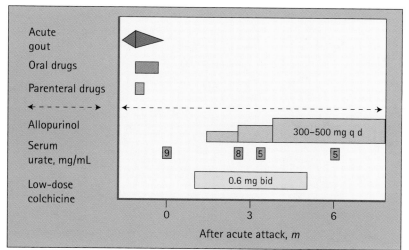

**FIGURE 2-56.** Timeline for treatment. Long-term control of hyperuricemia is required to avoid the risk of chronic or tophaccous gout and secondary osteoarthritis. This figure shows the temporal relationship between the treatment of acute gout with oral or parenteral anti-inflammatory agents (above the dashed line), and the subsequent management of hyperuricemia (below the line). In this example the baseline serum urate was 9 mg/dL. Most attacks of acute gout are managed effectively with an oral anti-inflammatory agent. Parenteral therapies, such as intravenous colchicine, intra-articular or intramuscular corticosteroid, or corticotropin, may be preferable in some patients with complicated medical conditons [14]. Colchicine, 0.6 mg bid is commonly prescribed after the acute attack, but before allopurinol is given, to reduce the risk of recurrent attacks during this period. Allopurinol should be administered only after the acute attack has resolved, and stepwise adjustments in the initial dose (in this example, 100 mg/d) are made to lower the serum urate to < 7mg/dL.

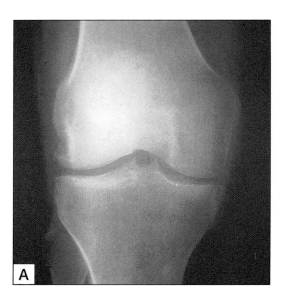

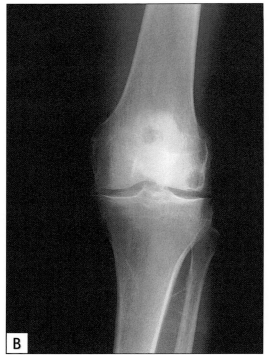

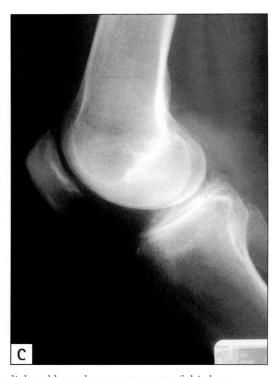

**FIGURE 2-57.** Chondrocalcinosis. **A,** This knee radiograph shows chondrocalcinosis, a faint white line parallel to the contours of the femoral condyle midway between the femur and tibial plateau, in a patient with pseudogout. The lateral tibial femoral compartment is slightly narrowed on this standing view, indicating concomitant osteoarthritis. Because deposits of nonbirefringent calcium-containing crystals (ie, basic calcium phosphate or apatite) also produce chondrocalcinosis, it is necessary to find calcium pyrophosphate dihydrate crystals in the synovial fluid to diagnose pseudogaut. **B,** Severe chondrocalcinosis is present in both the medial and lateral compartments of this knee. The medial and lateral tibiofemoral joint spaces are preserved, but a small marginal osteophyte on the medial femoral condyle and a subchondral cyst visible in the lateral femoral condyle indicate that osteoarthritis is present. **C,** In calcium pyrophosphate dihydrate arthropathy, chondrocalcinosis of the posterior horns of the menisci can be seen best on lateral views of the knee. The small "whisker" osteophytes at the upper and lower poles of the patella are common in this condition.

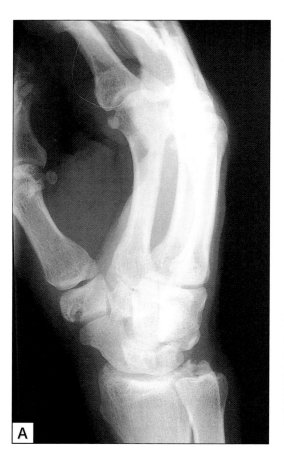

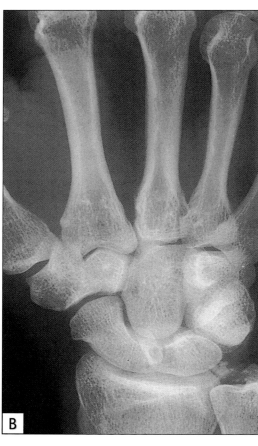

**FIGURE 2-58.** Chondrocalcinosis of the wrist. Chondrocalcinosis of the triangular fibro-cartilage distal to the ulna is seen in both lateral (**A**) and anteroposterior (**B**) views of the wrist. Large cysts, or geodes, are seen in the trapezium at the first carpometacarpal joint, and in the lunate bone.

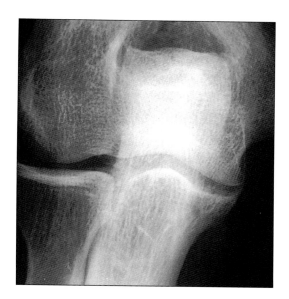

**FIGURE 2-59.**
Chondrocalcinosis of the humerus and radius. Chondrocalcinosis is visible on the lateral condyle of the humerus and on the head of the radius in a man with idiopathic calcium pyrophosphate deposition disease.

## CONDITIONS ASSOCIATED WITH CALCIUM PYROPHOSPATE OR APATITIE CRYSTAL DEPOSITION IN CARTILAGE, MENISCUS, TENDON, AND LIGAMENT

Aging
Articular trauma
Hyperparathydoidism
Hypothyroidism
Hemochromatosis
Hypomagnesemia
Gout

**FIGURE 2-60.** Conditions associated with crystal deposition. Aging and joint trauma increase the likelihood that calcium pyrophosphate dihydrate (CPPD) or apatite will be present in the joint. CPPD arthropathy has also been associated with hyperparathyroidism, hypothyroidism, hemochromatosis, and hypomagnesemia. Occasionally, CPPD and urate crystals are identified in the same joint.

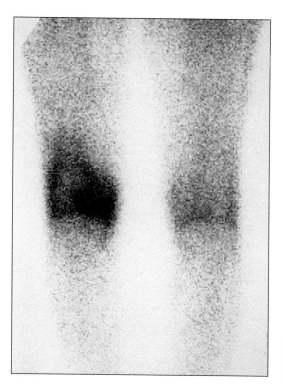

**FIGURE 2-61.** CPPD arthropathy and fever of the knee. A 74-year-old man was hospitalized for evaluation of recurrent fever. After a thorough evaluation for occult malignancy, a gallium scan was obtained and revealed an inflammatory synovial effusion (*right*). This directed the physician's attention to the effusion in the patient's knee, which contained numerous intracellular calcium pyrophosphate dihydrate crystals. A knee radiograph showed extensive chondrocalcinosis of the menisci.

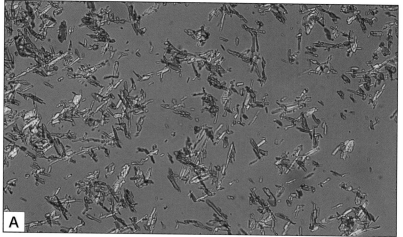

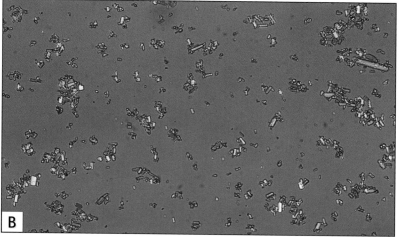

**FIGURE 2-62.** Corticosteroid ester crystal birefringence. **A,** Crystals of corticosteroids that are injected into joints are birefringent, and in specimens of synovial fluid they can be confused with urate or calcium pyrophosphate dihydrate. Typically, these crystals vary in size because they have been milled into a fine powder by the manufacturer. Many of the crystals in this specimen of prednisolone tebutate are needle-shaped and so resemble monosodium urate crystals. When photographed with a red compensator filter in place (50×), the majority of these crystals show positive birefringence instead of the negative birefringence expected of monosodium urate crystals. **B,** Crystals of triamcinolone diacetate that are injected into joints are birefringent, and some of these crystals closely resemble rhomboid-shaped calcium pyrophosphate dihydrate (CPPD) crystals. The triamcinolone crystals in this photograph (50×) show negative birefringence that distinguishes them from positively birefringent crystals of CPPD.

# References

1. Felson D: The course of osteoarthritis and factors that affect it. *Rheum Dis Clin North Am* 1993, 19:607–615.
2. Ike R: The role of arthroscopy in the differential diagnosis of osteoarthritis of the knee. *Rheum Dis Clin North Am* 1993, 19:673–696.
3. Knowlton RG, Katzenstein PL, Moskowitz RW, *et al.*: Genetic linkage of a polymorphism in the type II procollagen gene (COL2A1) to primary osteoarthritis associated with mild chondrodysplasia. *N Engl J Med* 1990, 322:526–530.
4. Mann RA, Coughlin M, DuVries HL: Hallux rigidus: a review of the literature and a method of treatment. *Clin Orthop* 1979, 142:57–63.
5. Buckland-Wright C: *Osteoarthritis Cartilage* 1995, 3(Suppl A):71–80.
6. Rozing PM, Insall J, Bohne WH: Spontaneous osteonecrosis of the knee. *J Bone Joint Surg* 1980,62A:2–7.
7. Harris WH: Etiology of osteoarthritis of the hip. *Clin Orthop* 1986, 213:20–33.
8. Towhead T, Hochberg M: A systematic review of randomized controlled trials of pharmacological therapy in osteoarthritis of the knee, with an emphasis on trial methodology. *Semin Arthritis Rheum* 1997, 26:755–770.
9. Lussier A, Cividino AA, McFarlane CA, *et al.*: Viscosupplementation with hylan for the treatment of osteoarthritis: findings from clinical practice in Canada. *J Rheumatol* 1996, 23:1579–1585.
10. Adams ME, Atkinson MH, Lussieri AJ, *et al.*: The role of viscosupplementation with hylan G-F 20 (Synvisc®) in the treatment of osteoarthritis of the knee: a Canadian multicenter trial comparing hylan G-F 20 alone, hylan G-F 20 with non-steroidal anti-inflammatory drugs (NSAIDs) and NSAIDs alone. *Osteoarth Cartilage* 1995, 3:213–226.
11. Neustadt, DH: Intraarticular steroid therapy. In *Osteoarthritis: Diagnosis and Medical/Surgical Management*, edn. 2. Edited by Moskowitz RW, Howell DS, Goldberg VM, Mankin HJ. Philadelphia: WB Saunders; 1992: pp 493–510.
11. George GT, Mandell BF: Individualizing the treatment of gout. *Cleve Clin J Med* 1996, 63:150–155.
13. Rozenberg S, Lan T, Laatar A, *et al.*: Diversity of opinions on the management of gout in France. A survey of 750 rheumatologists. *Rev Rhum Engl Ed* 1996, 63:255–261.
14. Siegel LB, Alloway JA, Nashel DJ: Comparison of adrenocorticotropic hormone and triameinolone acetonide in the treatment of acute gouty arthritis. *J Rheumatol* 1994, 21:1325–1327.

# Selected Bibliography

Altman RD, Hochberg M, Murphy WA Jr, Wolfe F, Lesquene M: Atlas of individual radiographic features in osteoarthritis. *Osteoarthritis Cartilage* 1995, 3 (Suppl A):3–70.

Bellamy N, Wells G, Campbell J: Relationship between severity and clinical importance of symptoms in osteoarthrtis. *Clin Rheumatol* 1991, 10:138–143.

Bulloch PG: The pathology of osteoarthritis. In *Osteoarthritis, Diagnosis and Medical/Surgical Mangement*, edn 2. Edited by Moskowitz RW, Howell DS, Goldberg VM, Mankin HJ. Philadelphia: WB Saunders; 1992:pp 39–69.

Halverson PB: Calcium crystal-associated diseases. *Curr Opin Rheumatol* 1996, 8:259–265.

Ike RW: The role of arthroscopy in the differential diagnosis of osteoarthritis of the knee. *Rheum Dis Clin North Am* 1993, 19:673–696.

Peterson I, Jacobsson L, Silman A, Croft P (eds): EULAR Workshop: The epidemiology of osteoarthritis in the peripheral joints. *Ann Rheum Dis* 1996, 55:651–688.

Schumacher HR: Secondary osteoarthritis: In *Osteoarthritis, Diagnosis and Medical/Surgical Mangement*, edn 2. Edited by Moskowitz RW, Howell DS, Goldberg VM, Mankin HJ. Philadelphia: WB Saunders; 1992:367–398.

Star VL, Hochberg MC: Prevention and management of gout. *Drugs* 1993, 45:212–222.

Uri DS, Martel W: Radiologic manifestations of the crystal-related arthropathies. *Semin Roentgenol* 1996, 31:229–238.

Wortmann RL: Management of hyperuricemia. In *Arthritis and Allied Conditions*, edn 12. Edited by McCarty DJ, Koopman WJ. Philadelphia: Lea & Febiger; 1993:1807–1818.

# 3

# Systemic Lupus Erythematosus, Antiphospholid Syndrome, Scleroderma, and Inflammatory Myopathies

## GRAHAM R. V. HUGHES and MUNTHER A. KHAMASHTA

**Systemic lupus erythematosus** (lupus, LE, SLE) is a genetically determined disease characterized by diverse clinical features [1].

Defective suppressor T cell function allows the proliferation of B cell clones producing a variety of antibodies. These antibodies are predominantly (notably in fact) nonorgan specific and may contribute to disease either directly (e.g., Coombs' positive hemolytic anemia) or indirectly through mediation of immune complexes. A number of the antibodies have significant diagnostic importance. These include anti-DNA which is highly specific for SLE, antiphospholid (lupus anticoagulant), which is associated with thrombosis and anti-Ro (anti SSA) which is associated with Sjögren's, photosensitivity, less renal disease, and congenital heart block. Others appear to vary in different populations (eg, anti-Sm—common in blacks, 10% to 15% only in whites).

The disease affects females nine times more frequently than males and is most common in child-bearing years. New cases are unusual under the age of 14 and over age 50 [2]. Factors that appear to exacerbate the disease are ultraviolet light, certain drugs (notably Septrin and sulphonamides), postpregnancy, and marked stress.

Systemic features include fatigue, fever, mood swings, myalgia, and arthralgia. Skin lesions are present in up to 80% of cases and include cutaneous vasculitis (especially on the hands, feet, and elbows), facial "butterfly" rash, and alopecia. Recognizably distinct cutaneous lesions include discoid lupus, subacute cutaneous LE (associated with anti-Ro antibodies), lupus profundus, and urticarial vasculitis. Raynaud's phenomenon is common but generally less severe than in scleroderma or mixed connective tissue disease.

Other organs prominently involved are the joints and tendons (usually nondestructive), lungs and heart (especially pleurisy and pericarditis), kidney (in about 50% of cases depending on the clinical referral patterns), and brain. Neurologic lupus is probably underdiagnosed, with features including the whole spectrum of neurologic and psychiatric disease.

The disease is masked by remission and exacerbation. Treatment ranges from no treatment through antimalarials and steroids to immunosuppressives. In the majority of cases, the disease can be controlled.

An important subset of patients carries antibodies directed against phospholipids (or, more commonly, phospholipid-protein complexes) [3–5]. These patients have a strikingly increased risk of both venous and arterial thrombosis, including strokes. Clearly, treatment of this group is very different and directed primarily toward anticoagulation [6].

A much rarer disease than lupus and the antiphospholipid syndrome, **scleroderma** also has a wide variety of forms with differing prognoses [7].

In scleroderma, Raynaud's sydnrome is prominent and early. The skin and subcutaneous tissues are initially inflamed, but subsequently become progressively fibrosed. Spreading from the hands, the thickening and fibrosis can involve the arms, chest wall, face, and all parts of the body.

The process can extend to internal organs, notably the esophagus (with reflux, dystonia, and rigidity), small and large bowel, lungs (pulmonary fibrosis), and kidney (resulting in severe renovascular hypertension).

The earliest clinical changes are shininess and tightness of the skin of the fingers, pigmentation especially of the foreams, and abnormal nail-fold capillaries seen either with the naked eye or by nail-fold capillaroscopy.

A number of variants of scleroderma are recognized clinically. These include morphea, an inflammatory and scarring form of the disease confined to the skin, and CREST syndrome (calcinosis, Raynaud's, esophagitis, sclerodactyly, and telangiectasia)—a chronic and often debilitating disease less likely to develop into systemic sclerosis but carrying the distinct risk of pulmonary hypertension.

A number of classifications of **myositis** and **dermatomyositis** have been proposed [8]. A simple clinical categorization is: inclusion body myositis (resistant to treatment); autoimmune myositis, often associated with circulating autoantibodies, notably those directed at synthetases (such as Jo1); and (rare) myositis or dermatomyositis associated with malignancy.

The characteristic feature of myositis is weakness rather than pain. Muscle biopsy reveals an inflammatory cell infiltrate with muscle necrosis. The skin rash of dermatomyositis is characteristically purple (heliotrope) and affects the periorbital regions, the V neck, and the hands, especially the dorsum of the knuckles.

Many connective tissue diseases show clinical **overlap** with each other. Thus, patients with myositis may develop sclerodactyly and Raynaud's, and have dry eyes demonstrated on Schirmer testing or Rose Bengal conjunctival staining. Autoantibody testing has helped to define some of these "overlap" conditions more precisely, e.g., anti-Jo1 is associated with myositis, pulmonary fibrosis and tenosynovitis; anti-Scl 70 (topoisomerase) with systemic sclerosis; anticentromere with CREST; and anti-Ro with Sjögren's syndrome and subacute cutaneous LE.

Perhaps the most important antibody-disease association in this group is anti-ribonucleoprotein (RNP) and mixed connective tissue disease (MCTD) [9]. MCTD, despite the doubts expressed by some, is one of the most distinct "overlap" connective tissue diseases. With severe Raynaud's, synovitis and tenosynovitis ("sausage fingers"), and frequent muscle inflammation, it is clinically distinct. Although the prognosis is good, since renal disease is unusual, it often proves difficult to treat, because Raynaud's can be especially refractory.

Immunologically, it is one of the most interesting connective tissue diseases. Unlike lupus it is characterized by a single antibody, anti-RNP, often present in extraordinarily high titers.

# Systemic Lupus Erythematosus

## Clinical Features

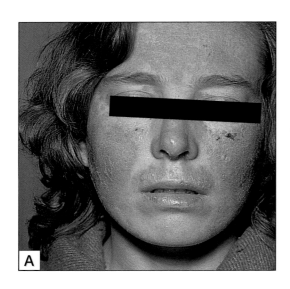 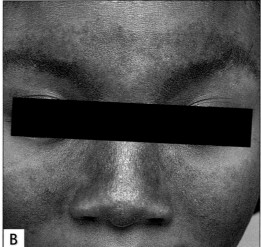

**FIGURE 3-1.** **A**, Butterfly rash. Classic lupus rash on the cheeks, nose, and forehead. The distribution varies and the classic rash is now seen in a minority of patients as milder cases of lupus are diagnosed. **B**, Rash and hyperpigmentation in active lupus. In addition to the classic butterfly rash on the nose and cheeks, note the marked involvement of the eyebrows and skin above the eyebrows. In pigmented skin, hyper- or hypopigmentation can occur.

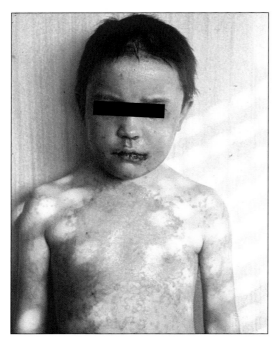

**FIGURE 3-2.** Lupus in childhood. Widespread lupus rash in a child. Distribution is on the face as well as on the anterior chest and arms. A more common distribution is on the "V-neck" area of the anterior chest.

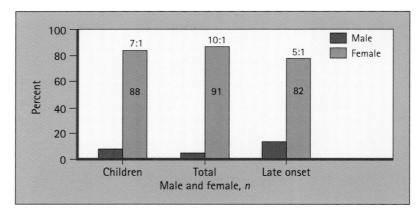

**FIGURE 3-3.** Sex and age distribution. This figure shows the distribution in a multicentered European lupus project. At all age groups, females outnumber males with the disease in the region of 9:1 or 10:1. It has been said that in children and in older age groups the figure is more equal but in this study there is still a large female preponderance in every age group studied [2].

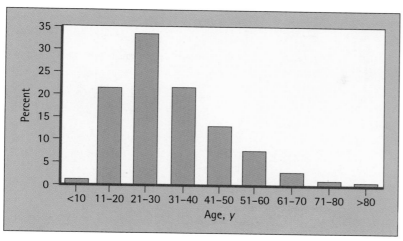

**FIGURE 3-4.** Age at diagnosis. The peak age of diagnosis is in the twenties. In females the majority of cases are diagnosed in the child-bearing years. New cases of lupus are uncommon in patients over age 60. In many of these patients the diagnosis is more likely to be Sjögren's rather than lupus.

## ETIOLOGY OF SLE

| Host factors | Environmental factors |
|---|---|
| Sex | Infection |
| Race | Ultraviolet radiation |
| Genetic factors | Drugs and chemicals |
| Immunologic abnormalities | Geographic factors |
| | Diet |

**FIGURE 3-5.** Etiology. All factors listed here play a part. Clearly, genetic factors underline the development of lupus with hormonal factors playing a major role. The influence of environmental factors (other than ultraviolet irradiation) has only recently been studied in depth and may well play a greater role than had hitherto been thought [10].

## PRINCIPAL PATHOLOGIC FEATURES

### General

Fibrinoid necrosis
Hematoxylin bodies
Deposition of immune complexes
    along basement membranes

### Skin

Discoid-follicular plugging and
    scarring
Systemic - Immune complexes in
    dermal/epidermal junction

### Kidneys

Immune complex deposition
Focal or diffuse glomerulonephritis
Fibrinoid necrosis of arterioles or
    arteries

### Cerebral

Microinfarcts
Choroid plexus immune complexes

### Heart

Pericarditis
Myocarditis
Libman-Sacks endocarditis

### Blood vessels

Arteriolitis and capillaritis
Microthrombi

### Spleen

"Onion-skin" thickening

### Joints

Fibrinoid deposition

### Lungs and Pleura

Fibrinoid adhesions
Effusions
Interstitial pneumonitis
Recurrent atelectasis

**FIGURE 3-6.** Principal pathologic features. The most striking histologic feature is the so-called fibrinoid necrosis, which affects particularly the small arteries, arterioles, and capillaries (as distinct from polyarteritis nodosa, which affects predominantly medium-sized vessels such as the coronary and mesenteric arteries) [1].

## Cutaneous Lesions and Vasculitis

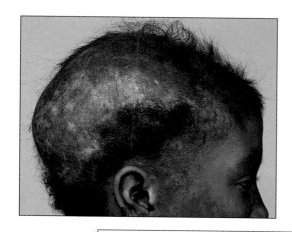

**FIGURE 3-7.** Scalp lesions and alopecia. Hair loss is a common feature of lupus. Most commonly it is diffuse and subtle but occasionally, as in this patient, it can be widespread. This kind of lupus in particular produces severe alopecia on occasion. Normally, unless scarring occurs, regrowth is expected.

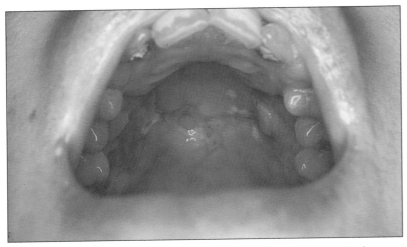

**FIGURE 3-8.** Mouth ulcers. A variety of mouth ulcers occur in lupus. They are nonspecific and usually not as painful as those seen in Behçet's disease, for example.

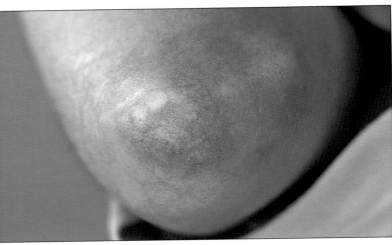

**FIGURE 3-9.** Elbow lesions. Vasculitic lesions of the elbow are common in lupus. Examination of the elbow is extremely important in this disease especially in the extremely ill patient where the telltale signs of blood vessel inflammation are often seen.

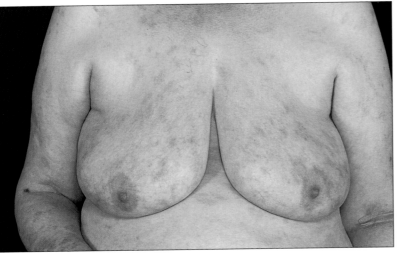

**FIGURE 3-10.** Vasculitis. Vasculitic lesions can affect all parts of the body skin. In this patient there are widespread vasculitic lesions in the skin and subcutaneous tissues of the breasts.

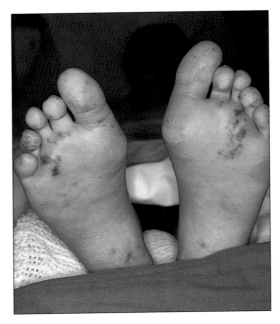

**FIGURE 3-11.** Vasculitis in the feet. In this patient the diagnosis was compounded by septicemia and the differential diagnosis was difficult. Distribution in vasculitis is more commonly on the toes and lateral sides of the sole.

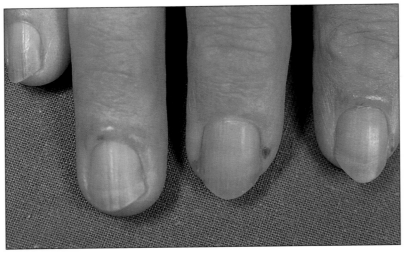

**FIGURE 3-12.** Nail-fold vasculitis. A variety of vasculitic lesions beside the nail can occur. In this example the vasculitic lesions are more reminiscent of those of rheumatoid arthritis periungal lesions.

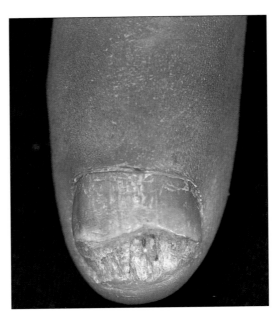

**FIGURE 3-13.** Nail changes. The nails are commonly affected in SLE with mild changes varying to severe psoriasis-like nail lesions as in this patient.

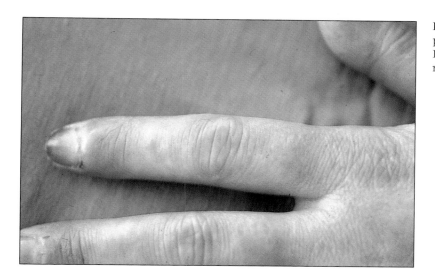

**FIGURE 3-14.** Finger lesions. This shows a number of lesions in a patient with lupus and overlap features. This patient suffers from Raynaud's phenomenon, ischemia of the digits, nail-fold infarcts, and rashes.

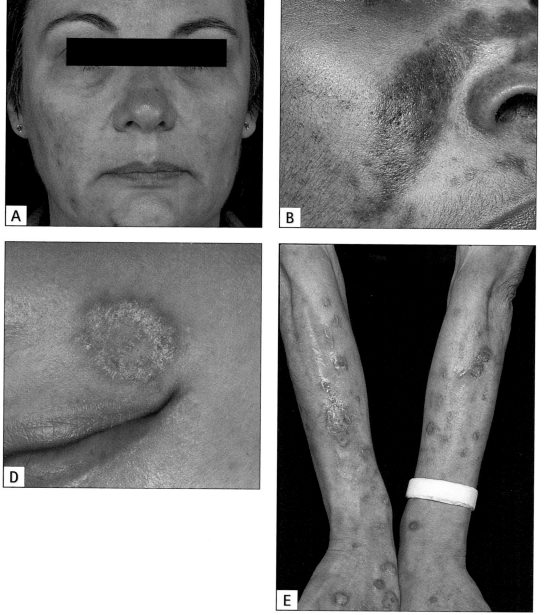

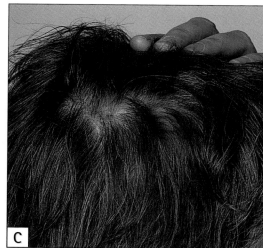

**FIGURE 3-15.** Discoid lupus. This causes a variety of lesions and is much more prone to scarring of the skin than SLE. **A**, Patient has severe lesions in the photosensitive areas of the forehead, nose, and cheeks. **B**, This patient presented with lesions on the cheeks and nose with marked hyperpigmentation and early scarring. **C**, Scalp alopecia. Scarring is much more a feature than in SLE and if not treated can lead to permanent patches of alopecia. **D**, Lesion on the upper lip. Annular lesions of discoid lupus as shown here can present diagnostic difficulties. Sometimes they are only confirmed on biopsy. **E**, Patient has widespread active discoid lesions on the forearms.

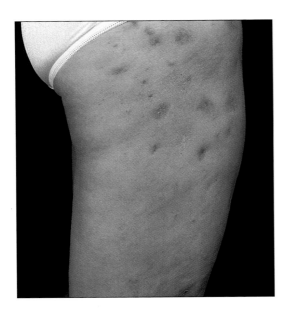

**FIGURE 3-16.** Lupus profundus. This title is given to a rare cutaneous form of lupus with deep scarring and fat necrosis. A predominantly cutaneous and subcutaneous disease, this is not usually associated with SLE. Commonly, the patient is anti-Ro (anti SSA) positive. Differential diagnosis is from other forms of fat necrosis including self-inflicted lesions.

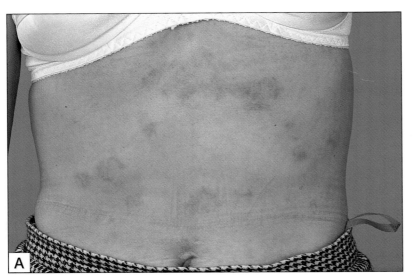

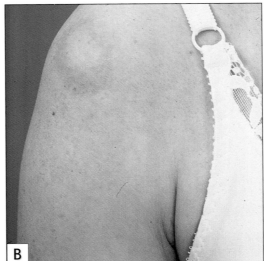

**FIGURE 3-17.** Subacute cutaneous lupus erythematosus (SCLE). **A,** Papulo-squamous and annular lesions shown on the abdomen of this patient are typical examples of this condition. It is strongly associated with anti-Ro antibodies and photosensitivity [11]. **B,** Annular lesion on the shoulder of this patient. These lesions usually respond well to antimalarial therapy.

## Tendons, Joints, and Organs Affected

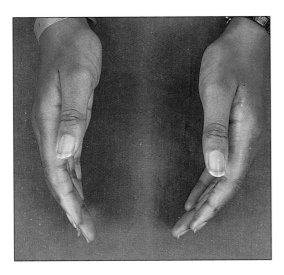

**FIGURE 3-18.** Tendon lesions. Tendon lesions are common and vary from mild to severe. This patient had difficulty flattening the fingers owing to inflammation of the flexor tendons.

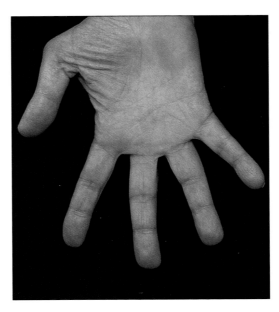

**FIGURE 3-19.** Classic hand deformity. In addition to palmar erythema shown dramatically in this patient there is the classic thumb deformity of lupus— the "hitch-hiking" thumb.

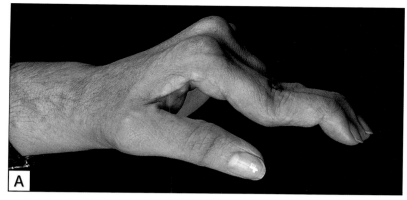

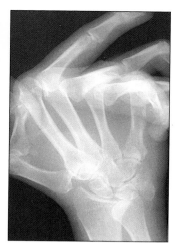

**FIGURE 3-20.** Jaccoud's arthropathy. **A,** Lateral view of hand shows finger deformities. The lesions are rarely extreme, but in some cases there can be rheumatoid-like deformity. This is nondestructive, however. **B,** A radiograph of a patient with severe deformity shows that the ends of the bones are not eroded despite the severe deformities seen.

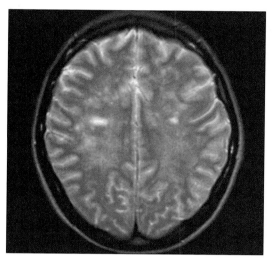

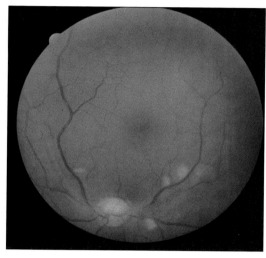

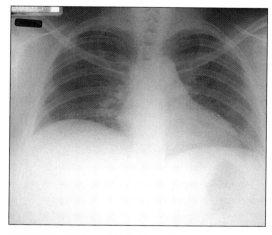

**FIGURE 3-21.** Cerebral vasculitis. Cerebral disease presents a major management problem in lupus because there are no diagnostic criteria, no reliable tests, and no ensured response to treatment. This patient had widespread vasculitis, and small lesions are seen in the brain on magnetic resonance imaging. The differentiation of vasculitis from infarction in the antiphospholipid syndrome is extremely difficult [12].

**FIGURE 3-22.** Cytoid bodies. Cytoid bodies in the fundus in lupus is pathognomonic of vascular inflammation in this disease and a vital sign in examination of the patient with lupus.

**FIGURE 3-23.** "Shrinking" lungs. A rare manifestation of lupus is elevation of the diaphragm associated with pleurisy and plate-like atelectasis with diminution of lung volumes and normal gas transfer. This severe lesion in lupus was originally thought to be irreversible but is now known to reverse to normal, possibly with more aggressive treatment.

## Nephritis

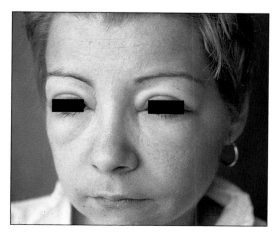

**FIGURE 3-24.** Nephrotic syndrome. Nephritis is a presenting feature of lupus in a small proportion of patients, although 40% to 75% develop this complication at some stage. Nephritis may be an occult manifestation in some patients, emphasizing the need for regular urinalysis and monitoring of blood pressure. Most patients present with proteinuria, sometimes leading to nephrotic syndrome with peripheral edema and edema of the periorbital tissues.

## MODIFIED WORLD HEALTH ORGANIZATION CLASSIFICATION OF RENAL PATHOLOGY OF LUPUS NEPHRITIS

I. Normal glomeruli
II. Mesangial glomerulonephritis
III. Focal proliferative glomerulonephritis
IV. Diffuse proliferative
    A. Hypercellularity only (without segmental necrotizing lesions)
    B. With active necrotizing lesions
    C. With active and sclerosing lesions
    D. With sclerosing lesions
V. Membranous nephropathy
VI. Sclerosing nephropathy

**FIGURE 3-25.** Modified World Health Organization (WHO) classification of renal pathology. Renal biopsy is initially important in differentiating patients with potentially reversible or steroid-responsive lesions (mesangial or focal proliferative) from those with diffuse proliferative disease requiring more aggressive immunosuppression and those minimally or unresponsive to therapy (membranous nephropathy). Follow-up biopsy is sometimes helpful in guiding changes in or withdrawal of treatment. Management of terminal chronic renal failure does not differ from that of other causes and SLE is not usually a contraindication to transplantation.

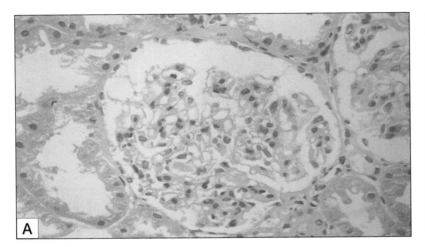

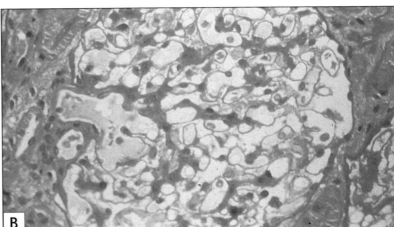

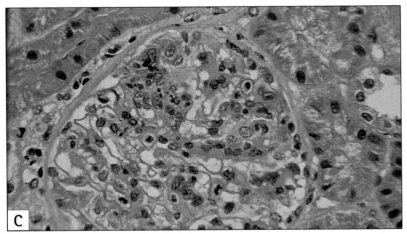

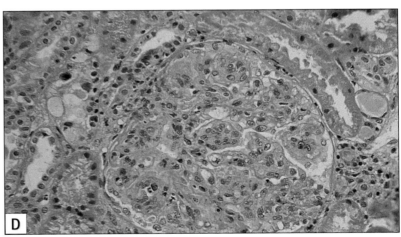

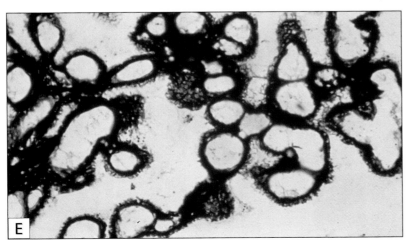

**FIGURE 3-26.** Light microscopy of the major World Health Organization (WHO) classes of lupus nephritis. **A**, No renal lesions (minimal changes), WHO class 1. (Hematoxylin and eosin) **B**, Mesangial lupus nephritis, WHO class II. (Hematoxylin and eosin) **C**, Focal proliferative lupus nephritis, WHO class III. (Hematoxylin and eosin) **D**, Diffuse proliferative lupus nephritis, WHO class IV. (Hematoxylin and eosin) **E**, Membranous lupus nephritis, WHO class V. (Silver methenamine)

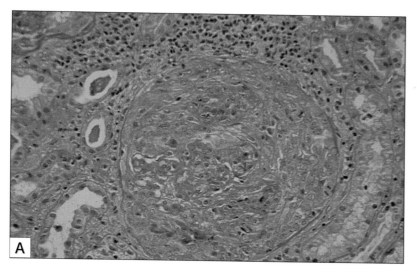

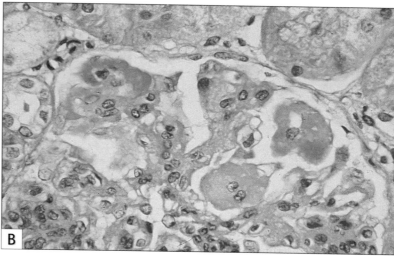

**FIGURE 3-27.** Light microscopy of specific lesions in lupus nephritis. **A**, Cellular crescent in a case of severe, rapidly progressive lupus nephritis (hematoxylin and eosin). **B**, "Wire-loop" lesions in a case of diffuse proliferative lupus nephritis (hematoxylin and eosin).

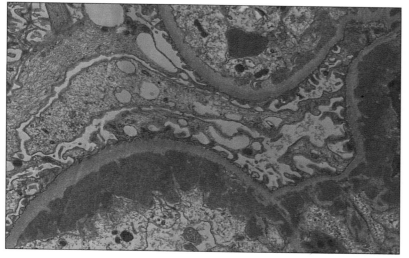

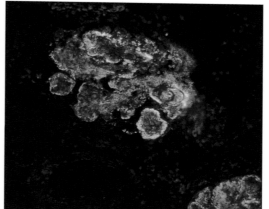

**FIGURE 3-29.** IgG immune deposits in lupus nephritis (photomicrograph). The basement membrane of the glomerulus is partly outlined by irregular "lumpy and bumpy" deposits of antigen-antibody complex (cryostat section, stained with fluorescent human anti-IgG).

**FIGURE 3-28.** Electron microscopy of lupus nephritis. This electron photomicrograph of a glomerular capillary wall shows a large granular subendothelial deposit, characteristic of diffuse proliferative lupus nephritis. These deposits are the ultrastructural counterpart of the light microscopic "wire-loop" lesion.

## Diagnostic Tests and Criteria

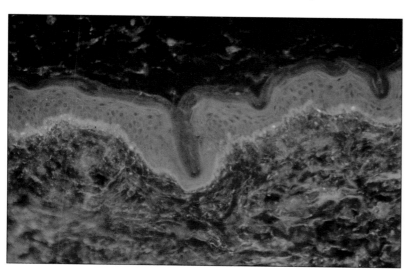

**FIGURE 3-30.** Lupus "band" test. In this photomicrograph, a strong, positive fluorescence at the dermoepidermal junction is owing to the deposition of immune complexes in this region of the skin in a patient with SLE. This is often used as a diagnostic test for SLE. Similar deposits are frequently demonstrable in nonlesional skin of patients with SLE. In discoid lupus, lesional skin biopsies show a positive hand test, but the test is generally negative in biopsies of nonlesional skin.

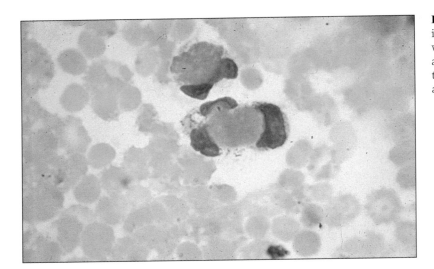

**FIGURE 3-31.** Lupus cell photomicrograph. This cell, first observed in 1948, led to the more widespread diagnosis of lupus. It is no longer widely used because it takes time and is less clinically useful than newer antinuclear and anti-DNA antibody measurements. It is less sensitive than the fluorescent antinuclear antibody test and less specific than the anti-DNA antibody test.

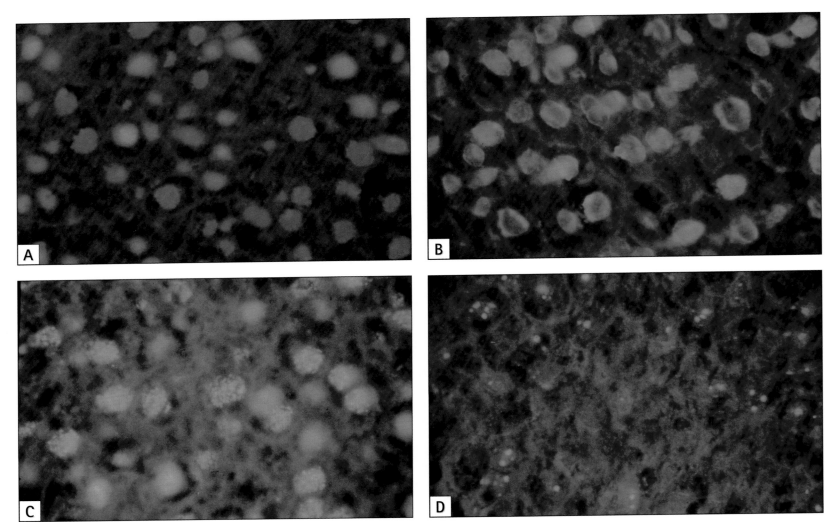

**FIGURE 3-32.** Antinuclear antibody (ANA) testing. This is the most useful method for screening for lupus. It is very sensitive (more than 95% of lupus) but is not specific and may be found in rheumatoid disease, primary Sjögren's, scleroderma, fibrosing alveolitis, chronic hepatitis, thyroiditis, and myasthenia gravis. The pattern of immunofluorescence may indicate the origin of the antigen. In SLE, the pattern and titer of ANA results are variable and do not necessarily reflect disease activity. **A,** Diffuse pattern (photomicrograph). This is the most common pattern in lupus. **B,** Peripheral pattern (photomicrograph) common in active lupus. **C,** Speckled pattern (photomicrograph). This pattern is commonly found in patients with antibodies to ribonucleoprotein and features of overlap. **D,** Nucleolar pattern (photomicrograph). This pattern is commonly found in patients with scleroderma but seldom in lupus and Sjögren's syndrome.

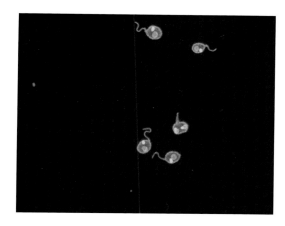

**FIGURE 3-33.** Crithidia DNA (photomicrograph). The use of a noninfective trypanosome crythidia in diagnostic testing allows DNA antibodies to be measured simply. Part of this organism is a structure of double-stranded DNA. Immunofluorescence of this is highly specific for the presence of antibodies to double-stranded DNA. This is much more specific for the diagnosis of SLE but less sensitive (50% to 70%). Positive tests are uncommon in other connective tissue diseases. The presence of the double stranded-DNA antibody correlates generally (though not specifically) with renal disease. A reasonable correlation exists between the levels of ds-DNA antibodies and lupus disease activity.

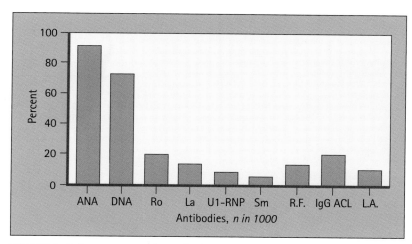

**FIGURE 3-34.** Immunologic findings in 1000 patients. This graph represents the variety of antibodies found in 1000 patients with lupus scattered throughout Europe in a major collaborative study. ANA are seen in the vast majority of patients, as are DNA antibodies. Antibodies to Ro are found in a quarter of lupus patients. Antibodies to RNP and Sm are found more rarely, though much more commonly in black individuals [2]. ACL—anticardiolipin; ANA—antinuclear antibodies; LA—lupus anticoagulant; RF—rheumatoid factor; RNP—ribonucleoprotein.

## REVISED CRITERIA OF THE AMERICAN COLLEGE OF RHEUMATOLOGY FOR THE CLASSIFICATION OF SYSTEMIC LUPUS ERYTHEMATOSUS

1. Malar rash
2. Discoid rash
3. Photosensitivity
4. Oral ulcers
5. Arthritis
6. Serositis (pleuritis or pericarditis)
7. Renal disorders (proteinuria >0.5 g/day or cellular casts)
8. Neurologic disorder (seizures or psycosis)
9. Hematologic disorder (hemolytic anemia or leukopenia <4.0 × 10⁹/L or lymphopenia <1.5 × 10⁹/L or thrombocytopenia <100 × 10⁹/L)
10. Immunologic disorder (positive LE cell or anti-native DNA antibodies or anti-Sm antibodies or chronic false-positive test for syphilis)
11. Antinuclear antibodies

**FIGURE 3-35.** Classification criteria. Lupus is diagnosed on the basis of four or more criteria present serially or simultaneously during any interval of observation [13]. These criteria, drawn up by the American College of Rheumatology, are strictly intended for classification use only. Unfortunately, they have often been used for diagnostic purposes and severely limit the spectrum of SLE if used in this way. New classification criteria are currently being determined by the American College of Rheumatology.

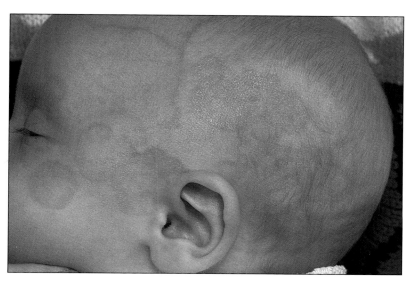

**FIGURE 3-36.** Skin rash in neonatal lupus erythematosus syndrome. Annular lesions on the face of a neonate are reminiscent of those seen in the adult with anti-Ro (anti-SSA) antibodies and subacute cutaneous lupus erythematosus. These are associated with transfer of maternal anti-Ro across the placenta and are usually benign, disappearing within a few weeks of birth.

*Systemic Lupus Erythematosus, Antiphospholid Syndrome, Scleroderma, and Inflammatory Myopathies*

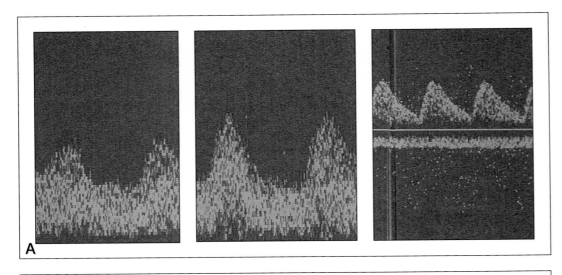

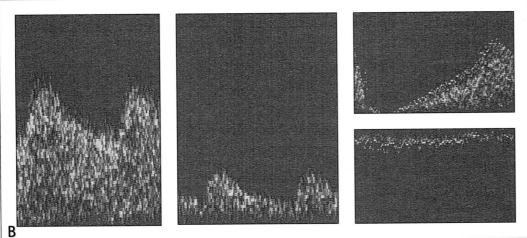

**FIGURE 3-37.** Fetal heart block in neonatal lupus erythematosus syndrome. A rare manifestation of anti-Ro (anti-SSA) antibodies in the mother is the development of congenital heart block in the infant during pregnancy. This is thought to be direct damage caused by anti-Ro antibodies on the conducting tissue in the fetal heart and is (at the present time) irreversible. The child is born with a heart rate of 40 to 50 and the majority of infants require subsequent pacemaking [14]. **A,** Normal fetal heartbeat: normal Doppler blood-flow studies at 19 weeks' gestation. The left and center windows show umbilical artery blood flows. The right-hand window shows the flow in the umbilical artery. The overall picture is of a normal fetal rate in the umbilical artery of 140 beats per minute and normal end-diastolic blood flow. **B,** Fetal heart block: Doppler blood flow studies detecting heart block in a fetus at 23 weeks' gestation. The fetal heart rate is 60 beats per minute and shows complete heart block combined with absent end-diastolic flow. The infant was subsequently delivered at 34 weeks' gestation uneventfully and is alive and well.

## *Sjögren's Syndrome*

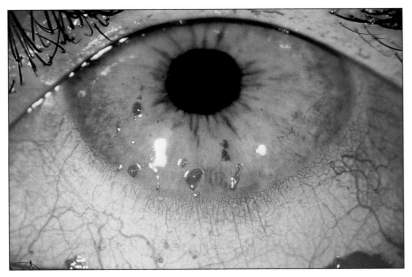

**FIGURE 3-38.** Sjögren's syndrome with keratoconjunctivitis sicca. Severe Sjögren's syndrome (dry eyes, dry mouth, and a connective tissue disease) is associated in some cases with secondary problems in the conjunctiva. In the majority of patients with SLE, severe sicca syndrome is unusual.

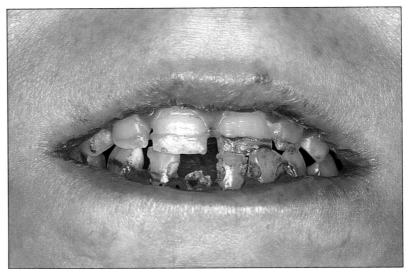

**FIGURE 3-39.** Sjögren's syndrome with xerostomia associated with dental caries. Dryness of the mouth and inadequate saliva formation result in a tendency to dental caries. For patients with primary Sjögren's syndrome and those with lupus and sicca, dental care must be fastidious.

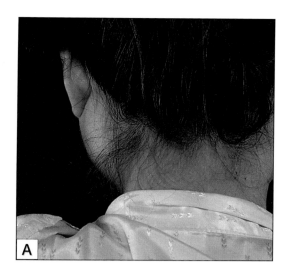

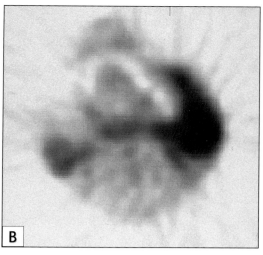

**FIGURE 3-40.** Sjögren's syndrome with parotid gland enlargement. In some patients with primary Sjögren's syndrome, there is massive enlargement of the parotid or submandibular glands. Differential diagnosis includes lymphoma. Lymphoma is an uncommon manifestation of primary Sjögren's syndrome and extremely rare in patients with primary lupus and secondary Sjögren's syndrome. **A**, Primary Sjögren's syndrome in a 30-year-old patient, in whom lymphomatous change had occurred, shows a bilateral enlargement of the parotid gland. **B**, Positron emission tomography (PET) scan of the same patient shows increased uptake in the parotid gland. We believe PET scanning is useful in the differentiation of benign and malignant salivary disease in Sjögren's syndrome.

## Drug-induced Lupus

### DRUG-INDUCED LUPUS: DRUGS IMPLICATED IN INDUCTION

| Common | Rare | Possible |
|---|---|---|
| Hydralazine | Isoniazid | Methyl-dopa |
| Procainamide | Chlorpromazine | Carbamazepin |
| | Phenytoin | D-Penicillamine |
| | Atenolol | Captopril |
| | Primidone | Gold salts |
| | Quinidine | Sulfasalazine |
| | | Lithium carbonate |
| | | Reserpine |
| | | Methylthiouracil |
| | | Minocycline |

**FIGURE 3-41.** Drug-induced lupus. Drugs implicated in induction. Although drugs have been suggested as one of the causes of the apparent increase in the prevalence of lupus, drug-induced lupus is not common. Some of the drugs more frequently implicated are listed. The clinical features closely resemble those of idiopathic lupus though renal and cerebral disease are uncommon in drug-induced lupus. Remission after withdrawal of the offending drug may take several months but a conservative therapeutic approach is required [10].

### DRUG-INDUCED AND IDIOPATHIC LUPUS: AUTOANTIBODY–DISEASE ASSOCIATIONS

| | Idiopathic Lupus, % | Drug-induced Lupus, % |
|---|---|---|
| ANA | >95 | 100 |
| LE cells | 75 | 90 |
| Anti-histone | 60 | >95 |
| Anti-dsDNA | 60 | <5 |
| Anti-Sm | 25 | <5 |
| Anti-RNP | 35 | <5 |
| Anti-Ro | 30 | <5 |
| Anti-La | 15 | <5 |

**FIGURE 3-42.** Drug-induced and idiopathic lupus, autoantibody–disease associations. ANA tests are almost invariably positive in patients with drug-induced lupus and lupus cells are plentiful. However, Anti-ds-DNA antibodies are usually absent or in low titer. Anti-histone antibodies are positive in most patients with drug-induced lupus. ANA—antinuclear antibodies.

## Treatment, Complications, and Prognosis

### DRUG THERAPY IN SYSTEMIC LUPUS ERYTHEMATOSUS

| Drug | Indications |
|---|---|
| Nonsteroidal anti-inflammatories* | Synovitis and mild systemic illness |
| Antimalarials* | Synovitis and cutaneous disease |
| Corticosteroids | Moderate to severe systemic disease, including nephritis, vasculitis, neuropathy and other vital organ involvement |
| Immunosuppressives* | Severe disease including nephritis |
| Plasma exchange (use still not proven) | Severe vasculitis and nephritis; used in combination with corticosteroids and immunosuppressives |

*Useful steroid-sparing agents

**FIGURE 3-43.** Therapeutic approach. Patients must be evaluated fully to determine the extent of organ involvement, so that treatment can be tailored to individual needs.

---

*Systemic Lupus Erythematosus, Antiphospholid Syndrome, Scleroderma, and Inflammatory Myopathies*

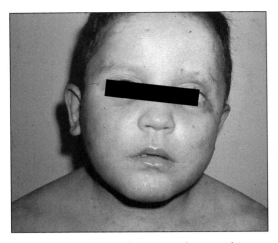

**FIGURE 3-44.** Cushing's syndrome. This complication of SLE is now less common as treatment has become more conservative.

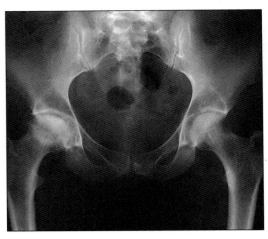

**FIGURE 3-45.** Avascular necrosis of bone. Avascular necrosis of the hip is strongly associated with high-dose corticosteroid therapy. Recently there has been a suggestion that this may also be accelerated in patients with the prothrombotic disorder antiphospholid syndrome (Hughes' syndrome lupus anticoagulant syndrome), with thrombosis and vasculopathy affecting the blood supply to the femoral heads [15].

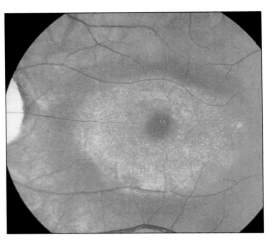

**FIGURE 3-46.** Antimalarial-induced retinal lesions. Antimalarial retinal toxicity "bull's eye" was once regarded as common but now with lower doses (especially 200 mg hydroxychloroquine daily), retinopathy is rare. In a recent 5-year follow-up study in our hospital, no cases of retinopathy were noted in patients taking this dosage [16].

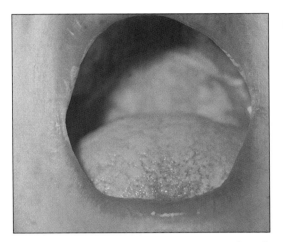

**FIGURE 3-47.** Immunosuppressive-induced fungal infection. Immunosuppressive and steroid therapy as well as general malaise and poor nutrition associated with active disease predispose to candida infections in many cases. In this case it is seen at the back of the mouth and oropharynx.

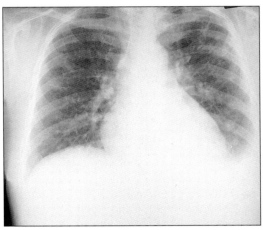

**FIGURE 3-48.** Pulmonary tuberculosis. Tuberculosis was seen in a patient who developed a cough while receiving immunosuppressive therapy for SLE. Secondary infection is still a major problem even with the more conservative regimens now used in the treatment of lupus.

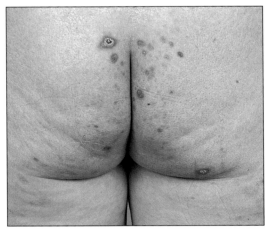

**FIGURE 3-49.** Herpes zoster. Herpes is common both in lupus itself and especially in patients with lupus who receive prolonged immunosuppressive therapy.

| SURVIVAL RATES IN SLE | | |
|---|---|---|
| | 5 y, % | 10 y, % |
| 1950s | 50 | — |
| 1960s | 70 | 55 |
| 1970s | 85 | 75 |
| 1980s | 90 | 80 |
| 1990s | 95 | 90 |

**FIGURE 3-50.** Prognosis. Although there is an essential role for corticosteroids in severe disease, a higher index of suspicion and better diagnostic tests have revealed benign variants of the disease and resulted in an apparently improved prognosis. The 10-year survival rate in a recent series was 90% [17].

# Antiphospholipid (Hughes') Syndrome

## Definition and Diagnosis

### ANTIPHOSPHOLIPID SYNDROME: CLINICAL FEATURES

| Feature | Patients, % |
| --- | --- |
| Venous thrombosis | 48 |
| Arterial thrombosis | 38 |
| Thrombocytopenia | 32 |
| Recurrent pregnancy loss | 55 |

**FIGURE 3-51.** Definition—Hughes' syndrome. In 1983, a distinct syndrome was described associated with both venous and (importantly) arterial thrombosis. The syndrome is marked by the presence of circulating antiphospholipid antibodies. A major feature of this syndrome in women is recurrent pregnancy loss and treatment in these patients is centered on anticoagulation rather than immunosuppression or anti-inflammatory therapy [18,19].

### CLINICAL ASSOCIATIONS

**Major features**

Venous thrombosis: Deep venous thrombosis, Budd-Chiari syndrome, and pulmonary thromboembolism

Arterial thrombosis: Strokes, transient ischemic attacks, multi-infart dementia, myocardial infarctions

Recurrent pregnancy loss

Thrombocytopenia

**Associated clinical features**

Leg ulcers, livedo reticularis, thrombophlebitis and Sneddon's syndrome

Migraine headaches

Heart valve lesions

Transverse myelitis, chorea and epilepsy

Hemolytic anaemia, Coombs positivity and Evans syndrome

Pulmonary hypertension

**Others (less common)**

Splinter haemorrhages

Labile hypertension and accelerated atherosclerosis

Ischaemic necrosis of bone

Addison's disease

Guillain-Barré syndrome and pseudo-multiple sclerosis

Renal artery and vein thrombosis and renal microangiopathy

Retinal artery and vein thrombosis

Amaurosis fugax

Digital gangrene

**FIGURE 3-52.** Clinical associations.

### DIAGNOSTIC CRITERIA FOR THE ANTIPHOSPHOLIPID SYNDROME

| Clinical | Laboratory |
| --- | --- |
| Venous thrombosis | IgG Anticardiolipin antibodies (moderate/high levels) |
| Arterial thrombosis | IgM Anticardiolipin antibodies (moderate/high levels) |
| Recurrent fetal loss | Positive lupus anticoagulant test |
| Thrombocytopenia | |

**FIGURE 3-53.** Diagnostic criteria [18]. Patients with this syndrome should have at least one clinical plus one laboratory finding during their disease. The antiphospholipid antibody test must be positive on at least two occasions more than 3 months apart [20]. Many of the patients reported to have the syndrome have lupus and can be regarded as having secondary antiphospholipid (Hughes') syndrome. Some patients do not have any underlying systemic disease. These patients may be regarded as having primary antiphospholipid (Hughes') syndrome [21].

## Clinical Features

**FIGURE 3-54.** Inferior vena cava thrombosis. The patient is a young woman with antiphospholipid antibodies who had started taking oral contraceptives. Note the dilated lower abdominal collateral vessels.

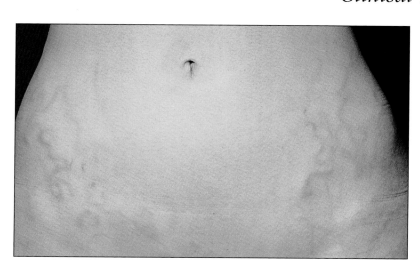

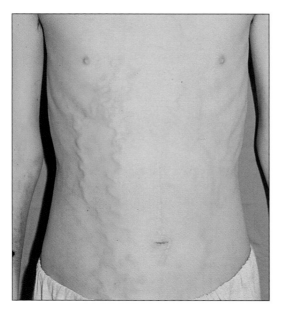

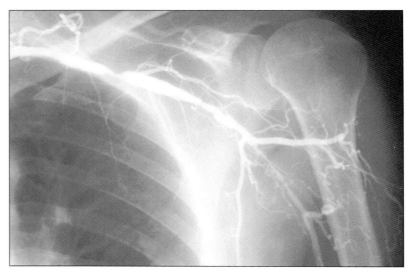

**FIGURE 3-55.** Antiphospholipid (Hughes') syndrome and Budd-Chiari syndrome. A 16-year-old male patient developed hepatic vein thrombosis (Budd-Chiari syndrome) with prominent enlarged collateral veins on the upper abdomen and chest. (*Courtesy of* Lucio Pallares, MD, Palma de Mallorca, Spain.)

**FIGURE 3-56.** Venous thrombosis. Major venous thrombosis is seen in the arm of a young woman with antiphospholipid antibodies.

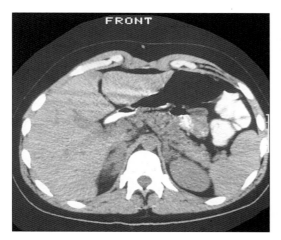

**FIGURE 3-57.** Bilateral adrenal hemorrhage. Infarction of the adrenal glands leading to Addison's disease in a young man with widespread thrombosis was associated with antiphospholipid antibodies.

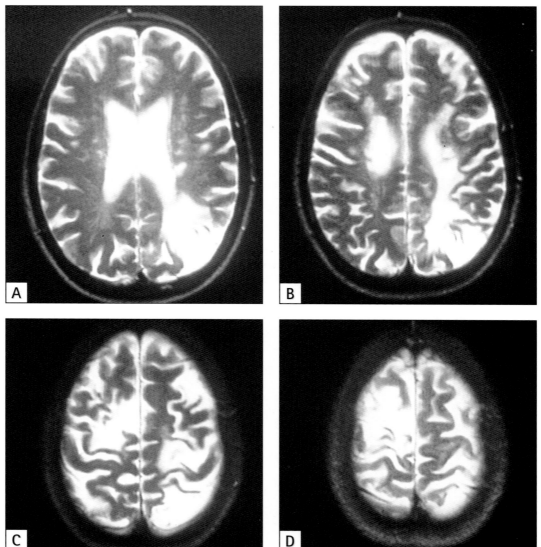

**FIGURE 3-58.** Multi-infarct dementia. **A**, **B**, **C**, and **D**, Magnetic resonance imaging scan shows recurrent cerebral thrombosis in a 35-year-old patient with Hughes' syndrome leading to multi-infarct dementia and subsequent death.

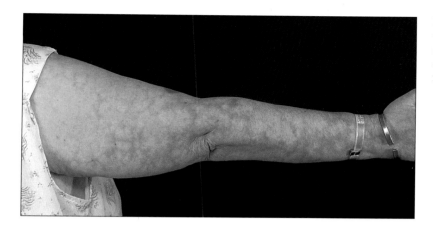

**FIGURE 3-59.** Prominent livedo reticularis of the arm in a woman with antiphospholipid antibodies. Livedo is a major feature in a number of patients with this syndrome and commonly affects the arms, especially the wrists, and the knees but may be more widespread as shown in this patient.

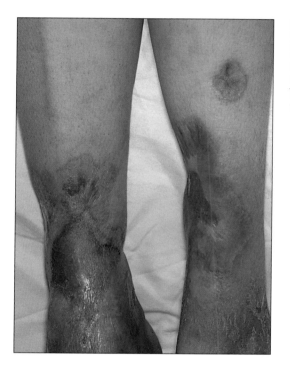

**FIGURE 3-60.** Leg ulcers. Chronic leg ulcerations developed in a patient with antiphospholipid antibodies and recurrent venous thrombosis.

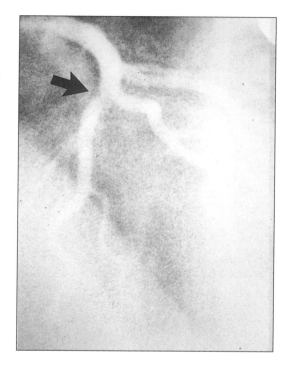

**FIGURE 3-61.** Coronary artery thrombosis. Coronary angiogram shows localized stenosis of left anterior descending coronary artery (*arrow*) in a woman with antiphospholipid antibodies and myocardial infarction.

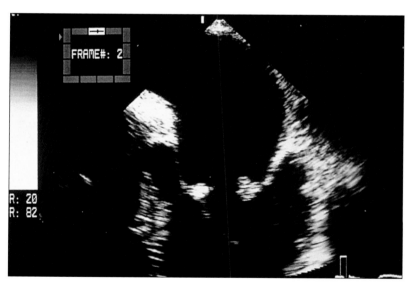

**FIGURE 3-62.** Heart valve disease. This transesophageal echocardiogram of a 32-year-old woman with primary antiphospholipid syndrome demonstrates nodules over the free edge of both mitral leaflets. Valvular disease of the heart is a major feature in some patients with this syndrome [22]. (*Courtesy of* Mary-Carmen Amigo, MD, Mexico.)

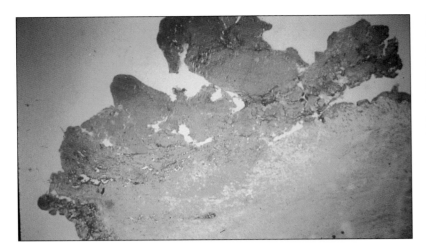

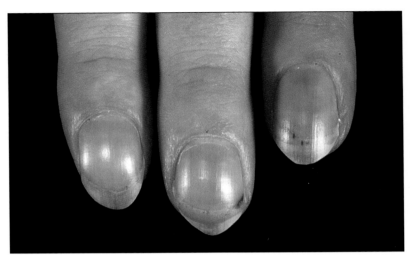

FIGURE 3-63. Heart valve disease (histology). A 45-year-old woman with florid primary antiphospholipid syndrome (venous thrombosis, recurrent fetal loss, cerebrovascular accident, thrombocytopenia, lupus anticoagulant, and IgG anticardiolipin antibodies) presented with moderate to severe aortic regurgitation requiring valve replacement. The histopathologic study of the excised aortic valve showed enlarged fibrin vegetation over the fibrotic valvular tissue. The absence of inflammation differentiates this lesion from Libman-Sacks endocarditis. (*Courtesy of* Mary-Carmen Amigo, MD and Romeo Garcia-Torres, MD, Mexico.)

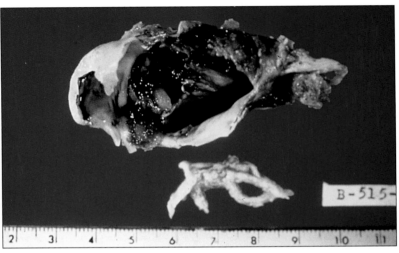

FIGURE 3-64. Subungual splinter hemorrhage. Some patients with valvular disease and with the antiphospholipid syndrome have recurrent splinter hemorrhages making this a major differential diagnosis from infectious endocarditis.

FIGURE 3-65. Pulmonary embolism. Surgical specimen removed during thromboendarterectomy in a 40-year-old patient with a history of pulmonary hypertension and massive pulmonary embolism associated with the procoagulant tendency of this syndrome. (*Courtesy of* Mary-Carmen Amigo, MD, and Romeo Garcia-Torres, MD, Mexico.)

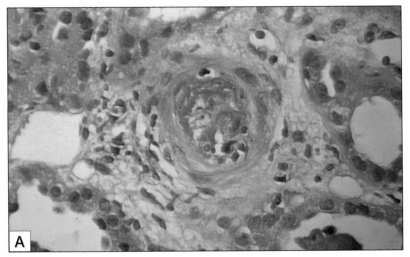

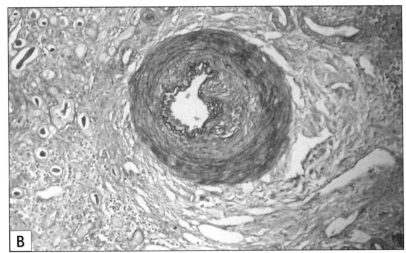

FIGURE 3-66. Thrombotic microangiopathy. Renal biopsy shows thrombotic microangiopathy in a 34-year-old woman with primary antiphospholipid syndrome. **A**, An afferent arteriole with hyperplastic wall and a recent intraluminal nonocclusive thrombus are shown by light microscopy. **B**, An interlobular arteriole shows marked medial hyperplasia, subendothelial fibrosis, and severe excentrical luminal narrowing under light microscopy. Immunofluorescence studies were negative. Electron microscopy showed basal membrane thickening and electron-lucent subendothelial deposits characteristic of thrombotic microangiopathy. (*Courtesy of* Mary-Carmen Amigo, MD, and Romeo Garcia-Torres, MD, Mexico.)

## TREATMENT OF THE DIFFERENT ANTIPHOSPHOLIPID-ASSOCIATED CLINICAL MANIFESTATIONS

| Clinical situation | Suggested Treatment |
| --- | --- |
| Asymptomatic individuals | Observation ± low-dose aspirin |
| Recurrent deep venous thrombosis ± pulmonary embolism | Life-long oral anticoagulants (INR ≥ 3) |
| Large vessel arterial occlusion (i.e., stroke) | Life-long oral anticoagulants (INR ≥ 3) ± low-dose aspirin |
| Transient ischemic attack | Low-dose aspirin |
| Recurrent transient ischemic attacks | Life-long oral anticoagulants (INR ≥ 3) ± low-dose aspirin |
| Catastrophic antiphospholipid syndrome | Oral anticoagulants (INR ≥ 3) + plasmapheresis ± corticosteroids or immunosuppressives |
| History of first trimester pregnancy loss | Low-dose aspirin |
| History of second or third trimester fetal loss | Low-dose aspirin ± subcutaneous heparin |
| Severe thrombocytopenia (< 20,000) | Corticosteroids |

**FIGURE 3-67.** Therapeutic approach to the different clinical manifestations of antiphospholid syndrome. INR—International normalized ratio.

# Scleroderma

## *Clinical Features*

### CLASSFICATION OF SCLERODERMA

**Systemic Scleroderma**
  Diffuse cutaneous scleroderma
  Limited cutaneous scleroderma
  CREST syndrome
**Localized Scleroderma**
  Morphea
  Linear scleroderma
**Overlap syndromes**
**Scleroderma–like syndromes**

**FIGURE 3-68.** Classification [7]. CREST—calcinosis, Raynaud's esophageal dysmotility, sclerodactyly, telangiectasia.

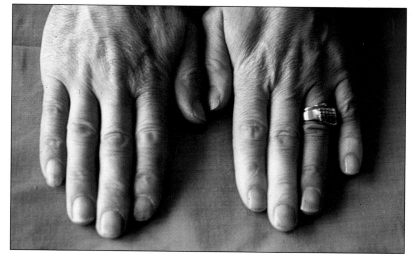

**FIGURE 3-69.** Raynaud's phenomenon. Mild to moderate Raynaud's phenomenon occurs in over 75% of patients with scleroderma and may precede other disease manifestations. It should arouse syspicion in women over the age of 35 years, especially when there is considerable edema. The Raynaud's may be confined to a single digit or, as shown in this case, to two or three digits.

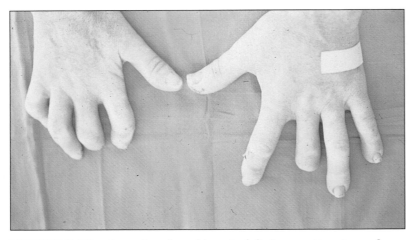

**FIGURE 3-70.** Acrosclerosis and terminal digit resorption. Loss of terminal parts of the digits and sclerodactyly are seen in a patient with scleroderma. Flexion contractures and tightened indurated skin are also shown.

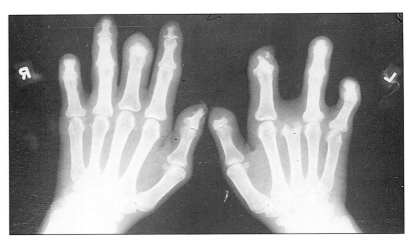

**FIGURE 3-71.** Acrolysis. A radiograph of the hands of this patient shows severe loss of the terminal phalanges with resorption of bone. This is a rare but well recognized feature of scleroderma and its variants.

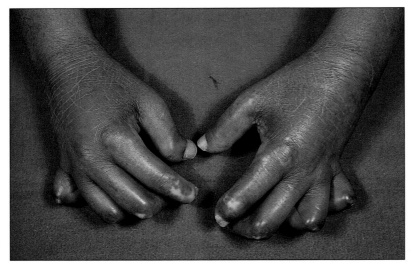

**FIGURE 3-72.** Skin thickening and shininess. The hands show an alteration in pigment and loss of shape on the terminal aspects of the fingers in severe scleroderma. Flexion contractures of the fingers are secondary to a tightened indurated skin.

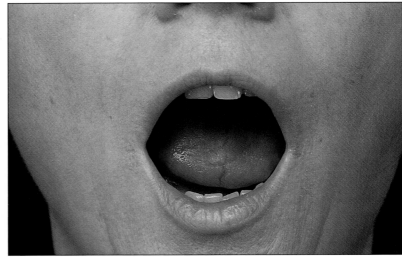

**FIGURE 3-73.** Facial changes. Tightness of the skin is apparent around the mouth in a patient with scleroderma.

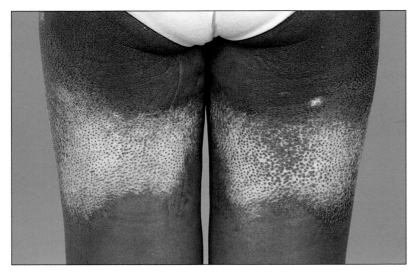

**FIGURE 3-74.** Hypopigmentation. In black skin hypopigmentation and vitiligo can occur in scleroderma.

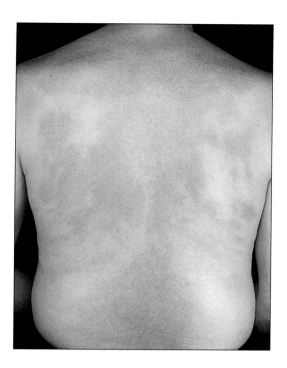

**FIGURE 3-75.**
Superficial morphea. This is scleroderma localized to areas of the skin. There is marked change in color and thickness of the skin. Distribution is patchy and sometimes widespread.

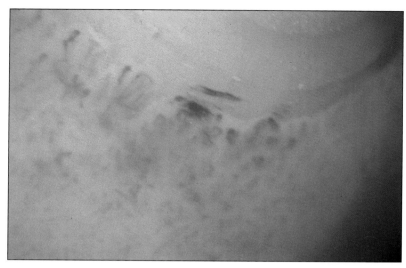

**FIGURE 3-76.** Nail-fold capillaroscopy. Microscopic examination of the capillary nail folds at the nail bed often reveals abnormalities in scleroderma, dermatomyositis, and related conditions. The abnormalities as shown here are sometimes gross and visible to the naked eye. Tortuous, dilated capillary loops are seen at the base of the nail in this patient.

## Other Organ Involvement

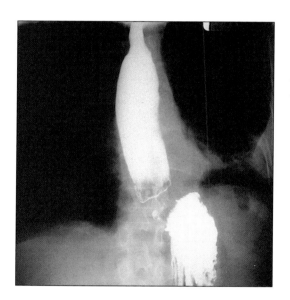

**FIGURE 3-77.** Hypomotility and dilation of the esophagus. Scleroderma affects both the upper and lower gastrointestinal tract. The esophagus is involved in 90% of patients of whom approximately half are symptomatic. Hypomotility may be accompanied by reflux esophagitis, a hiatal hernia and, in late-stage disease, by stricture formation that may require surgical intervention. Although the diagnosis of esophageal disease may be made on contrast radiography, esophageal manometry is more sensitive in detecting early disturbances in motility.

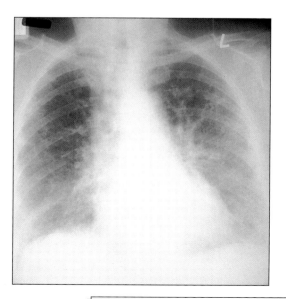

**FIGURE 3-78.** Pulmonary fibrosis. Pulmonary involvement in scleroderma may result in pleural disease (but rarely effusion), pulmonary hypertension, and diffuse interstitial pulmonary fibrosis "honeycomb lung." Dense reticular fibrosis of the lungs, especially the lower lobes, typical of scleroderma is shown here on chest radiography. Pulmonary function tests, particularly the diffusing capacity, become deranged well in advance of any radiographic evidence of disease.

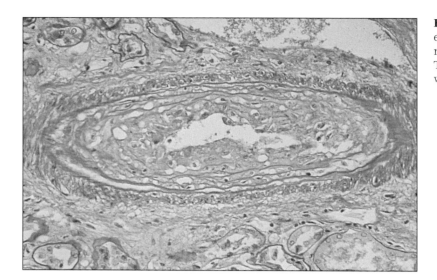

**FIGURE 3-79.** Severe arterial disease on renal biopsy. A rare and extremely serious manifestation of scleroderma is accelerated, often malignant, hypertension associated with arterial disease in the kidney. The figure shows marked thickening in the renal arteriole in a patient with scleroderma.

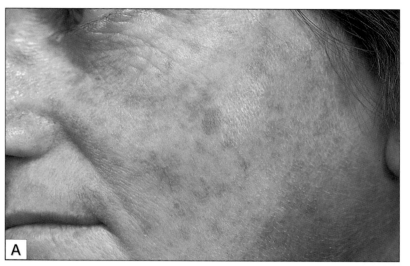

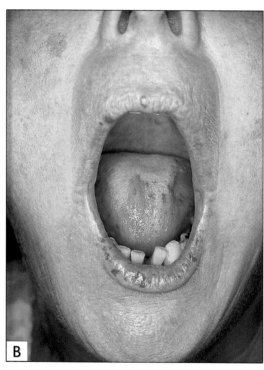

**FIGURE 3-80.** Telangiectasia. **A**, In some patients (notably those with CREST syndrome) telangiectasia is a major feature. CREST is an acronym for calcinosis, Raynaud's, esophageal dysmotility, sclerodactyly, and telangiectasia. Anticentromere antibodies are particularly common in this syndrome (90% of cases). **B**, This patient demonstrates telangiectasia of the lips and tongue characteristic of CREST syndrome. They may be confused with hereditary hemorrhagic telangiectasia (Osler-Weber-Rendu disease).

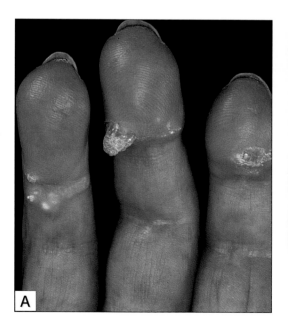

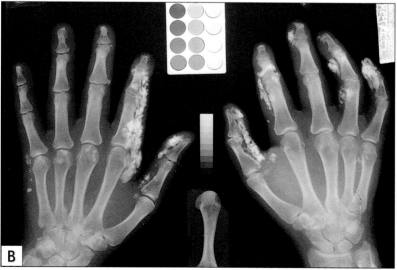

**FIGURE 3-81.** Calcinosis cutis. **A**, Calcinosis resulting in skin ulceration in a patient with CREST syndrome. Note also the widespread telangiectasia. **B**, Radiograph shows widespread subcutaneous calcification in the hands of a patient with CREST syndrome. CREST—calcinosis, Raynaud's esophageal dysmotility, sclerodactyly, telangiectasia.

## Classification and Diagnostic Criteria

### CLASSIFICATION OF THE IDIOPATHIC INFLAMMATORY MYOPATHIES

Major Forms

Dermatomyositis (DM)
  Adult form
  Juvenile form
Polymyositis (PM)
Inclusion body myositis (IBM)

Other Forms

Polymyositis associated with other
  connective tissue diseases
Sarcoid myopathy
Myositis in graft-versus-host disease
Eosinophilic polymyositis
Focal myositis
Proliferative myositis
Myositis ossificans

**FIGURE 3-82.** Classification of the idiopathic inflammatory myopathies [8].

### DISTINCTIVE CLINICAL FEATURES OF THE MAJOR FORMS OF THE IDIOPATHIC INFLAMMATORY MYOPATHIES

|  | DM | PM | IBM |
|---|---|---|---|
| Male/female ratio | 1/2 | 1/1 | 3/1 |
| Age | Juvenile/adult | Adult | Older adult |
| Course | Subacute | Chronic | Very chronic |
| Distribution of weakness | Proximal | Proximal | Proximal/distal/asymmetrical |
| Muscle pain with exercise or to palpation | Yes | No | No |
| Cutaneous lesions | Yes | No | No |
| Response to treatment | Yes | Yes | No |

**FIGURE 3-83.** Idiopathic inflammatory myopathies. Distinctive clinical features of the major forms [8]. DM—dermatomyositis; IBM—inclusion body myositis; PM—polymyositis.

### DIAGNOSTIC CRITERIA FOR POLYMYOSITIS/DERMATOMYOSITIS

Symmetric proximal muscle weakness
Elevated muscle enzymes
Myopathic EMG abnormalities
Typical changes on muscle biopsy
Typical rash of dermatomyositis

**FIGURE 3-84.** Proposed diagnostic criteria for polymyositis/dermatomyositis. Polymyositis diagnosed as definite with four of five criteria or probable with three of five criteria. Dermatomyositis diagnosed as definite with rash plus three of four criteria or probable with rash plus two of four criteria [23].

### DIAGNOSTIC CRITERIA FOR MIXED CONNECTIVE TISSUE DISEASE

Serological: positive anti-ribonucleoprotein antibodies at a
  hemagglutination titer of 1:1600 or higher
Clinical:
  Edema of the hands
  Synovitis
  Myositis
  Raynaud's Phenomenon
  Acrosclerosis

**FIGURE 3-85.** Proposed diagnostic criteria for mixed connective tissue disease (MCTD). Requirements for diagnosis: 1) serologic; 2) at least three clinical features; 3) the association of edema of the hands, Raynaud's phenomenon, and acrosclerosis requires at least one of the other two criteria [9].

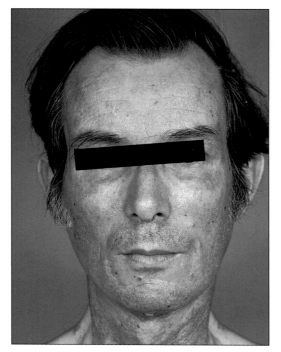

**FIGURE 3-86.** Facial rash and violaceous (heliotrope) discoloration of the eyelids are seen in a male with dermatomyositis.

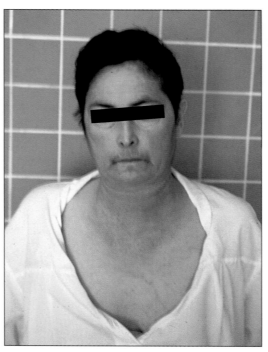

**FIGURE 3-87.** This woman has acute onset dermatomyositis. Note the classic rash over light-exposed areas on the neck, upper chest, and cheeks.

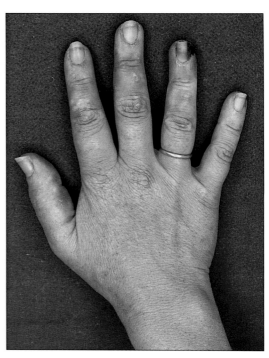

**FIGURE 3-88.** Gottron's papules. Typical appearance of dermatomyositis with thickened patches on the dorsal surface of the knuckles.

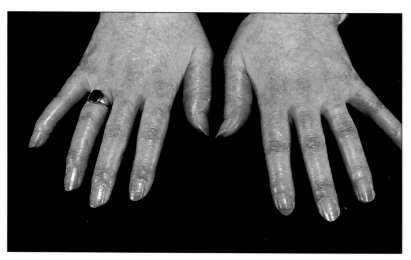

**FIGURE 3-89.** Typical dermatomyositis shows the overlap features with early scleroderma-marked shininess and erythema on the knuckles.

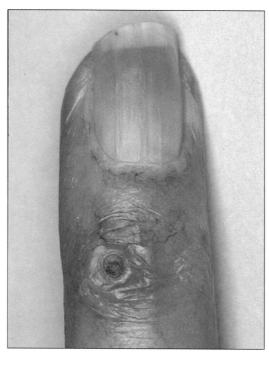

**FIGURE 3-90.** Finger lesions. Rash of dermatomyositis with prominent nail-fold capillaries, purple discoloration of the skin, and ulceration.

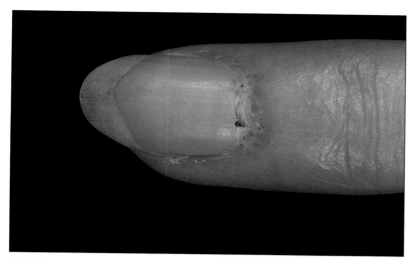

**FIGURE 3-91.** Nail-fold capillary lesions clearly visible to the naked eye in a patient with low-grade dermatomyositis.

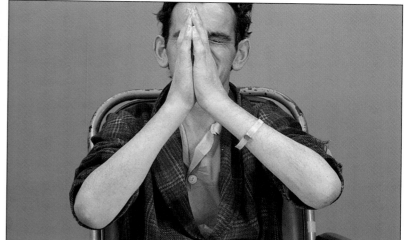

**FIGURE 3-92.** This patient had a variant associated with Jo-1 antibody. This is characterized by recurrent myositis, lung fibrosis, and, in this case, prominent tenosynovitis with flexor tendon deformities and limitation of movement in the wrists and hands. Serum anti-Jo-1 is diagnostically helpful. It is notably specific for this syndrome, rarely being found, for example, in SLE, and was the first of the precipitating antibodies to be demonstrated against an intracellular enzyme, in this case histidyl-tRNA synthetase.

## Polymyositis

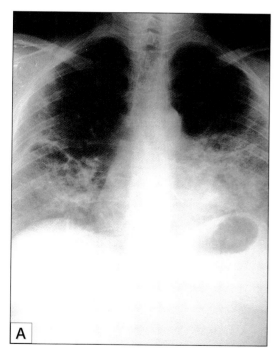

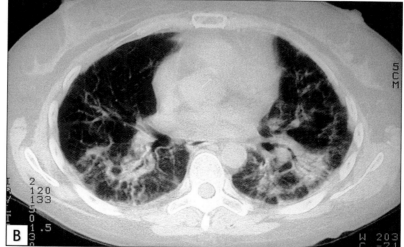

**FIGURE 3-93.** Polymyositis with pulmonary fibrosis. Widespread pulmonary fibrosis is seen in a patient with the Jo-1 syndrome. **A,** Chest radiograph. **B,** Chest computed tomography scan.

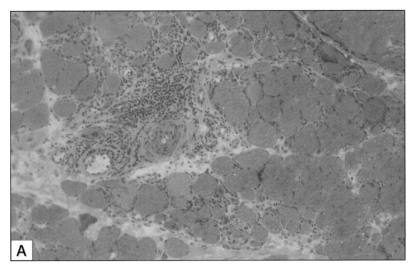

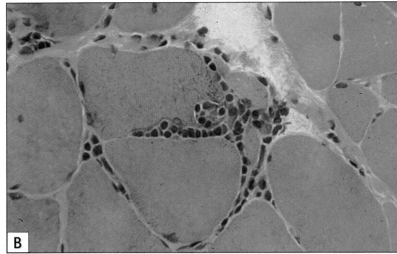

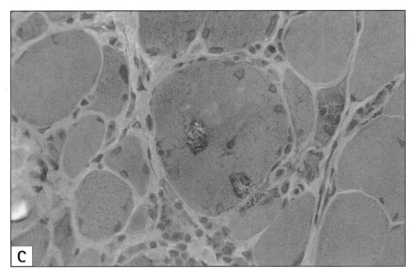

**FIGURE 3-94.** Idiopathic Inflammatory Myopathies. Muscle biopsy (photomicrographs). Care must be taken in the selection of the location, processing, and interpretation of the muscle biopsy. A muscle selected for biopsy should be moderately weak, without marked atrophy, and free of recent trauma, such as intramusclular injection or electromyographic testing. Selection of a biopsy site is also aided by choosing the corresponding muscle on the opposite side of the body of one showing EMG changes or use of MRI. **A**, Severe perivascular inflammatory infiltrate, muscle necrosis, and perifascicular atrophy in a patient with dermatomyositis (hematoxylin and eosin, ×140). **B**, Marked variability in the size of the muscle cells and mononuclear inflammatory infiltrate in the endomysial space in a patient with polymyositis. Note the typical "partial cellular invasion" phenomenon, characterized by the presence of inflammatory cells beneath the basal membrane of otherwise normal appearing muscle cells (trichrome stain, ×350). **C**, Marked variability in the size of the muscle cells and mononuclear inflammatory infiltrate in the endomysial space in a patient with inclusion body myositis. Note the distinctive rimmed vacuoles in the myofibers (hematoxylin and eosin, ×350). (*Courtesy of* Jose-Maria Grau, MD, Barcelona, Spain.)

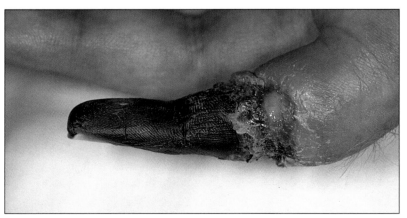

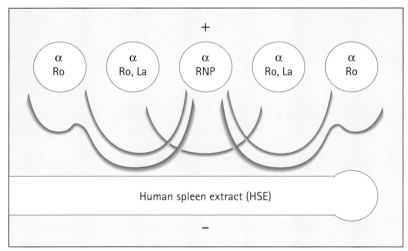

**FIGURE 3-95.** Mixed connective tissue disease (MCTD). Digital gangrene in a patient with anti-ribonucleoprotein antibodies and MCTD. The reason for the severe acute occlusion remained obscure.

**FIGURE 3-96.** Extractable nuclear antigen (ENA) antibody system measured by counterimmunoelectrophoresis. This figure shows the principle involved with spleen extract containing a variety of ENA and various precipitin lines seen in known and in test sera. Lines of identity show the nature of the ENA and test serum.

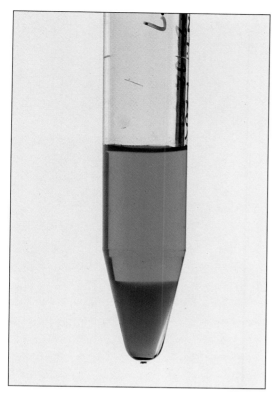

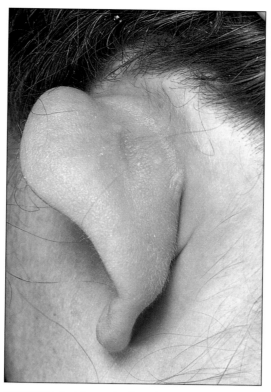

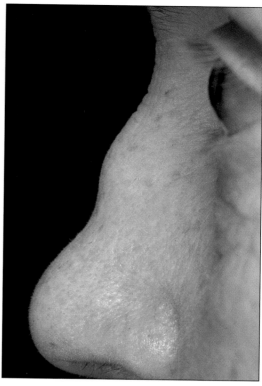

**FIGURE 3-97.** Cryoprecipitate. One of the more useful tests in rheumatology in which 15 to 20 mL of blood is taken and immediately transferred from the warm (37°C) syringe to a warmed plain tube (37°C). The blood is then allowed to clot. After this, it is separated and the serum stored for 48 hours. If correctly performed, this test is one of the simplest tests for immune complexes.

**FIGURE 3-98.** Polychondritis. In acute polychondritis, the ear may become swollen, inflamed, and tender. If untreated the hyaline cartilege is destroyed and the ear becomes floppy and distorted.

**FIGURE 3-99.** Polychondritis. In chondritis (either idiopathic or associated with Wegener's granulomatosis or other vasculitis) acute collapse of the cartilage of the nose can occur, as in this patient.

# References

1. Hughes GRV: Systemic lupus erythematosus. In *Connective Tissue Diseases*, edn 4. Edited by Hughes GRV. Oxford: Blackwell Scientific Publications; 1994:4–74.

2. Cervera R, Khamahsta MA, Font J, *et al*.: Systemic lupus erythematosus: clinical and immunologic patterns of disease expression in a cohort of 1,000 patients. *Medicine (Baltimore)* 1993, 72:113–124.

3. Hughes GRV: The antiphospholipid syndrome: ten years on. *Lancet* 1993, 342:341–344.

4. Khamashta MA, Asherson RA: Hughes syndrome—antiphospholipid antibodies move closer to thrombosis in 1994. *Br J Rheumatol* 1995, 34:493–494.

5. Roubey RAS: Autoantibodies to phospholipid-binding plasma proteins: a new view of lupus anticoagulants and other "antiphospholipid" antibodies. *Blood* 1994, 84:2854–2867.

6. Khamashta MA, Cuadrado MJ, Mujic F, *et al*.: The management of thrombosis in the antiphospholipid-antibody syndrome. *N Engl J Med* 1995, 332:993–997.

7. LeRoy EC, Black C, Fleischmajer R, et al: Scleroderma (systemic sclerosis): classification, subsets and pathogenesis. *J Rheumatol* 1988, 15:202–205.

8. Grau JM, Casademont J, Urbano-Marquez A: Polymyositis-dermatomyositis. In *Autoimmune Connective Tissue Diseases*. Edited by Khamashta MA, Font J, Hughes GRV. Barcelona: Doyma, 1993:73–84.

9. Alarcon-Segovia D, Cardiel MH: Comparison between 3 diagnostic criteria for mixed connective tissue disease. Study of 593 patients. *J Rheumatol* 1989, 16:328–334.

10. Hess EV: Drug and environmental lupus syndromes. *Lupus* 1994, 3:441–491.

11. Sontheimer RD: Skin disease in lupus erythematosus. *Lupus* 1997, 6:75–217.

12. Toubi E, Khamashta MA, Panarra A, Hughes GRV: Association of antiphospholipid antibodies with central nervous system disease in systemic lupus erythematosus. *Am J Med* 1995, 99:397–401.

13. Tan EM, Cohen AS, Fries JF, et al: The 1982 revised criteria for classification of systemic lupus erythematosus. *Arthritis Rheum* 1982, 25:1271–1277.

14. Buyon JP, Waltuck J, Kleinman C, Copel J: In utero identification and therapy of congenital heart block. *Lupus* 1995, 4:116–121.

15. Asherson RA, Liote F, Page B, *et al*.: Avascular necrosis of bone and antiphospholipid antibodies in systemic lupus erythematosus. *J Rheumatol* 1993, 20:284–288.

16. Spalton DG, Verdon Roe GM, Hughes GRV: Hydroxychloroquine, dosage parameters and retinopathy. *Lupus* 1993, 2:355–358.

17. Gladman DD: Prognosis and treatment of systemic lupus erythematosus. *Curr Opin Rheumatol* 1996, 8:430–437.

18. Khamashta MA, Mackworth-Young C: Antiphospholipid (Hughes) syndrome—a treatable cause of recurrent pregnancy loss. *Br Med J* 1997, 314:244.

19. Hunt BJ, Khamashta MA: Management of the Hughes syndrome. *Clin Exp Rheumatol* 1996, 14:115–117.

20. Harris EN, Khamashta MA, Hughes GRV: Antiphospholipid syndrome. In *Arthritis and Allied Conditions*, edn 12. Edited by McCarty DJ, Koopman WJ. Philadelphia: Lea & Febiger; 1993:1201–1212.

21. Asherson RA, Khamashta MA, Ordi-Ros J, *et al*.: The primary antiphospholipid syndrome: major clinical and serological features. *Medicine (Baltimore)* 1989, 68:366–374.

22. Khamashta MA, Cervera R, Asherson RA, *et al*.: Association of antiphospholipid antibodies with heart valve disease in systemic lupus erythematosus. *Lancet* 1990, 335:1541–1544.

23. Bohan A, Peter JB, Bowman BS, *et al*.: A computer assisted analysis of 153 patients with polymyositis and dermatomyositis. *Medicine (Baltimore)* 1977, 56:255–286.

# 4

# Vasculitides

## LOÏC GUILLEVIN

Vasculitides are heterogeneous disorders, with diverse and overlapping clinical manifestations and types of blood vessels involved, all of which have prevented the development of a universally acceptable classification. Distinguishing subsets of vasculitis may be justifed by recognizing new symptoms that are not consistent with the usual presentation of the disease, differences in prognosis, requirements for different therapeutic strategies, and unique pathogenic mechanisms. Treatment may be optimized by recognizing specific therapeutic alternatives for each entity, based on the clinical symptoms, laboratory investigations, and predictible outcome. This optimization should be the ultimate incentive for designation of subsets.

Detailed classification [1-8] or diagnostic [9] criteria of each type of vasculitis and their main characteristics are given below.

It is important to specify differences between classic polyarteritis nodosa and microscopic polyangiitis. In Fauci's classification [10], the polyarteritis nodosa group comprised polyarteritis nodosa, Churg-Strauss syndrome, and overlap angiitis. This pragmatic classification has been useful for clinicians but, recently, the recognition of a form of systemic vasculitis distinct from classic polyarteritis nodosa—microscopic polyangiitis—has been generally accepted. This distinction did not appear in the criteria for classification of polyarteritis nodosa developed in 1990 by the American College of Rheumatology [4]. Classification criteria are not appropriate for the diagnosis of individual patients but provide a standard way to evaluate and describe patients with vasculitis included in therapeutic trial or epidemiologic studies.

## CRITERIA FOR CLASSIFICATION OF POLYARTERITIS NODOSA

| Criterion | Definition |
|---|---|
| 1. Weight loss ≥ 4 kg | Loss of 4 kg or more of body weight since illness began, not due to dieting or other factors |
| 2. Livedo reticularis | Mottled reticular pattern over the skin of portions of the extremities or torso |
| 3. Testicular pain or tenderness | Pain or tenderness of the testicles, not due to infection, trauma, or other causes |
| 4. Myalgias, weakness, or leg tenderness | Diffuse myalgias (excluding shoulder and hip girdle) or weakness of muscles or tenderness of leg muscles |
| 5. Mononeuropathy or polyneuropathy | Development of mononeuropathy, multiple mononeuropathies, or polyneuropathy |
| 6. Diastolic BP >90 mm Hg | Development of hypertension with the diastolic BP higher than 90 mm Hg |
| 7. Elevated BUN or creatinine | Elevation of BUN >40 mg/dL (14.3 μ—/L) or creatinine >1.5 mg/dL (132 μM/L), not due to dehydration or obstruction |
| 8. Hepatitis B virus | Presence of hepatitis B surface antigen or anti-HBs antibody in serum |
| 9. Arteriographic abnormality | Arteriogram showing aneurysms or occlusions of the visceral arteries, not due to arteriosclerosis, fibromuscular dysplasia, or noninflammatory causes |
| 10. Biopsy of small- or medium-sized artery containing PMN | Histologic changes showing the presence of granulocytes or granulocytes and mononuclear leukocytes in the artery wall |

**FIGURE 4-1.** American College of Rheumatology 1990 classification criteria for polyarteritis nodosa [1]. For classification purposes, a patient with vasculitis shall be said to have polyarteritis nodosa when at least three of these criteria are present. The presence of any three or more critieria yields a sensitivity of 82.2% and a specificity of 86.6%. BP—blood pressure; BUN—blood urea nitrogen; PMN—polymorphonuclear neutrophils.

## PRACTICAL CLASSIFICATION OF VASCULITIDES

### Primary vasculitides

Affecting large-, medium-, and small-sized blood vessels
- Takayasu arteritis
- Giant cell (temporal) arteritis
- Isolated angiitis of the central nervous system

Affecting predominantly medium- and small-sized blood vessels
- Polyarteritis nodosa
- Churg-Strauss syndrome
- Wegener's granulomatosis

Affecting predominantly small-sized blood vessels
- Microscopic polyangiitis
- Henoch-Schönlein purpura
- Cutaneous leukocytoclastic angiitis

Miscellaneous conditions
- Buerger's disease
- Cogan's syndrome
- Kawasaki disease

### Secondary vasculitides

- Infection-related vasculitis
- Vasculitis secondary to connective tissue disease
- Drug hypersensitivity-related vasculitis
- Vasculitis secondary to mixed essential cryoglobulinemia
- Malignancy-related vasculitis
- Hypocomplementemic urticarial vasculitis
- Post-organ transplant vasculitis
- Pseudovasculitic syndromes (myxoma, endocarditis, Sneddon's syndrome)

**FIGURE 4-2.** Lie's classification of vasculitides [2]. This classification is based on clinical and pathologic criteria. We advocate the use of similar clinical and pathologic findings to classify the vasculitides, for example, lung and renal involvement to help separate polyarteritis nodosa and microscopic polyangitis, the use of laboratory tests (antineutrophil cytoplasmic antibodies, hepatitis B virus or hepatitis C virus infection), and angiographic data [11], and realizing that individual patients may have findings that overlap the clinical diagnostic categories. Frequency of antineutrophil cytoplasmic antibodies and their pathogenetic mechanisms are shown below [12,13].

## CHAPEL HILL CONSENSUS CONFERENCE NOMENCLATURE*

**Large-sized vessel vasculitis**

Giant cell (temporal) arteritis — Granulomatous arteritis of the aorta and its major branches, with a predilection for the extracranial branches of the carotid artery. *Often involves the temporal artery. Usually occurs in patients over 50 y and is often associated with polymyalgia rheumatica.*

Takayasus arteritis — Granulomatous arteritis of the aorta and its major branches. *Usually occurs in patients under 50 y.*

**Medium-sized vessel vasculitis**

Polyarteritis nodosa (classic polyarteritis nodosa) — Necrotizing inflammation of medium- or small-sized arteries, without glomerulonephiritis or vasculitis in arterioles, capillaries, or venules.

Kawasaki disease — Arteritis involving large-, medium-, and small-sized arteries, and associated with mucocutaneous lymph node syndrome. *Coronary arteries are often involved. Aorta and veins may be involved. Usually occurs in children.*

**Small-sized vessel vasculitis**

Wegener's granulomatosis † — Granulomatous inflammation involving the respiratory tract and necrotizing vasculitis affecting small- to medium-sized vessels (eg, capillaries, venules, arterioles, and arteries). *Necrotizing glomerulonephritis is common.*

Churg-Strauss syndrome † — Eosinophil-rich and granulomatous inflammation involving the respiratory tract, and necrotizing vasculitis affecting small- to medium-sized vessels, associated with asthma and eosinophilia.

Microscopic polyangiitis † (microscopic polyarteritis) — Necrotizing vasculitis, with few or no immune deposits, (ie, capillaries, venules, or arterioles). *Necrotizing arteritis involving small- and medium-sized vessels may be present. Necrotizing glomenuloephritis is very common. Pulmonary capillaritis often occurs.*

Henoch-Schönlein purpura — Vasculitis, with IgA-dominant immune deposits, affecting small-sized vessels (ie, capillaries, venules, or arterioles). *Typically involves skin, gut and glomeruli, and is associated with arthralgias or arthritis.*

Essential cryglobulinemia vasculitis — Vasculitis, with croglobulin immune deposits, affecting small-sized vessels (ie, capillaries, venules, or arterioles), and associated with cryoglogulins in serum. *Skin and glomeruli are often involved.*

Cutaneous leukocytoclastic angiitis — Isolated cutaneous leukocytoclastic angiitis without systemic vasculitis or glomerulonephritis.

*Large-sized vessels refers to the aorta and the largest branches directed toward major body regions (eg, to the extremities and the head and neck); medium-sized vessels refers to the main visceral arteries (eg, renal, hepatic, coronary and mesenteric arteries); small-sized vessels refers to venules, capillaries, arterioles and the intra-parenchymal distal arteries that connect with arterioles. Some small- and large-sized vessel vasculitides may involve medium-sized arteries, but large- and medium-sized vessel vasculitides do not involve vessels smaller than arteries. Essential components are represented by normal type; usual, but not essential, components, are in italics.*

*† Strongly associated with antineutrophil cytoplasmic autoantibodies.*

**FIGURE 4-3.** Names and definitions adopted by the Chapel Hill Consensus Conference on the nomenclature of systemic vasculitides [3]. This group attempted to define a standardized classification system for some of the most common forms of noninfectious systemic vasculitis and to construct root definitions for the vasculitides so named. The authors of the consensus assigned 10 selected entities of vasculitis to one of three categories: large-sized vessel vasculitis, medium-sized vessel vasculitis, or small-sized vessel vasculitis. The proposed distinguishing feature for polyarteritis nodosa versus microscopic polyangiitis (formerly microscopic polyarteritis) is the absence versus the presence of vasculitis in arterioles, venules, or capillaries. Small vessel involvement, when present, was the definitive diagnostic criterion of microscopic polyangiitis and excludes the diagnosis of polyarteritis nodosa even if medium-sized artery lesions were seen. This nomenclature has the advantage of emphasizing the existence of microscopic polyangiitis but the disadvantage of giving it too large a place in the family of vasculitides. Histologic findings of vasculitis, in nerve for instance, are often common to several necrotizing angiopathies.

**FIGURE 4-4.** Vasculitides classified according to vessel size.

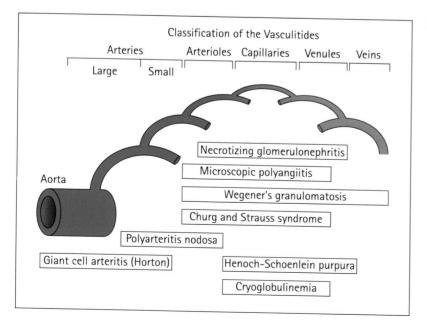

Classification of the Vasculitides

Arteries — Large / Small; Arterioles; Capillaries; Venules; Veins

Aorta

Necrotizing glomerulonephritis
Microscopic polyangiitis
Wegener's granulomatosis
Churg and Strauss syndrome
Polyarteritis nodosa
Giant cell arteritis (Horton)
Henoch-Schoenlein purpura
Cryoglobulinemia

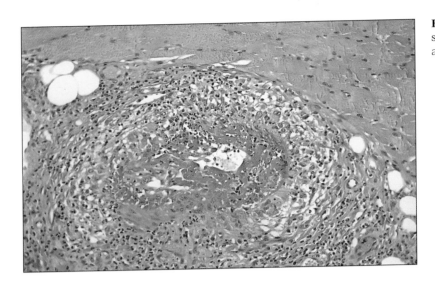

**FIGURE 4-5.** Muscle biopsy showing vasculitis involving a medium-sized muscular artery. Fibrinoid necrosis, endothelial modifications, and adventitial leukocyte infiltrate are seen (X100).

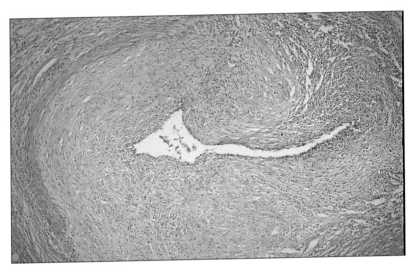

**FIGURE 4-6.** Kidney biopsy. Fibrous endarteritis, thickened intima, and segmental inflammation are apparent. This appearance is nonspecific and can be observed in every healed vasculitic process.

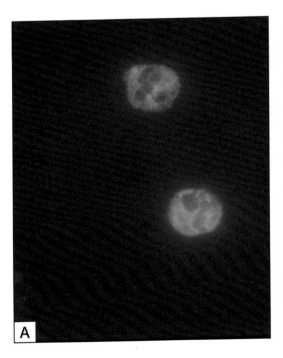

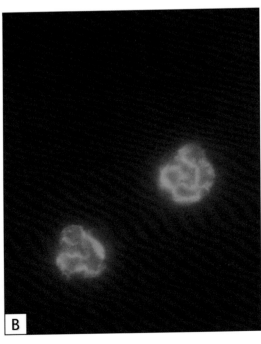

**FIGURE 4-7.** Antineutrophil cytoplasmic antibodies (ANCA). ANCA are implicated in several systemic vasculitides. They are found in approximatively 80% of systemic Wegener's (WG) granulomatosis, 50% of localized WG, 50% to 60% of microscopic polyangiitis (MPA), and Churg-Strauss syndrome (CSS) [12]. ANCA are present in less than 10% of classic polyarteritis nodosa. At present, ANCA should be considered as reflecting small-sized vessel involvement. In WG, a cytoplasmic (c) fluorescent staining pattern, **A**, is observed and antibodies directed against proteinase 3 (PR3) are responsible. These antibodies are also detected by enzyme-linked immunosorbent assay (ELISA). Anti-PR3 antibodies are highly specific to WG. Conversely, in MPA, CSS, and in rare cases of WG, the fluorescence pattern is perinuclear (p), **B**. Antibodies producing this pattern are directed against myeloperoxidase (MPO). These antibodies can also be detected by ELISA. p-ANCA are less specific for vasculitis than c-ANCA and can be found in other diseases (inflammatory colitis, infections).

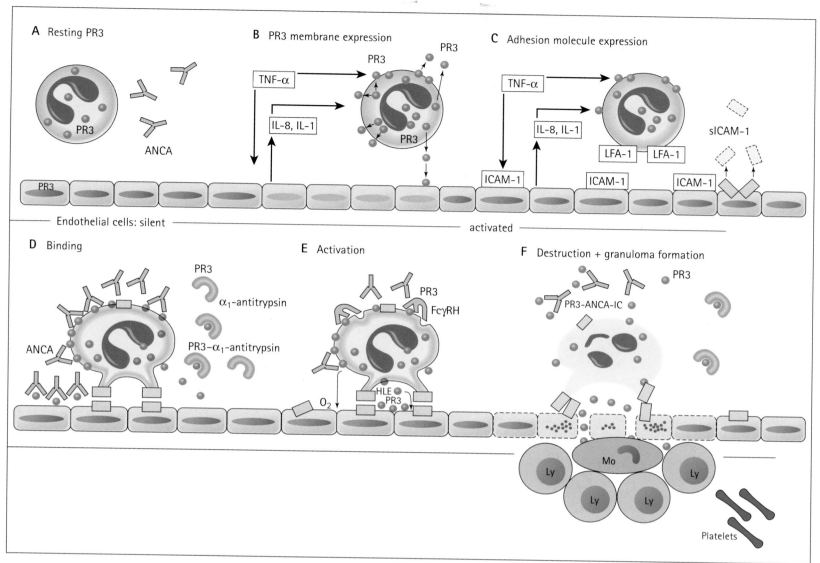

**FIGURE 4-8.** Pathogenetic mechanisms of antineutrophil cytoplasmic antibody (ANCA) according to ANCA–cytokine sequence
theory. **A**, Resting neutrophil proteinase 3 (RP3) is mostly sequestered
in azurophil granules. **B**, Priming of polymorphonuclear leukocytes
(PMN) by cytokines. Intracytoplasmic PR3 is translocated to the cell
surface and becomes accessible to ANCA. **C**, Membrane expression
of adhesion molecules. **D**, Adhesion of PMN to endothelial cells and
binding of ANCA to PR3 via F(ab')$_2$ fragments. **E**, Interaction between
ANCA and PR3 via FcγRII receptor leads to activation of neutrophils
with degranulation, generation of oxygen radicals, and endothelial cell
injury. **F**, The final results are intravascular lysis of PMN, necrotizing
vasculitis, and granuloma formation. HLE—human leukocyte elastase;
IC—immune complexes; ICAM-1—intercellular adhesion molecule 1;
IL—interleukin; LFA-1—leukocyte function associated antigen 1;
sICAM-1—soluble intercellular adhesion molecule 1; TNF-α—tumor
necrosis factor-α. It should be mentioned that the presence of activated
PR3 in endothelial cells has not been formally demonstrated and is
controversial. (*Adapted from* Gross and Csernok [13].)

## CLINICAL FEATURES OF POLYARTERITIS NODOSA

| | Frohnert* | Leib* | Cohen* | Guillevin* | Guillevin† | Fortin* |
|---|---|---|---|---|---|---|
| Reference | 1967 [17] | 1979 [14] | 1980 [19] | 1988 [16] | 1992 [15] | 1995 [18] |
| Number of patients | 130 | 64 | 53 | 165 | 182 | 45 |
| Age mean (y) | | 47 | 54 | 48 | | 54 |
| range | 6–75 | 17–80 | 17–78 | 11–65 | | 22–86 |
| Male/female ratio | 1.9 | 1.1 | 1.9 | 1.2 | 1 | 1.1 |
| **System involvement (%)** | | | | | | |
| General symptoms | 76 | | | | | |
| Fever | | 36 | 31 | 69 | 65 | |
| Weight loss | | | 16 | 66 | | |
| Peripheral nervous | 52 | 72 | 60 | 67 | 70 | 51 |
| Muscles | 30 | | | 53 | 54 | |
| Joints | 58 | | 55 | 44 | 46 | |
| Joints and muscles | 58 | 73 | | | | 51 |
| Cutaneous | 8 | 28 | 58 | 46 | 49 | 44 |
| Renal | 14 | 63 | 66 | 29 | 36 | 44 |
| Hypertension | | 25 | 14 | 31 | 33 | |
| Gastrointestinal | 38 | 42 | 25 | 31 | 26 | 53 |
| Respiratory | 3 | 47 | 13 | 29 | 20 | 40 |
| Central nervous system | 10 | 25 | | 17 | | 24 |
| Cardiac | | 30 | 4 | 23 | 9 | 18 |
| Eyes | | 3 | 8 | 44 | | |
| Ear, nose, and throat | | 3 | 0 | | | |

*Retrospective studies
† Prospective study

**FIGURE 4-9.** Main clinical manifestations of polyarteritis nodosa. Polyarteritis nodosa, first described by Küssmaul and Maier, is a necrotizing angiitis whose main manifestations are weight loss, fever, asthenia, peripheral neuropathy, renal involvement, musculoskeletal and cutaneous manifestations, hypertension, gastrointestinal tract involvement, and cardiac failure [14–19].

Polyarteritis nodosa is a rare disease. In studies [20,21] that considered biopsy-proven forms only, the annual incidence and prevalence of the disease were, respectively, 0.7/100,000 and 6.3/100,000 habitants. Estimates of the annual incidence rate for polyarteritis nodosa-type systemic vasculitis in a general population range from 4.6/1,000,000 in England [20], 9.0/1,000,000 in Olmsted County, Minnesota, to 77/1,000,000 in a hepatitis B hyperendemic Alaskan Eskimo population [22]. Polyarteritis nodosa affects men and women equally at every age, with a predominance between 40 and 60 years old. It is observed in all racial groups.

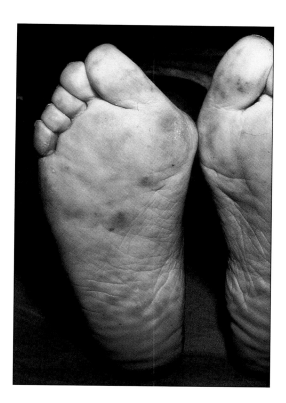

**FIGURE 4-10.** Skin nodule located on the foot. When a skin biopsy is performed, small-sized vasculitis is found. Biospy of the deep dermis may show affected medium-sized vessels.

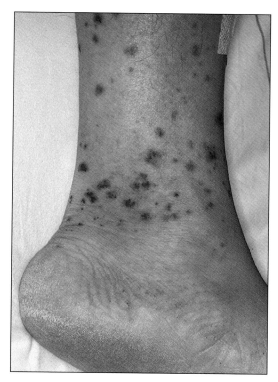

**FIGURE 4-11.** Purpura. Palpable purpura is frequent in vasculitis affecting vessels of the skin. It is frequent in microscopic polyangiitis and reflects small-sized vessel involvement. Infiltration of the purpuric area and local necrosis are the most characteristic features of vascular purpura.

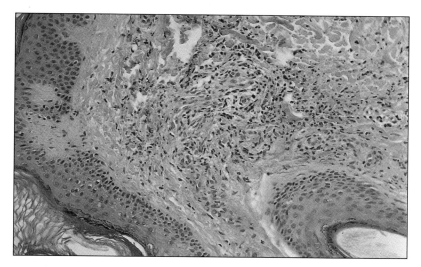

**FIGURE 4-12.** Kistopathologic appearance of palpable purpura, Leukocytoclastic vasculitis is seen. Neutrophil infiltration, leukocytoclasis, and nuclear fragmentation arae prominent. Other types of leukocytes may be present. Vessel wall neurosis with focal hemorrhage is typical.

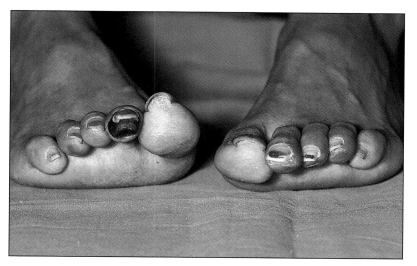

**FIGURE 4-13.** Gangrene. Gangrene is rarely observed (<10%) but suggests the diagnosis of vasculitis. Distal pulses are detected indicating the vascular lesions are more distal.

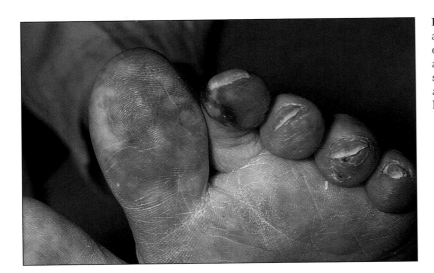

**FIGURE 4-14.** Vasculitis in toes. In young people, local ischemic areas and distal necrosis suggest inflammatory vasculitis. Conversely, in elderly people, cholesterol emboli are the most frequent diagnosis associated with toe gangrene. In such cases, cholesterol crystals are found in skin and muscle biopsies. Cholesterol emobolization is most common after an event such as arterial catheterization and usually is seen in the lower extremities.

## Renal Involvement

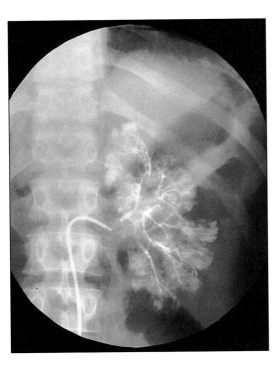

**FIGURE 4-15.** Renal angiogram. Renal vasculitis is characteristic of polyarteritis nodosa. The angiogram shows renal infarcts that result from the thromboses of arcuate arteries. When pathologic examinations are done months or years after disease onset, macroscopic examination shows a small bumpy kidney.

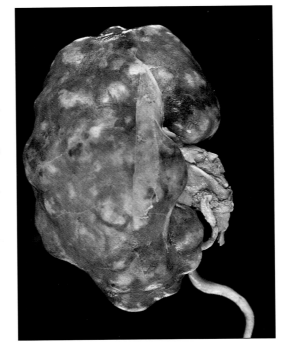

**FIGURE 4-16.** Pathology of kidney. Lumpy surface is secondary to previous infarctions of the kidney with scarring. Histologic examination shows that renal involvement is due to an ischemic process. Microaneurysms are also frequently observed in kidney and digestive tract arteries (*see* Fig. 4-19).

## Gastrointestinal Manifestations

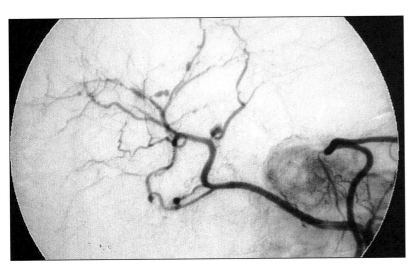

**FIGURE 4-17.** Gallbladder vasculitis. The gastrointestinal tract is affected in 25% of the cases [15]. Vasculitis is seen here in the gallbladder. Vasculitis can be also found in every digestive tract artery. When vasculitis is found in the bowel, especially the small intestines or stomach, necrosis may result in bowel perforation and subsequent peritonitis. The angiogram showed microaneurysms and multiple vessel stenoses.

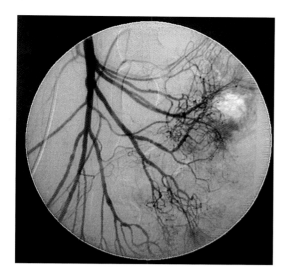

**FIGURE 4-18.** Vessel caliber changes. Modifications of vessel caliber often occur at bifurcations and in distal vessels, producing turbulence. Hemodynamic modifications and turbulence appear to facilitate immune-complex deposition, intimal lesions, and vasculitis lesions at these sites.

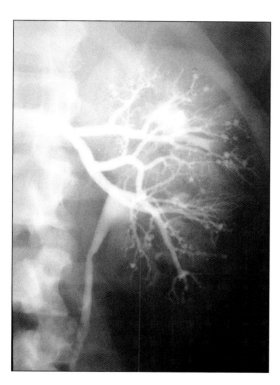

**FIGURE 4-19.** Renal angiogram. Multiple kidney aneurysms can be seen.

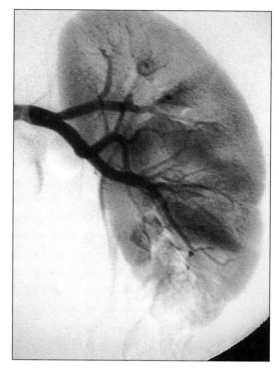

**FIGURE 4-20.** Renal angiography. The angiogram, performed 8 months after onset of treatment, shows that aneurysms observed in 4-19 have disappeared [23]. This evolution is probably the consequence of aneurysm thrombosis followed by arterial fibrosis. On this angiogram, only the renal infarct present in the inferior part of the kidney persists.

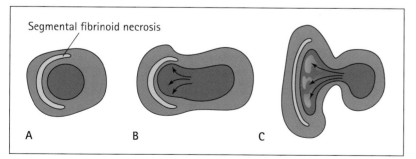

Segmental fibrinoid necrosis

A    B    C

**FIGURE 4-21.** Microaneurysm formation. A microaneurysm is the consequence of an immunopathologic process (left side of vessel) that weakens the vessel wall. When the vessel wall is not involved in the vasculitic process over its entire circumference, the local increase in blood pressure is responsible for parietal ballooning and aneurysm formation (**A** to **C**).

## CHARACTERISTICS OF HEPATITIS B VIRUS-RELATED POLYARTERITIS NODOSA

**Features**

Classic-polyarteritis nodosa

ANCA absent

No overlap with microscopic polyangiitis

**Distribution and localization**

Kidney

  Renal vasculitis with renovascular hypertension, renal infarcts
    and microaneurysms

  Rapidly progressive glomerulonephritis is never observed

Orchitis

Grastrointestinal tract involvement

  Bowel primarily small intestine perforation, hemorrhage

**Relapses**

Relapse in < 10% of the cases

**Laboratory data**

ANCA absent

HBV present

HBs, HBe positive, viral DNA reflecting replication

**Abnormal angiography (microneurysms, stenoses)**

**FIGURE 4-22.** Characteristics of hepatitis B virus (HBV)-related polyarteritis nodosa (PAN). PAN can be the consequence of viral infections [24]. Before the development of an effective vaccine and improved transfusion safety, HBV was responsible for more than 30% of classic PAN cases. Now, it is found in less than 5% of PAN. HBV-related PAN is related to immune-complex deposits. Some characteristics of this process are summarized here. They demonstrate clearly that etiology can influence the clinical expression of the disease. We can postulate that differences between vasculitis subsets could be due to different etiologies. Other viral etiologies have been demonstrated but are rare and sometimes anecdotal: hepatitis C virus (5%) [25], parvovirus (anecdotal), human immunodeficiency virus (discussed later). ANCA—antineutrophil cytoplasmic antibodies; HBs—hepatits B surface antigen; Hbe—hepatits B e antigen.

# Microscopic Polyangiitis

## DIFFERENTIAL DIAGNOSIS OF POLYARTERITIS NODOSA AND MICROSCOPIC POLYANGIITIS

| Criteria | PAN | MPA |
|---|---|---|
| Histology | | |
| • Type of vasculitis | Necrotizing with mixed cells, rarely granulomatous | Necrotizing with mixed cells, not granulomatous |
| • Type of vessels involved | Medium- and small-sized muscle arteries, sometimes arterioles | Small vessels (ie, capillaries, venules or arterioles) |
| | | Small- and medium-sized arteries may be also affected |
| Distribution and localization | | |
| Kidney | | |
| • Renal vasculitis with renovascular hypertension, renal infarcts and microaneurysms | Yes | No |
| • Rapidly progressive glomerulonephiritis | No | Very common |
| Lung | | |
| • Pulmonary hemorrhage | No | Yes |
| Peripheral neuropathy | 50%–80% | 10%–20% |
| Relapses | Rare | Frequent |
| Laboratory data | | |
| pANCA | Rare (< 10%) | Yes (50%–80%) |
| HBV infection present | Yes (uncommon) | No |
| Abnormal angiography (microaneurysms, stenoses) | Yes (variable) | No |

**FIGURE 4-23.** Differences between polyarteritis nodosa (PAN) and microscopic polyangiitis (MPA). MPA is now recognized as an entity distinct from PAN (or classic PAN) (*Adapted from* [26]). Glomerulonephritis and lung hemorrhage are the two manifestations that distinguish MPA from PAN because they are never observed in PAN.

According to the Chapel Hill criteria [3], MPA would not be limited to pulmonary-renal syndrome and every type of vasculitis respecting the Chapel Hill criteria could be considered MPA. ANCA—antineutrophil cytoplasmic antibodies; HBV—hepatitis B virus.

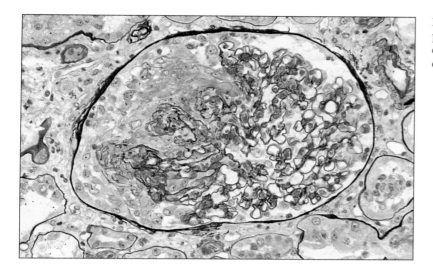

**FIGURE 4-24.** Glomerulonephritis occurring in microscopic polyangiitis (MPA). Rapidly progressive glomerulonephritis is frequently observed in MPA. A fibrinoid crescent covering a large part of the outer circumference of the glomerulus is present.

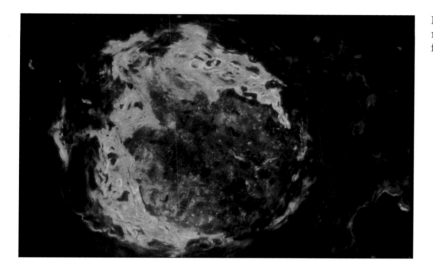

**FIGURE 4-25.** Fibrinoid crescent. Immunofluorescence labeling is negative for immunoglobulins and complement but shows an intense fluorescence of the fibrinoid crescent.

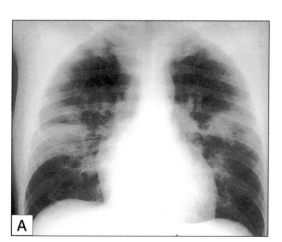

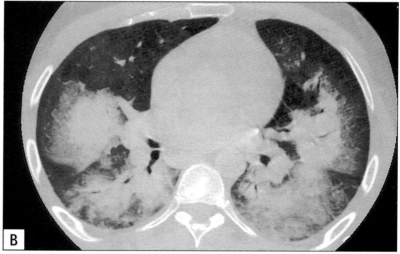

**FIGURE 4-26.** Pulmonary infiltrates. **A**, Pulmonary infiltrates are noted in a patient who presented with hemoptysis. This symptom associated with anemia suggests lung hemorrhage. **B**, A computed tomography scan of the same patient shows more precisely the extensive bilateral lung infiltrates. Lung hemorrhage is also better visualized on this scan.

## CRITERIA FOR CLASSIFICATION OF WEGENER'S GRANULOMATOSIS

| Criterion | Definition |
|---|---|
| 1. Nasal or oral inflammation | Development of painful oral ulcers or purulent or bloody nasal discharge |
| 2. Abnormal chest radiograph | Chest radiograph showing the presence of nodules, fixed infiltrates or cavities |
| 3. Urinary sediment | Microhematuria (>5 red blood cells per high power field) or red cell casts in urine sediment |
| 4. Granulomatous inflammation on biopsy | Histologic changes showing granulomatous inflammation within the wall of an artery or in the perivascular or extravascular area (artery or arteriole) |

**FIGURE 4-31.** American College of Rheumatology 1990 classification criteria for Wegener's granulomatosis [5]. Wegener's granulomatosis is characterized by involvement of lung (nodules and infiltrates), ear, nose, throat, and kidneys (rapidly progressive glomerulonephritis); the necrotizing vasculitis involves medium- and small-sized arteries, veins, and capillaries; extravascular granulomas are present [5]. The association between antibodies directed against components of neutrophil cytoplasm and Wegener's granulomatosis has been demonstrated [29] and these autoantibodies may be involved in the pathophysiology of the disease [30]. Indirect immunofluorescence labeling of antineutrophil cytoplasmic antibodies usually gives a diffuse cytoplasmic staining pattern. Enzyme-linked immunosorbent assay usually detects antibodies directed against proteinase 3 in patients whose antibodies give a cytoplasmic staining pattern (against myeloperoxidase perinuclear staining pattern). Antibodies are rare in Wegener's granulomatosis. The sensitivity of antineutrophil cytoplasmic antibodies, mainly those recognizing the cytoplasm, is about 90% in active Wegener's granulomatosis and 40% when the disease is in remission or in those with localized disease. The specificity of cytoplasm-staining autoantibodies in the diagnosis of Wegener's granulomatosis is about 90% [12]. For classification purposes, a patient shall be said to have Wegener's granulomatosis when at least two of the above four criteria are present. The presence of any two or more criteria yields a sensitivity of 88% and a specificity of 92%. Not all patients in the classification study had ANCA tests performed so the test was not included as a criteria.

## FREQUENCY OF CLINICAL MANIFESTATIONS OF WEGENER'S GRANULOMATOSIS (PERCENTAGE)

| | Walton | Cordier | Hoffman | Anderson |
|---|---|---|---|---|
| Year | 1958 | 1990 | 1992 | 1992 |
| Reference | [34] | [32] | [33] | [31] |
| Patients, n | 56 | 77 | 158 | 265 |
| Age, y (range) | 45 (12–75) | 46.5 (17–80) | 41 (9–78)] | 50 (10–83) |
| Sex ratio (M/F) | 1.5 | 1 | 1 | 1.2 |
| Fever, weight loss | | 83 | 50 | |
| Lung manifestations | 100 | 100 | 85 | 73 |
| Ear, nose, throat symptoms | 89 | 75 | 92 | 87 |
| Kidney involvement | 90 | 74 | 77 | 60 |
| Arthritis | 34 | 34 | 67 | 20 |
| Skin manifestations | 46 | 29 | 46 | 25 |
| Neurologic manifestations | 29 | 30 | 15 | |
| Ocular manifestations | 41 | 29 | 52 | 14 |

**FIGURE 4-32.** Main clinical symptoms of systemic Wegener's granulomatosis [31–34].

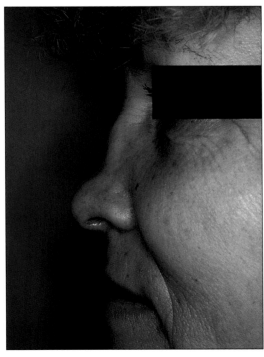

**FIGURE 4-33.** Saddle nose. Cartilage neurosis and collapse occurs in systemic or localized Wegener's granulomatosis. This symptom often causes a disfiguring sequel to the disease.

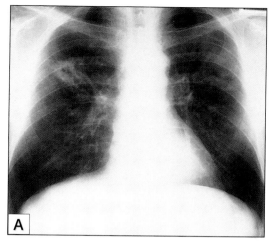

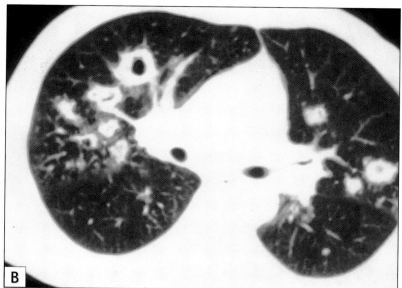

**FIGURE 4-34.**
Nodules. **A**, A nodule is located in the right lung with cavitation and bronchial drainage. **B**, In the same patient a computed tomography scan of the lungs shows several nodules, some with thick-walled cavities. Some nodules were not visible on a standard radiograph. Computed tomography scanning with thin slices is the major radiologic investigation for diagnosis and follow-up of Wegener's granulomatosis.

**FIGURE 4-35.** Characteristics of lung manifestations in Wegener's granulomatosis (WG) [32].

| LUNG MANIFESTATIONS OF WEGENER'S GRANULOMATOSIS | | |
|---|---|---|
| | At time of diagnosis | During the course of WG |
| Lung manifestations | 45 | 87 |
| Radiologic symptoms | | |
| Infiltrates | 25 | 67 |
| Nodules | 23 | 58 |
| Respiratory symptoms | | |
| Cough | 19 | 46 |
| Hemoptysis | 12 | 30 |
| Thoracic pain | 10 | 28 |

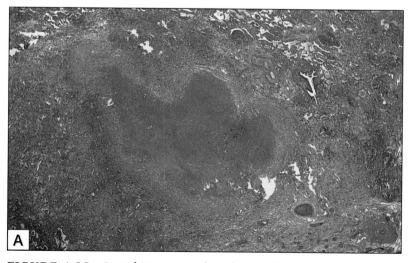

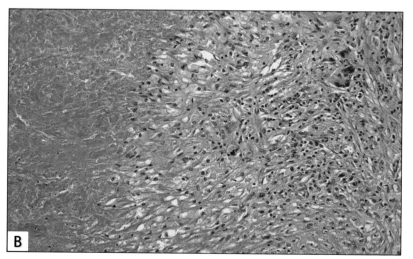

**FIGURE 4-36.** Lung biopsy. **A**, A lung biopsy shows a large focus of granulomatosis inflammation and neurosis with a clearly outlined contour (X40). **B**, In another region of the same biopsy, a granuloma with giant cells is close to the area of necrosis (X200).

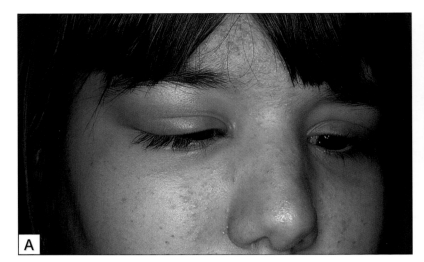

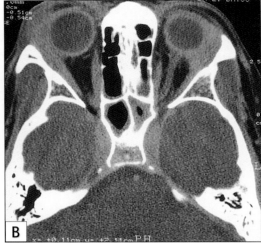

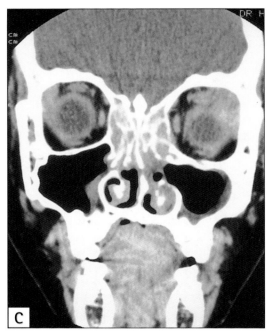

**FIGURE 4-37.** Orbital involvement. **A**, The orbital involvement, which was the first symptom of Wegener's granulomatosis in this patient, is responsible for the inflammatory pseudotumor. **B** and **C**, Computed tomography scans of the same patient show the ``tumor'' that was responsible for motor nerve palsy. An orbital biopsy was not performed and is not usually recommended because of its invasive and destructive nature; other biopsy sites should be preferred. The scan shows a minor left maxillary sinusitis.

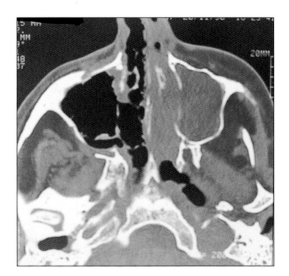

**FIGURE 4-38.** Sinusitis. Facial computed tomography scan shows sinusitis affecting maxillar sinusitis, associated with bone destruction.

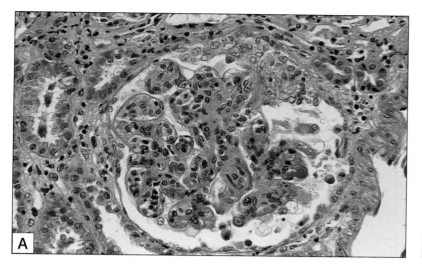

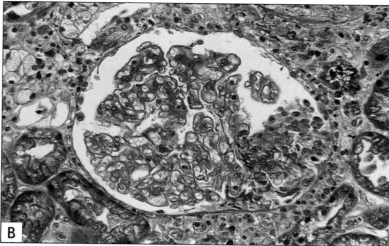

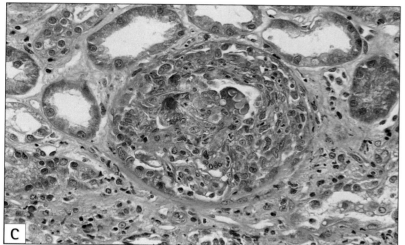

**FIGURE 4-39.** Glomerulonephritis. Extracapillary glomerulonephritis at 3 different stages of its evolution, from the early stage with bleeding into the Bowman's capsule **A**, to crescent formation **B**, and finally complete glomerular involvement preceding "pain à cacheter" scarring **C**.

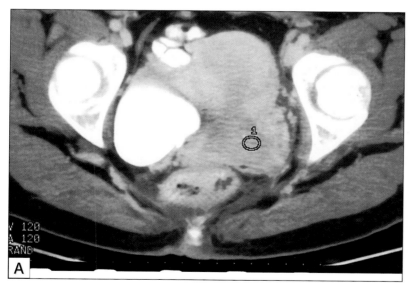

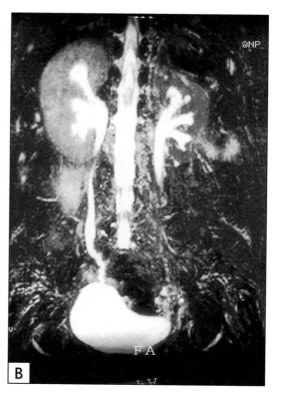

**FIGURE 4-40.** Ureteral stenosis. **A**, This rare complication was responsible for renal failure and anuria. A pelvic granulomatous tumor was responsible for the painless atrophy of the left kidney and was the first manifestation of the disease. **B**, After diagnosis, made during surgery, anuria occurred and was reported to be the consequence of ureteral stenosis in its pelvic trajectory. Anuria disappeared and creatininemia returned to normal after three pulses of methylprednisolone.

## CRITERIA FOR DIAGNOSIS OF BEHÇET'S DISEASE

| Criterion | Definition |
|---|---|
| 1. Recurrent oral ulceration | Minor aphthous, major aphthous, or herpetiform ulceration observed by physician or patient, which recurred at lest three times I one 12-mo period |
| *Plus two of:* | |
| 2. Recurrent genital ulceration | Aphthous ulceration scarring, observed by physician or patient |
| 3. Eye lesions | Anterior uveitis, posterior uveitis, or cells in the vitreous humor on slit-lamp examination or retinal vasculitis observed by an ophthalmologist |
| 4. Skin lesions | Erythema nodosum observed physician or patient, pseudofolliculitis or papulopustular lesions; or acneiform nodules observed by a physician in post adolescent patients not on corticosteroid treatment |
| 5. Positive pathergy test | Read by physician at 24–48 h |

**FIGURE 4-41.** Diagnostic criteria for Behçet's disease [9]. Behçet's disease is a systemic vasculitis affecting either veins or arteries. The main clinical manifestations are oral and genital ulcers, which can be associated with other systemic symptoms (*ie*, skin, arthritic, neurologic, pulmonary). The association of various suggestive clinical symptoms in patients living mainly around the Mediterranean sea and Japan favors the diagnosis. Nevertheless, in the absence of a biologic marker of the disease, these diagnostic criteria have been established. The findings are, however, applicable only in the absence of another clinical explanation.

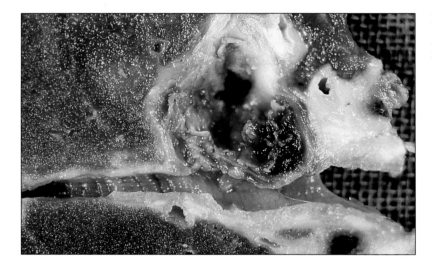

**FIGURE 4-42.** Pulmonary aneurysm. Aneurysms are one of the most severe pulmonary manifestations of Behçet's disease. They involve pulmonary arteries, often proximal to a thrombosis. On this macroscopic view of an autopsy specimen, the aneurysm ruptured in a bronchus. The aneurysm was also partially thrombosed.

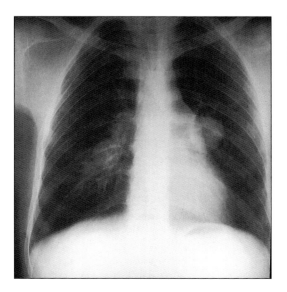

**FIGURE 4-43.** Pulmonary artery aneurysm. The aneurysm(s) can be several centimeters in diameter and several can be seen on this chest radiograph. This is a severe manifestation and rupture may occur. Hemoptysis and thrombosis are often the main clinical manifestations of lung involvement in Behçet's disease.

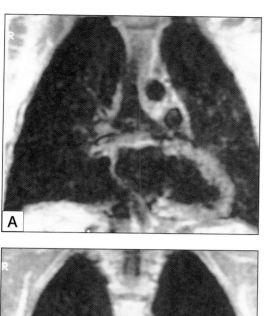
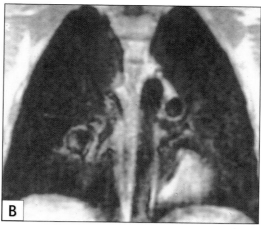

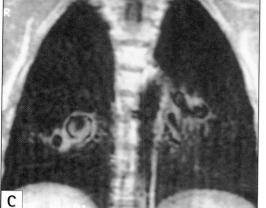
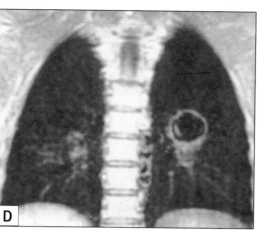

**FIGURE 4-44.** Magnetic resonance imaging. **A** through **D** show the structure, size, and anatomic relationships between the pulmonary aneurysm and the other vascular and bronchial structures.

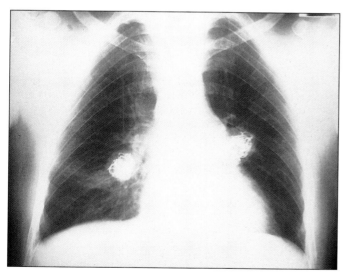

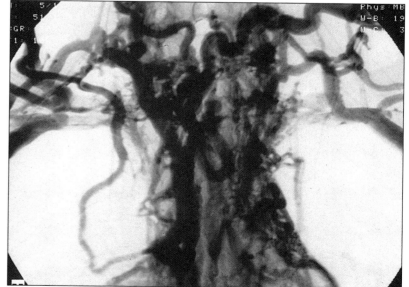

**FIGURE 4-45.** Coil embolization. To prevent rupture, aneurysms should be subjected to coil embolization. This local treatment should be combined with steroids, cytotoxic agents, and sometimes anticoagulants, which effectively treat the disease, control its evolution, and prevent further flares. Aneurysms containing radiopaques coils are visible on this chest radiograph.

**FIGURE 4-46.** Vena cava thrombosis complicating Behçet's disease. The association of thrombosis and pulmonary aneurysms is called Hughes-Stovin syndrome.

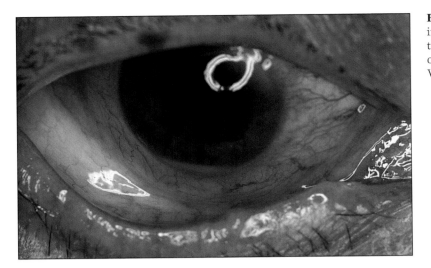

**FIGURE 4-47.** Anterior uveitis with hypopyon. Commonly observed in Behçet's disease, hypopyon is the consequence of leukocyte infiltration into the anterior chamber of the eye. Ophthalmologic examination can also show retinal involvement with arteriolar or venular vasculitis. Venular thrombosis can also be observed.

# Takayasu Arteritis

## CRITERIA FOR CLASSIFICATION OF TAKAYASU ARTERITIS

| Criterion | Definition |
|-----------|------------|
| 1. Age at disease onset 40 y | Development of symptoms or findings related to Takayasu arteritis at age of 40 y |
| 2. Claudication of extremities | Development and worsening of fatigue and discomfort in muscles of one or more extremity while in use, especially the upper extremities |
| 3. Decreased brachial artery pulse | Decreased pulsation of one or both brachial arteries |
| 4. Blood pressure difference >10 mm Hg | Difference of >10 mm Hg in systolic blood pressure between arms |
| 5. Bruit over subclavian arteries or aorta | Bruit audible on auscultation over one or both subclavian arteries or abdominal aorta |
| 6. Arteriogram abnormality | Arteriographic narrowing or occlusion of the entire aorta, its primary branches, or large arteries in the proximal upper or lower extremities, not due to atherosclerosis, fibromuscular dysplasia, or similar causes; changes usually focal or segmental |

**FIGURE 4-48.** American College of Rheumatology 1990 classification criteria for Takayasu arteritis [8]. Takayasu arteritis is a primary inflammatory vasculitis that affects large vessels, mainly the aorta and its major branches [8,35]. This rare disease, also called "pulseless disease," is usually observed in young women. It is difficult to diagnose because many nonspecific symptoms are present, including fever, myalgias, arthralgias, weight loss, and anemia. Vasculitis comprises granulomatous changes in the media and adventitia. The disease progresses slowly to intimal hyperplasia, medial degeneration, and fibrosis. For the purpose of classification, a patient shall be said to have Takayasu arteritis when at least three of the six criteria are present. The presence of any three or more criteria yields a sensitivity of 90.% and a specificity of 97.8%.

**FIGURE 4-49.** Classification of angiograms in Takayasu arteritis [35]. C—involved coronary artery; P—involved pulmonary artery.

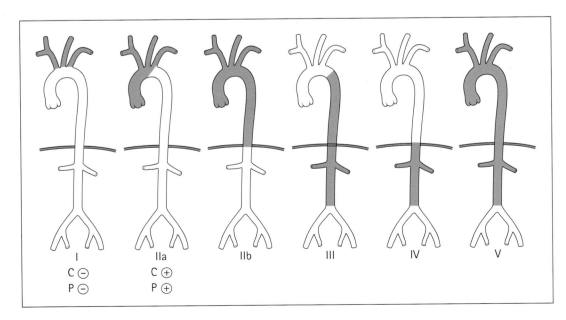

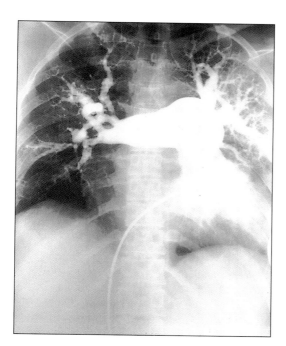

**FIGURE 4-50.** Takayasu arteritis of the pulmonary arteries. Hemoptyses were the revealing symptom in this patient. This distal location of vasculitis cannot be effectively treated with steroids. Lung transplantation could be the most reasonable therapy in this uncommon complication. This patient died of lung hemorrhage shortly after diagnosis.

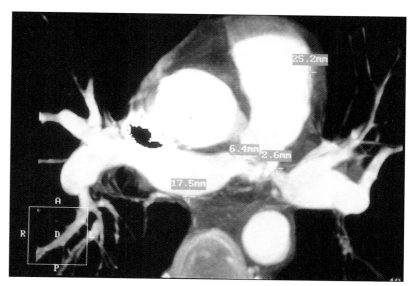

**FIGURE 4-51.** Spiral scan. In this patient with multiple vessel sites of Takayasu arteritis, the spiral scan shows distal stenoses of the branches of pulmonary arteries.

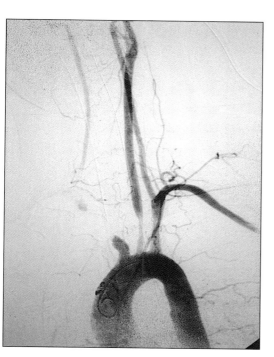

**FIGURE 4-52.** Angiography. This angiogram of the aortic arch shows the long stenosis of the left carotid artery and the obstruction of the brachiocephalic arterial trunk. The right vertebral artery is seen after a few centimeters of total obstruction of the subclavian artery. The right carotid artery appears to have been obstructed and is not seen on this angiogram.

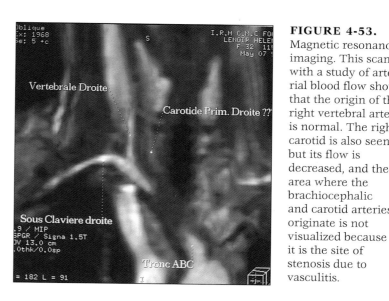

**FIGURE 4-53.** Magnetic resonance imaging. This scan with a study of arterial blood flow shows that the origin of the right vertebral artery is normal. The right carotid is also seen but its flow is decreased, and the area where the brachiocephalic and carotid arteries originate is not visualized because it is the site of stenosis due to vasculitis.

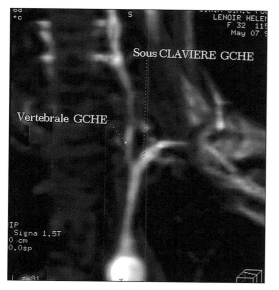

**FIGURE 4-54.** Magnetic resonance imaging. This scan shows that the left vertebral artery is normal and the beginning of left subclavian artery is probably stenosed.

## CRITERIA FOR CLASSIFICATION OF GRANT CELL (TEMPORAL) ARTERITIS

| Criterion | Definition |
|---|---|
| 1. Age at disease onset 50 y | Development of symptoms or findings beginning at age of 50 or older |
| 2. New headache | New onset of or new type of localized pain in the head |
| 3. Temporal artery abnormality | Temporal artery tenderness to palpation or decreased pulsation, unrelated arteriosclerosis of cervical arteries |
| 4. Elevated ESR | ESR 50 mm/h by the Westergren method |
| 5. Abnormal artery biopsy | Biopsy specimen with artery showing vasculitis characterized by a predominace of mononuclear cell infiltration or granulomatous inflammation, usually with multinucleated giant cells |

**FIGURE 4-55.** American College of Rheumatology 1990 classification criteria for giant cell (temporal) arteritis [6]. Giant cell arteritis is considered to be the most common vasculitis. It is recognized most frequently in people over age 50 years. Its incidence rate is 15 to 30 cases per year per 100,000 persons over the age of 50 [36,37]. Clinical findings are attributable to the involved arteries, mainly cephalic. Symptoms of polymyalgia rheumatica occur initially in 30% of cases [38]. For the purpose of classification, a patient shall be said to have giant cell arteritis when at least three of these five criteria are present. The presence of any three or more criteria yields a sensitivity of 93.5% and a specificity of 91.2%. ESR—erythrocyte sedimentation rate.

## PERCENTAGE OF SYMPTOMS IN GIANT CELL ARTERITIS

| | Godeau (1982) [40] | Smith (1983) [39] | Machado (1988) [36] | Varin (1994) [41] |
|---|---|---|---|---|
| Number of Patients | 47 | 24 | 14 | 29 |
| Headache | 91.4 | 83 | 71 | 88.9 |
| Scalp tenderness | 38.2 | 62 | 42 | 75 |
| Myalgia | 51 | 25 | 29 | NS |
| Malaise | NS | 62 | 45 | NS |
| Fatigue | NS | 62 | NS | NS |
| Anorexia | NS | NS | NS | NS |
| Weight loss | 89.3 | 21 | 29 | 71.4 |
| Fever | 80.8 | 29 | 3 | 100 |
| Vision changes | 31.9 | 12 | 6 | 21.4 |
| Loss vision | 27.6 | 21 | 42 | 0 |
| Jaw claudication | 46.8 | 25 | NS | 75 |
| Arthralgia | NS | NS | 16 | NS |
| Anemia | 85.1 | NS | NS | NS |
| Other | NS | 29* | NS | NS |
| First symptom to diagnosis | – | NS | NS | NS |
| Dizziness | – | – | – | – |

**FIGURE 4-56.** Main clinical manifestations of giant cell arteritis [36,39–41]. NS—not significant.

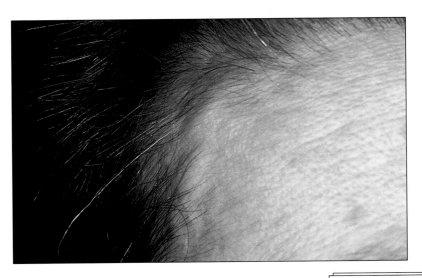

**FIGURE 4-57.** Temporal artery. The right temporal artery is visible and inflamed; palpation of the hard vessel is painful for the patient. The temporal artery is the usual localization, but other superficial cranial arteries and, less frequently, other large- and medium-sized arteries can be involved.

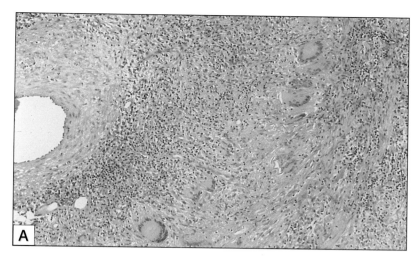

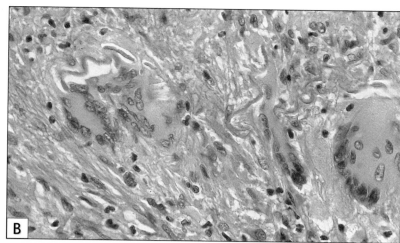

**FIGURE 4-58.** Temporal artery biopsy. **A**, This biopsy shows extensive infiltration of the media with lymphocytes and macrophages (granulomatous inflammation). Several multinucleated giant cells are seen.

**B**, Higher magnification of the same specimen shows fragmentation of the internal elastic lamina next to multinucleated giant cells.

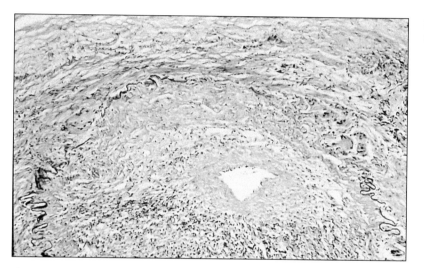

**FIGURE 4-59.** Orcein staining. This temporal artery biopsy shows fragmentation of the internal elastic lamina.

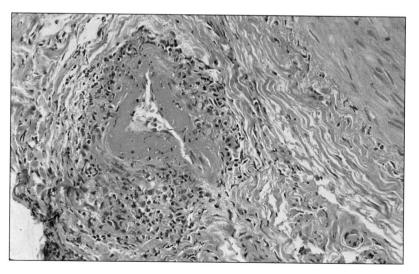

**FIGURE 4-60.** Acute necrotizing angiitis in a branch of the temporal artery. Any necrotizing angiitis can occasionally involve the temporal artery or its branches. It may mimic the clinical symptoms of giant cell arteritis. Histologic examination of temporal artery biopsies shows fibrinoid necrosis but no giant cells. In the present case, the final diagnosis was polyartertis nodosa initially revealed by the unusual temporal localization.

# Henoch–Schönlein Purpura

## CRITERIA FOR CLASSIFICATION OF HENOCH-SCHÖLEIN PURPURA

| Criterion | Definition |
|---|---|
| 1. Palpable purpura | Slightly raised "palpable" hemorrhagic skin lesions not related to thrombocytopenia |
| 2. Age 20 at disease onset | Patient 20 y or younger at onset of first symptoms |
| 3. Bowel angina | Diffuse abdominal pain, worse after meals, or the diagnosis of bowel ischemia, usually including bloody diarrhea |
| 4. Wall granulocytes on biopsy | Histologic changes showing granulocytes in the walls of aterioles or venules |

**FIGURE 4-61.** American College of Rheumatology 1990 classification criteria for Henoch-Schönlein purpura [7]. More frequent in children than adults, this disease occurs predominantly in children between the ages of 2 and 10. Clinical symptoms are cutaneous palpable purpura, arthritis, acute abdominal symptoms, and glomerulonephritis. Abdominal pain often accompanies the rash. Melena and symptoms of peritonitis can be present. In most cases it is a benign disease; surgery is rarely necessary. Although rare, complications like intussusception may occur and require surgery. Proteinuria and hematuria are the first symptoms of glomerulonephritis. Its outcome is good in most cases but can progress despite the resolution of other symptoms. In adults, Henoch-Schönlein purpura is rare but can be more severe because of acute digestive complications and glomerulonephritis. For the purpose of classification, a patient shall be said to have Henoch-Schönlein purpura when at least two of these four criteria are present. The presence of any two or more criteria yields a sensitivity of 87.1% and a specificity of 87.7%.

## TYPES OF GLOMERULONEPHRITIS OCCURRING IN HENOCH-SCHÖLEIN PURPURA

| Nephritis | Description |
|---|---|
| Mesangiopathic glomerulonephritis | Nearly normal glomeruli, enlargement of mesangial stalks |
| Focal and segmental glomerulonephritis | Crescents or synechiae on Bowman's capsule superimposed on a mesangiopathic glomerulonephritis |
| Diffuse proliferative endocapillary glomerulonephritis | Cellular proliferation composed of mesangial cells, increase in mesangial matrix with more or less "double contours." |
| Endo- and extracapillary glomerulonephritis | Variable proportions of crescents superimposed on diffuse proliferative glomerulonephritis |

**FIGURE 4-62.** Main renal manifestations of Henoch-Schönlein purpura [42]. Renal manifestations are present in 25% of cases.

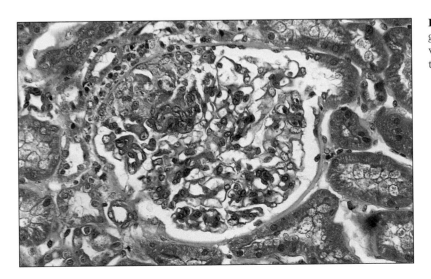

**FIGURE 4-63.** Renal biopsy. Glomerular involvement is a mesangiopathy characterized by the presence of mesangial deposits with various degrees of hypercellularity and of superimposed crescent formation. This slide shows crescent associated with mesangial proliferation.

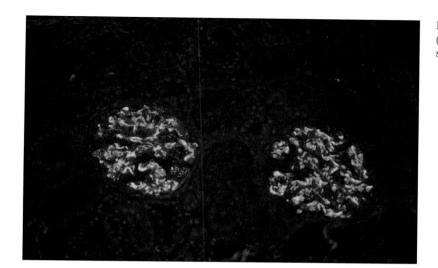

**FIGURE 4-64.** Renal biopsy immunofluorescence. IgA deposits (mainly IgA1) are characteristic of Henoch-Schönlein purpura. In this specimen deposits were in the mesangium.

# Cryoglobulinemia

## MAIN CHARACTERISTICS OF CRYOGLOBULINEMIA

| Type | Immunoglobin characteristics | Associated Disease | Immunoglobulin Type | Etiology |
|------|------------------------------|---------------------|---------------------|----------|
| I | Monoclonal only | Mulitple myeloma | Mainly IgG | Unknown |
| | | Walderström's macroglobulinemia | IgM | HCV? (47) |
| II | Monoclonal Ig and polyclonal Ig | Essential cryoglobulinemia | IgG and IgM | HCV (>80%^) |
| III | Polyclonal Ig | Essential cryoglobulinemia | Polyclonal, all types | Other virus unknown |

**FIGURE 4-65.** Classification and etiologies of cryoglobulinemia. Cryoglobulinemia is characterized by the presence of abnormal proteins that precipitate when plasma is cooled at temperatures below 37°C. Cryoglobulinemias are classified into three groups [43]. The main clinical manifestations consist of a systemic vasculitis, arthralgia, myalgias, vascular purpura, Raynaud's phenomenon, glomerulonephritis, peripheral neuropathy, and cardiac involvement [44–46]. The disease is thought to develop secondary to vascular deposition of immune complexes and may be triggered by viral antigens. Hematologic malignancies are always present in type I cryoglobulinemia. Type III, formerly called essential cryoglobulinemia, is, in most cases, caused by hepatitis C virus (HCV) infection. Type II is an intermediate situation in which benign or malignant neoplasic disease can be found. In type II HCV-related cryoglobulinemia, IgM κ are found in most patients [43].

**FIGURE 4-66.** Main clinical manifestations of cryoglobulinemia [44–46].

## MAIN CLINICAL CHARACTERISTICS OF CRYOGLOBULINEMIA

| | Gorevic 1980 [44] | Ferri 1993 [45] | Cohen 1996 [46] |
|------|------|------|------|
| Patients, n | 40 | 26 | 20 |
| Age mean (y) | 50.7 | 54 | 61.6 |
| range | 21–72 | | 46–80 |
| Female/male ratio | 2 | 1.36 | 2.3 |
| Purpura | 100 | 88 | 70 |
| Raynaud phenomenon | 25 | 15 | 30 |
| Peripheral neuropathy | 12.5 | 77 | 30 |
| Glomerulonephritis | 55 | 4 | 25 |
| Arthralgia | 72.5 | 92 | 35 |
| Myalgia | – | – | 15 |
| Sjögren's | 15 | 31 | 25 |
| Skin ulcers | 30 | – | 35 |
| Fatigue | – | 96 | 15 |

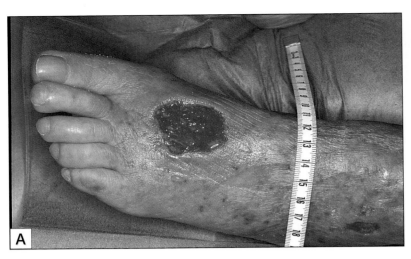

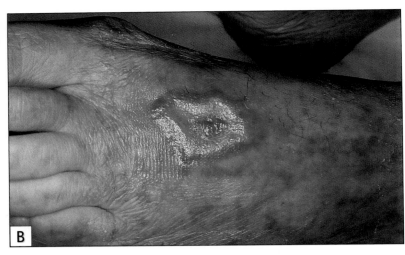

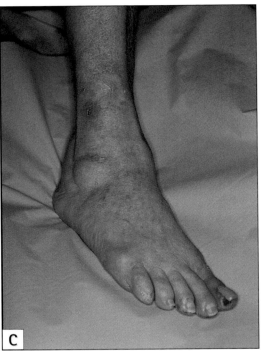

**FIGURE 4-67.** Skin ulcers. Skin ulcers arise as the consequence of small-sized vessel obliteration. They are a severe, painful, and chronic manifestation of cryoglobulinemia. They can appear in a few days but regress slowly under treatment. **A**, In this patient with hepatitis C virus-related cryoglobulinemia, treatment was with a combination of interferon-α, 3 million units, three times a week and plasma exchanges, three sessions a week for 3 weeks then progressively tapered. The treatment is effective for ulcers, but relapses are frequent because, in the majority of patients, no presently available therapy is able to eradicate the virus. **B**, After 1 month of treatment, the ulcer shows partial regression. **C**, The skin ulcer is healed with a pale area of atrophie blanche.

**FIGURE 4-68.** Digital gangrene occurring in type I cryoglobulinemia. This complication is observed more rarely in type II and III cryoglobulinemias.

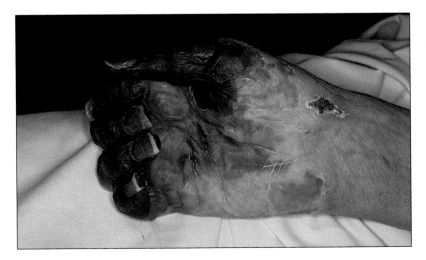

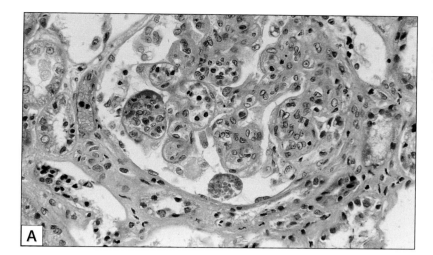

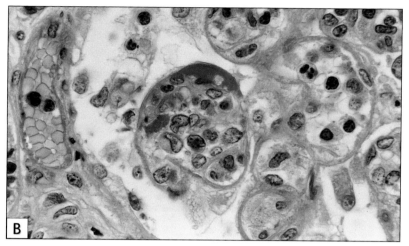

**FIGURE 4-69.** Renal biopsy in patient with cryoglobulinemia. **A**, Masson's trichrome stain shows a glomerulus with endocapillary proliferative changes. **B**, Higher magnification of the same section shows many mononuclear cells with endomembranous fibrinoid deposits in the lumen of a capillary loop.

**FIGURE 4-70.** Renal biopsy in patient with cryoglobulinemia. Jones' staining of a renal biopsy illustrates a "double contour" aspect reflecting interposition of mesangial cells.

*Vasculitides*

## MAIN ETIOLOGIES AND TYPE OF VASCULITIS OCCURRING IN VIRUS-ASSOCIATED VASCULITIDES

| Virus | Type of Vasculitis as a Function of the Size Vessels Involved | | | |
| --- | --- | --- | --- | --- |
| | Large | Medium | Small | Capillaries, venules |
| Hepatitis B | | PAN | Cryoglobulinemia | Cryoglobulinemia |
| Hepatitis C | | PAN | Cryoglobulinemia | Cryoglobulinemia, other systemic vasculitides |
| Human immunodeficiency | Giant cell arteritis (?) | PAN | Cryoglobulinemia | Cryoglobulinemia, leukocytoclastic vasculitis |
| Cytomegalovirus (CMV) | | | Vasculitis* | Vasculitis* |
| Parvovirus | | PAN | Rare vasculitis | |
| Epstein-Barr virus | | | Rare vasculitis | |
| Hantavirus | | | Rare vasculitis | |
| Hepatitis A virus | | | Rare vasculitis | |
| Herpes simplex virus | | | Rare vasculitis | |
| Influenza virus | | | Rare vasculitis | |
| Rubella virus | | | Rare vasculitis | |

*This form of vasculitis has generally come to be known as CMV vasculitis.*

**FIGURE 4-71.** Virus-associated vasculitides. Infectious etiologies have been demonstrated in several systemic vasculitides. Viral infections have been found in polyarteritis nodosa (PAN) [24], cryoglobulinemia [45,47], and in a broad spectrum of vasculitides [48–50]. Their responsibility for the vasculitic process is now accepted and supported by epidemiologic data and the demonstration of viral antigens in immune complexes or endothelial cells. Nevertheless, the implication of viruses in vasculitides seems limited to a selected group of diseases that should be clearly identified because the development of specific therapeutic approaches is based on the differences observed in the etiologies and pathogenetic mechanisms of viral and nonviral vasculitides. This table includes the main vasculitides and the viruses considered to be responsible for them. Viruses have been described in association with every type of vasculitis and vessels of every size; those listed are considered the major associations.

## MAIN CHARACTERISTICS OF HUMAN IMMUNODEFICIENCY VIRUS–RELATED VASCULITIDES

| | |
| --- | --- |
| Vessel size | Small-sized, rarely medium-sized artery |
| Number of flares | Usually one |
| Vasculitis type | Polyarteritis nodosa |
| | Leukocytoclastic vasculitis |
| | Other vasculitides have been rarely described |
| Pathogenesis | CD8 cells |
| | HIV |
| | Opportunistic infections |
| | (CMV, *Pneumocystis carinii*...)* |
| Outcome/treatment | Recovery under antiviral treatment ± plasma exchanges |
| | Steroids and cytotoxic agents not recommended |

*only in patients with <200 CD4+ T lymphyocytes*

**FIGURE 4-72.** Characteristics of vasculitides associated with human immunodeficiency virus (HIV) [48]. Vasculitis can occur early before the first manifestations of acquired immunodeficiency syndrome (stage A or B) or later, at the time the syndrome manifests itself. In this circumstance, vasculitis can be the consequence of opportunistic infections (viruses or parasites). CMV—cytomegalovirus.

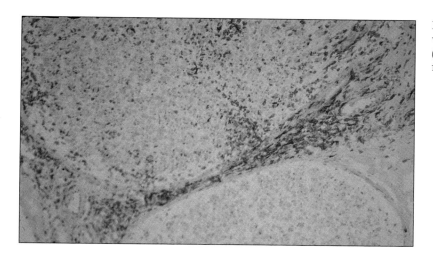

**FIGURE 4-73.** Vasculitis associated with human immunodeficiency virus (HIV). Anti-CD8 antibodies recognize one bundle of nerve fibers (*upper half*) but not another, which explains the asymmetric neurologic manifestations of HIV vasculitis.

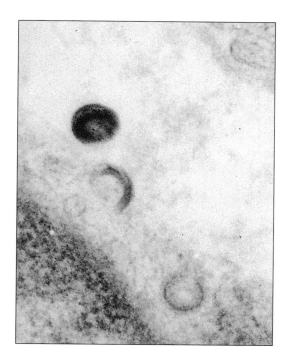

**FIGURE 4-74.** Muscle biopsy. This muscle biopsy from a patient with human immunodeficiency virus vasculitis shows virus replication in endothelial cell (dense oval bodies).

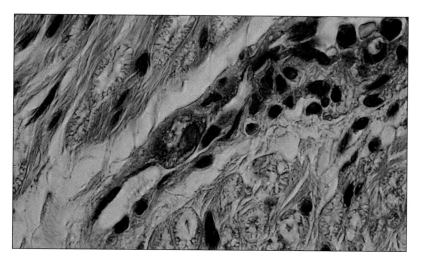

**FIGURE 4-75.** Cytomegalovirus inclusion in the venous wall (dense round bodies) of a patient presenting with vasculitis-complicating acquired immunodeficiency syndrome. In this case, treatment should be specifically antiviral and steroids are contraindicated. In the case of severe clinical manifestations of vasculitis, plasma exchanges can be prescribed as for other virus-related vasculitides [50].

## VASCULITIS–ASSOCIATED HEMATOLOGICAL MALIGNANCIES

**Cutaneous Vasculitis**

1. Leukocytoclastic vasculitis
   - Lymphocytic lymphoma
   - B-lymphocytic leukemia
   - T-cell lymphoma, including angioimmunoblastic lymphadenopathy
   - Cutaneous lymphoma, Sézary's syndrome
   - Hairy cell leukemia
   - Myelodysplastic syndrome
   - Chronic myeloid leukemia, polycythemia vera
   - Acute myeloblastic leukemia
   - Multiple myeloma, Waldenström's macroglobulinemia
2. Granulomatous vasculitis
   - T-cell lymphoma, including angioimmunoblastic lymphadenopathy
   - Myelodysplastic syndrome

3. Cutaneous polyarteritis nodosa
   - Chronic myelomonocytic leukemia

**Systemic Vasculitis**

1. Cryoglobulinemia
   - T-cell lymphoma, including angioimmunoblastic lymphadenopathy
   - Lymphocytic lymphoma
   - Waldenström's macroglobulinemia
   - Chronic lymphocytic leukemia

2. Polyarteritis nodosa
   - Hairy cell leukemia
   - Acute myeloblastic leukemia
   - Myelodysplasia
   - Multiple myeloma
   - Waldenström's macroglobulinemia
   - Hodgkin's disease
   - Lymphocytic lymphoma
3. Wegener's granulomatosis
   - Hodgkin's disease
4. Granulomatous angiitis of the central nervous system
   - Hodgkin's disease
   - Lymphocytic lymphoma
   - Leukemia
5. Giant cell arteritis
   - Lymphocytic lymphoma
   - B-lymphocytic leukemia
   - Hairy cell leukemia
6. Henoch-Schönleins purpura
   - Non-Hodgkin's lymphoma
   - Myeloma
7. Leukocytoclastic vasculitis
   - Myelodysplastic syndrome

**FIGURE 4-76.** Vasculitis and hematologic malignancies. Vasculitis can be present in assocation with malignant diseases or precede them. Such conditions are considered to be paraneoplastic syndromes and recovery from vasculitis requires essentially the specific treatment of malignancy rather than steroids, which are less effective. Malignancy-associated vasculitis is usually observed in conjunction with hematologic diseases, but it has also been described albeit rarely, in association with solid tumors. The spectrum of vasculitides comprises leukocytoclastic vasculitis and, more generally, small-sized vessel vasculitis, but polyarteritis nodosa has also been reported in association with leukemias or lymphomas [51].

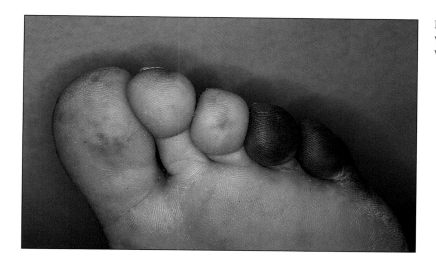

**FIGURE 4-77.** Toe gangrene. Painful gangrene of the toes, due to vasculitis in this patient with angioimmunoblastic lymphadenopathy, was the presenting symptom.

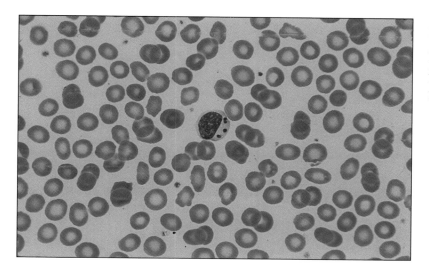

**FIGURE 4-78.** Immunophenotyping. Peripheral blood and bone marrow immunophenotyping should be done when a hematologic disorder is suspected as the underlying cause in a patient with vasculitis. Large granular lymphocytes (LGL) (CD56, CD57) can be observed on the hemogram. Relapses of vasculitis do not always correlate with LGL percentages on blood smears.

## Vasculitis Associated with Rheumatoid Arthritis

### CLINICAL AND HISTOLOGIC FEATURES OF RHEUMATOID ARTHRITIS–ASSOCIATED VASCULITIS

| System | Clinical/histologic features |
|---|---|
| Systemic | Malaise, weight loss, fever, hepatomegaly, splenomegaly |
| Cutaneous | Nail-fold vasculitis, nail-edge vasculitis, digital infarcts, ulcers, rash, nodules, gangrene |
| Neuropathy | Mononeuritis multiplex, polyneuropathy (sensorimotor) cerebrovascular accident |
| Cardiac | Pericarditis, arrhythmia, valve lesions, myocardial infarct |
| Pulmonary | Fibrosing alveolitis, pleuritis, nodules |
| Renal | Necrotizing glomerulitis, hematuria ± proteinuria |
| Ophthalmic | (Epi)scleritis |
| Gastrointestinal | Bowel ulcers or infarcts, colitis (ischemic) |
| Other viscera | Liver, spleen, pancreatic infarcts |

**FIGURE 4-79.** Clinical and histologic features of rheumatoid arthritis-associated vasculitis [52]. The term systemic rheumatoid vasculitis refers to patients with rheumatoid arthritis who have clinical or histologic evidence of vasculitis involving arteries. Rheumatoid arthritis vasculitis, like other connective tissue diseases, usually affects small-sized vessels. Its consequences are the clinical manifestations described here. Nevertheless, medium-sized vessels can also been involved and the clinical presentation of classic polyarteritis nodosa can be observed. Systemic rheumatoid vasculitis is a serious condition that is often relapsing and has a poor outcome and significant and cumulative mortality [53].

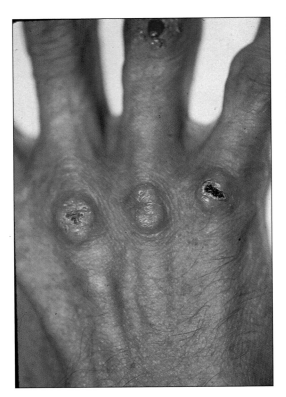

**FIGURE 4-80.** Subcutaneous nodule and necrosis in a patient presenting with vasculitis (polyarteritis nodosa type) and rheumatoid arthritis.

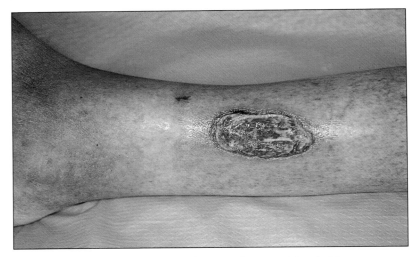

**FIGURE 4-81.** Leg ulcer complicating rheumatoid arthritis.

## Treatment of Vasculitis

| PREDICTIVE MORTALITY VALUE OF THE FIVE FACTOR SCORE AFTER FIVE YEARS | | | | |
|---|---|---|---|---|
| FFS | Death (%) | Survival (%) | Relative Risk (RR) | Patients, n |
| 0 | 12 | 88 | 0.63 | 217 |
| 1 | 26.25 | 73.75 | 1.38 | 80 |
| ≥2 | 45.95 | 54.05 | 2.4 | 37 |
| Total | 64 | 273 | | 337 |

**FIGURE 4-82.** Prognostic factors and treatment of the vasculitides. Vasculitis treatments should be chosen according to classification, etiology, pathogenetic mechanisms, severity, and predictible outcome. In virus-associated vasculitides, treatment is based on the combination of antiviral agents and symptomatic or immunomodulating therapies [24]. Hepatitis B virus-related polyarteritis nodosa and hepatitis C virus-related cryoglobulinemia [45] respond to interferon-α and plasma exchanges. Responses are excellent in hepatitis B virus-polyarteritis nodosa [24] but usually partial in hepatitis C virus-cryoglobulinemia and relapses occur in the majority of cases. Microscopic polyangiitis, classic polyarteritis nodosa, Wegener's granulomatosis, and other vasculitides respond to steroids and cytotoxic agents, mainly cyclophosphamide [54]. Optimal treatment duration and ways of administration can vary from one disease to another. Plasma exchanges are not recommended as the first-line treatment. Intravenous immunoglobulins and other immunomodulating treatments are indicated in some limited cases, and better definitions of their indications requires further prospective studies.

This table shows the prognostic factors of polyarteritis nodosa, microscopic polyangiitis, and Churg-Strauss syndrome. A prognostic five factor score (FFS) [55] was established and comprises the following items: levels of creatininemia (< and >1.58 mg/dL) and of proteinuria (< and >1 g/d), presence of severe gatrointestinal tract involvement, cardiomyopathy, and central nervous system involvement. The presence of each factor was accorded one point. Three classes of scores were defined to predict mortality after five years: 0, when no factor was noted; 1, when one factor was present; and 2, when two or more factors were present. The FFS can be correlated with outcome. $P < 0.0001$ for scores 0 versus 1 or 1 versus 2 [55].

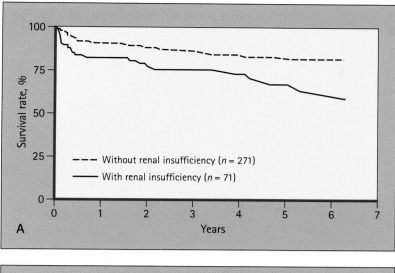

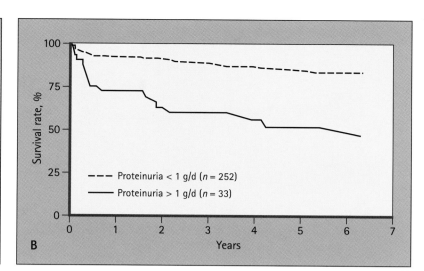

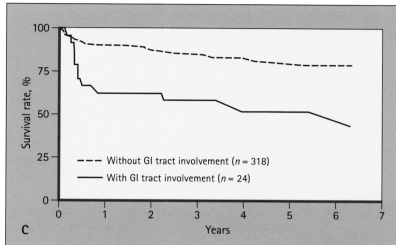

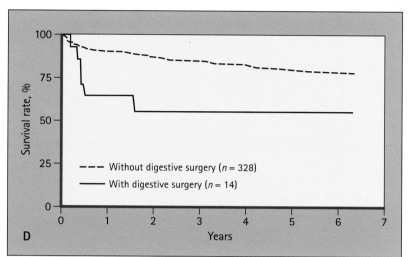

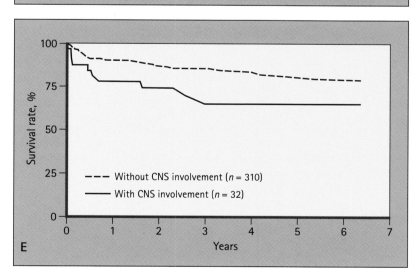

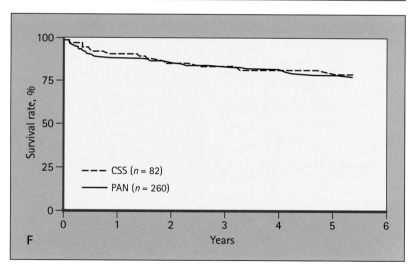

**FIGURE 4-83.** Outcome in 342 patients with polyarteritis nodosa, microscopic polyangiitis or Churg-Strauss syndrome based on manifestations included in the five factor score [55]. **A**, With and without renal insufficiency. **B**, Based on proteinura. **C**, With and without gastroin-testinal (GI) tract involvement. **D**, With and without digestive surgery. **E**, With and without central nervous system (CNS) involvement. **F**, Survival rates for Churg-Strauss syndrome (CSS) and polyarteritis nodosa (PAN).

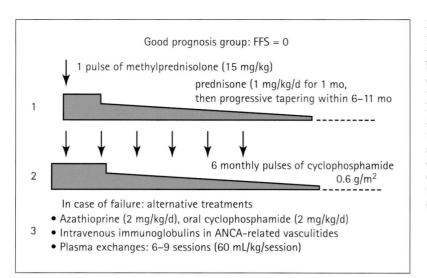

**FIGURE 4-84.** Treatment of good-prognosis (five factor score [FFS] = 0) polyarteritis nodosa without hepatitis B virus (HBV) infection, microscopic polyangiitis, and Churg-Strauss syndrome. 1) Considering the low probability of death and relapse, cytotoxic agents can be avoided and recovery obtained under steroid treatment alone. Duration of prednisone treatment varies from one disease and patient to another. In Churg-Strauss syndrome, low-dose prednisone (< 10 mg/d) often needs to be maintained to control asthma or to prevent a respiratory crisis. 2) Pulse cyclophosphamide is useful when prednisone alone fails (indication of cyclophosphamide as second-line treatment has not been demonstrated prospectively). 3) In case of above treatment failure, under certain conditions (*eg*, contraindications of other treatments) or when salvage therapy is necessary, the alternative treatments should be tried alone or in combination. ANCA—antineutrophil cytoplasmic antibodies.

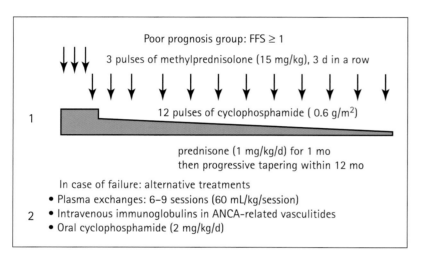

**FIGURE 4-85.** Treatment of poor-prognosis (five factor score [FFS] 1) polyarteritis nodosa without hepatitis B virus (HBV) infection, microscopic polyangiitis, and Churg-Strauss syndrome. 1) The combination of steroids and pulse cyclophosphamide should be prescribed in severe forms of vasculitis. This combination has been as effective and less toxic than oral cyclophosphamide [56]. 2) In the case of failure, oral cyclophosphamide can be replaced by pulses [57]. Plasma exchanges and high-dose intravenous immunoglobulins can be used in combination or replace to steroids and pulse cyclophosphamide.

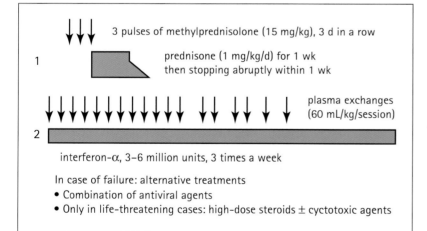

**FIGURE 4-86.** Treatment of polyarteritis nodosa with hepatitis B virus (HBV) infection [24]. 1) The first-line therapeutic regimen comprises short-term steroid treatment, which is necessary to control disease severity. It stimulates viral replication and favors the efficacy of subsequent antiviral treatment. 2) An intensive course of plasma exchanges (12 sessions within 3 weeks) tapers until ending plasma exchanges after 2 months. 3) At the same time, antiviral treatment (interferon-α) is administered and will be stopped when HBe/anti-HBe seroconversion occurs. Other antiviral treatments have been used in the past (vidarabine) or are presently being tested (lamivudine). The total treatment duration is 2 to 4 months.

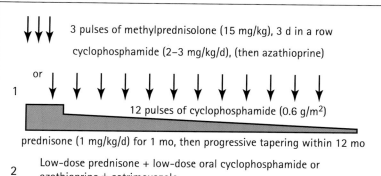

1  ↓↓↓  3 pulses of methylprednisolone (15 mg/kg), 3 d in a row

cyclophosphamide (2–3 mg/kg/d), (then azathioprine)

or ↓

↓ ↓ ↓ ↓ ↓ ↓ ↓ ↓ ↓ ↓ ↓ ↓

12 pulses of cyclophosphamide (0.6 g/m²)

prednisone (1 mg/kg/d) for 1 mo, then progressive tapering within 12 mo

2  Low-dose prednisone + low-dose oral cyclophosphamide or
azathioprine ± cotrimoxazole

In case of failure: alternative treatments

3
• Plasma exchanges: 6–9 sessions (60mL/kg/session)
• Intravenous immunoglobulins (1 g/kg/d) for 2 d, 1/mo
• Methotrexate 15–20 mg/wk, other cytotoxic or immunomodulating
  drugs

**FIGURE 4-87.** Treatment of systemic Wegener's granulomatosis. A consensus has been reached to combine steroids and cyclophosphamide [33]. The conventional treatment uses oral cyclophosphamide. Alternative treatments with triweekly pulses of cyclophosphamide are also effective to induce remission but do not always maintain it. The duration of treatment is debated: 1 to 3 years of cyclophosphamide or 6 to 12 months cyclophosphamide then azathioprine. Cotrimoxazole (Trimathoprim/sulfamethoazole combination) has also been effective in reducing relapses. Intravenous immunoglobulins should be infused more slowly (*eg*, over 5 days), or not be administered to patients with severe renal failure.

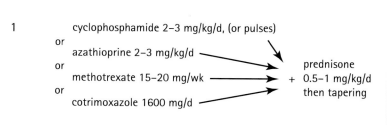

1  cyclophosphamide 2–3 mg/kg/d, (or pulses)

or

azathioprine 2–3 mg/kg/d

or

methotrexate 15–20 mg/wk       prednisone
                                + 0.5–1 mg/kg/d
or                                then tapering

cotrimoxazole 1600 mg/d

2  Local treatments if necessary: surgery for sinusitis, bronchial stenosis,
local medical treatments (steroids)

In case of failure: *see* Systemic Wegener's

3
• Intravenous immunoglobulins (1 g/kg/d for 2 d, 1/mo)
• Intensification or change and cytotoxic drug

**FIGURE 4-88.** Treatment of limited Wegener's granulomatosis. A consensus has not been reacted regarding the treatment of limited Wegener's granulomatosis (upper airway or upper airway and lungs). Usually, the same treatment as that for systemic Wegener's granulomatosis is given. Nevertheless, in limited forms without kidney involvement, less intensive treatments can be prescribed. Some therapeutic options are described here.

Type I   Treatment of multiple myeloma or
         Waldenstrom's macroglobulinemia

    +    Symptomatic treatment of ischemia:
         vasodilators, prostacyclins, local treatments

    +    Plasma exchanges: if hyperviscosity or chronic ulcers

Types II and III  ───────→  If malignant disease: see type I treatment

         ↓ ↘  If "essential cryoglobulinemia": steroids ± cytotoxic agents
                ± chronic plasma exchanges

If HCV-related cryoglobulinemia: interferon-α (3 million units, 3 times/wk)
+ plasma exchanges in the case of nephropathy, leg ulcers, neuropathy...
steroids ± cytotoxic agents only in the case of failure of "etiologic treatment"
± chronic plasma exchanges

**FIGURE 4-89.** Treatment of cryoglobulinemia. Treatment of cryoglobulinemia should be specifically adapted to its etiology: cytotoxic agents in the case of malignant disease or antiviral agents in case of hepatitis C virus (HCV)-related cryoglobulinemia [45,46]. Plasma exchanges are an effective safe, temporary treatment. Unfortunately, because relapses occur in the majority of patients, chronic treatments are often necessary.

Ophthalmologic symptoms

> 1 pulse of methylprednisolone then prednisone (1 mg/kg/d)
> +
> Heparin then low-dose aspirin

Without ophthalmologic symptoms

> Initial treatment: prednisone (0.7 mg/kg/d)

In the case of relapses or resistance to steroids: methotrexate can be tried

**FIGURE 4-90.** Treatment of giant cell arteritis. Different steroid doses are recommended depending on the presence or absence of ophthalmologic symptoms [58]. Steroids can be tapered according to different schedules, one of which is given here. Alternate-day steroid dosing is generally not effective early in the course of the disease [59].

## Ocular Vasculitis

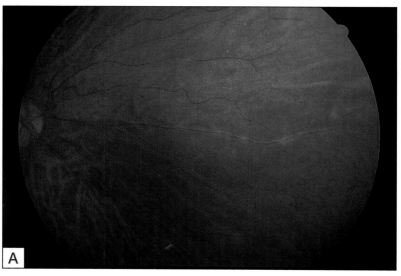

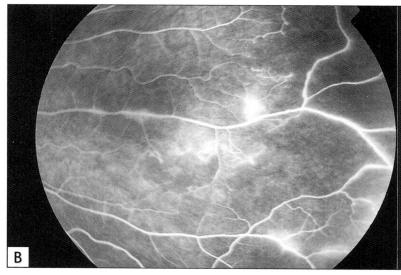

**FIGURE 4-91.** Ocular vasculitis. Ocular vasculitis can be primary or secondary to sysemic vasculitis. Ocular examination should be systematic during the course of a systemic disease. Conversely, when ocular vasculitis has been diagnosed, it is important to search carefully for extraocular manifestations before diagnosing primary ocular vasculitis.

**A**, Retinophotograph and angiogram **(B)** of right eye of the patient with retinal vasculitis. Nasal field show staining of vascular walls and leakage of fluorescein into the retina. Fluorescein angiography also shows an area of nonperfused capillaries.

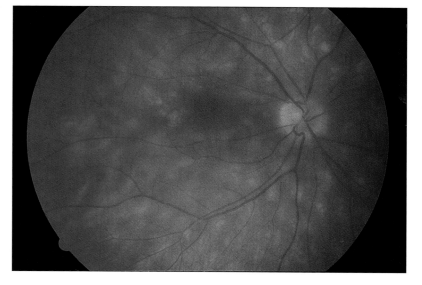

**FIGURE 4-92.** Retinophotograph. Deep white flecks are typical of birdshot chorioretinitis, an ocular vasculitis that is associated with HLA-A29.

# Acknowledgments

We are indebted to the followings colleagues for their help in preparing this section:

Professor Jacques Amouroux (Bobigny), Professor Olivier Blétry (Suresnes), Professor Patrice Callard (Paris), Professor Frédérique Capron (Clamart), Docteur Gilles Chaine (Bobigny), Professor Romain Ghérardi (Créteil), Doctor Geneviéve Le Roux (Bobigny), Doctor Marianne Kambouchner (Bobigny), Doctor Anne-Marie Piette (Suresnes).

# References

1. Lightfoot RJ, Michel BA, Bloch DA, *et al.*: The American College of Rheumatology 1990 criteria for the classification of polyarteritis nodosa. *Arthritis Rheum* 1990, 33:1088–1093.

2. Lie J: Nomenclature and classification of vasculitis: Plus ça change, plus c'est la même chose. *Arthritis Rheum* 1994, 37:181–186.

3. Jennette JC, Falk RJ, Andrassy K, *et al.*: Nomenclature of systemic vasculitides. Proposal of an international consensus conference. *Arthritis Rheum* 1994, 37:187–192.

4. Masi A, Hunder G, Lie J, *et al.*: The American College of Rheumatology 1990 criteria for the classification of Churg-Strauss syndrome (allergic granulomatosis angiitis). *Arthritis Rheum* 1990, 33:1094–1100.

5. Leavitt RY, Fauci AS, Bloch DA, *et al.*: The American College of Rheumatology 1990 criteria for the classification of Wegener's granulomatosis. *Arthritis Rheum* 1990, 33:1101–1107.

6. Hunder G, Bloch D, Michel B, *et al.*: The American College of Rheumatology 1990 criteria for the classification of giant cell arteritis. *Arthritis Rheum* 1990, 33:1122–1128.

7. Mills J, Michel B, Bloch D, *et al.*: The American College of Rheumatology 1990 criteria for the classification of Henoch-Schönlein purpura. *Arthritis Rheum* 1990, 33:1114–1121.

8. Arend W, Michel B, Bloch D, *et al.*: The American College of Rheumatology 1990 criteria for the classification of Takayasu arteritis. *Arthritis Rheum* 1990, 33:1129–1234.

9. International Study Group for Behçet's Disease: criteria for diagnosis of Behcet's disease. *Lancet* 1990, 335:1078–1080.

10. Fauci A, Haynes B, Katz P: The spectrum of vasculitis: clinical, pathologic, immunologic and therapeutic considerations. *Ann Intern Med* 1978, 89:660–676.

11. Guillevin L, Lhote F, Amouroux J, Gherardi R, *et al.*: Antineutrophil cytoplasmic antibodies, abnormal angiograms and pathological findings in polyarteritis nodosa and Churg-Strauss syndrome: indications for the classification of vasculitides of the polyarteritis nodosa group. *Br J Rheumatol* 1996, 35:958–964.

12. Kallenberg CG, Mulder AH, Tervaert JW: Antineutrophil cytoplasmic antibodies: a still-growing class of autoantibodies in inflammatory disorders. *Am J Med* 1992, 93:675–862.

13. Gross WL, Csernok E: Immunodiagnostic and pathophysiologic aspects of anti-neutrophil cytoplasmic antibodies in vasculitis. *Curr Opin Rheumatol* 1995, 7:11–19.

14. Leib E, Restivo C, Paulus H: Immunosuppressive and corticosteroid therapy of polyarteritis nodosa. *Am J Med* 1979, 67:941–947.

15. Guillevin L, Lhote F, Jarrousse B, Fain O: Treatment of polyarteritis nodosa and Churg-Strauss syndrome. A meta-analysis of 3 prospective controlled trials including 182 patients over 12 years. *Ann Med Interne (Paris)* 1992, 143:405–416.

16. Guillevin L, Le THD, Godeau P, *et al.*: Clinical findings and prognosis of polyarteritis nodosa and Churg-Strauss angiitis: a study in 165 patients. *Br J Rheumatol* 1988, 27:258–264.

17. Frohnert P, Sheps S: Long term follow-up study of polyarteritis nodosa. *Am J Med* 1967, 48:8–14.

18. Fortin PR, Larson MG, Watters AK, *et al.*: Prognostic factors in systemic necrotizing vasculitis of the polyarteritis nodosa group—a review of 45 cases. *J Rheumatol* 1995, 22:78–84.

19. Cohen R, Conn D, Ilstrup D: Clinical features, prognosis and response to treatment in polyarteritis. *Mayo Clin Proc* 1980, 55:146–155.

20. Scott D, Bacon P, Elliott P, *et al.*: Systemic vasculitis in a district general hospital 1972–1980: clinical and laboratory features, classification and prognosis in 80 cases. *Q J Med* 1982, 51:292–311.

21. Watts RA, Carruthers DM, Scott DG: Epidemiology of systemic vasculitis: changing incidence or definition? *Semin Arthritis Rheum* 1995, 25:28–34.

22. McMahon BJ, Heyward WL, Templin DW, *et al.*: Hepatitis B-associated polyarteritis nodosa in Alaskan Eskimos: clinical and epidemiologic features and long-term follow-up. *Hepatology* 1989, 9:97–101.

23. Darras Joly C, Lortholary O, Cohen P, *et al.*: Regressing microaneurysms in 5 cases of hepatitis B virus related polyarteritis nodosa. *J Rheumatol* 1995, 22:876–880.

24. Guillevin L, Lhote F, Cohen P, *et al.*: Polyarteritis nodosa related to hepatitis B virus. A prospective study with long-term observation of 41 patients. *Medicine Baltimore* 1995, 74:238–253.

25. Quint L, Deny P, Guillevin L, *et al.*: Hepatitis C virus in patients with polyarteritis nodosa. Prevalence in 38 patients. *Clin Exp Rheumatol* 1991, 9:253–257.

26. Lhote F, Guillevin L: Polyarteritis nodosa, microscopic polyangiitis, and Churg-Strauss syndrome. Clinical aspects and treatment. *Rheum Dis Clin North Am* 1995, 21:911–947.

27. Churg J, Strauss L: Allergic granulomatosis, allergic angiitis and periarteritis nodosa. *Am J Pathol* 1951, 27:277–294.

28. Guillevin L, Visser H, Noel LH, *et al.*: Antineutrophil cytoplasm antibodies in systemic polyarteritis nodosa with and without hepatitis B virus infection and Churg-Strauss syndrome—62 patients. *J Rheumatol* 1993, 20:1345–1349.

29. van der Woude F, Rasmussen N, Lobatto S, *et al.*: Autoantibodies against neutrophils and monocytes: tool for diagnosis and marker of disease activity in Wegener's granulomatosis. *Lancet* 1985, 1:425–429.

30. Cohen Tervaert J, Huitema MG, Hene RJ, *et al.*: Prevention of relapses in Wegener's granulomatosis by treatment based on antineutrophil cytoplasmic antibody titre. *Lancet* 1990, 336:709–711.

31. Anderson G, Coles ET, Crane M, *et al.*: Wegener's granuloma. A series of 265 British cases seen between 1975 and 1985. A report by a sub-committee of the British Thoracic Society Research Committee. *Q J Med* 1992, 83:427–438.

32. Cordier JF, Valeyre D, Guillevin L, *et al.*: Pulmonary Wegener's granulomatosis. A clinical and imaging study of 77 cases. *Chest* 1990, 97:906–912.

33. Hoffman GS, Kerr GS, Leavitt RY, *et al.*: Wegener granulomatosis: an analysis of 158 patients. *Ann Intern Med* 1992, 116: 488–498.

34. Walton E: Giant-cell granuloma of respiratory tract (Wegener's granulomatosis). *Br Med J* 1958, 2:265–270.

35. Hata A, Noda M, Moriwaki R, Numano F: Angiographic findings of Takayasu's arteritis: new classification. *Int J Cardiol* 1996, 54:S155–S163.

36. Machado EB, Michet CT, Ballard DJ, *et al.*: Trends in incidence and clinical presentation of temporal arteritis in Olmstead County, Minnesota, 1950–85. *Arthritis Rheum* 1988, 31:745–749.

37. Boesen P, Sörensen S: Giant cell arteritis, temporal arteritis and polymyalgia rheumatica in a Danish County: a prospective investigation, 1982–1985. *Arthritis Rheum* 1987, 30:294–299.

38. Wilke W: Large vessel vasculitis (giant cell arteritis, Takayasu arteritis). *Baillere's Clin Rheum* 1997, 11:285–313.

39. Smith CA, Fidler WI, Pinals RS: The epidemiology of giant cell arteritis. Report of a 10-year study in Shelby County, Tennessee. *Arthritis Rheum* 1983, 26:1214

40. Godeau P, Aubert I, Guillevin L, *et al.*: Aspect clinique, évolution et pronostic de la maladie de Horton. *Ann Mèd Interne (Paris)* 1982, 133:393–400.

41. Varin J, Guillot de Suduiraut C, Muffat-Joly M, *et al.*: Aspects cliniques et épidémiologiques de la maladie de Horton selon le milieu de recrutement, ophtalmologique ou de Médecine Interne. *Ann Méd Interne (Paris)* 1994, 145:398–404.

42. Niaudet P, Habib R: Schönlein-Henoch purpura nephritis: prognostic factors and therapy. *Ann Méd Interne (Paris)* 1994, 145:577–580.

43. Brouet J, Clauvel J, Danon F, *et al.*: Biologic and clinical significance of cryoglobulins: a report of 86 cases. *Am J Med* 1974, 57:775–788.

44. Gorevic P, Kassab H, Levo Y, *et al.*: Mixed cryoglobulinemia: clinical aspects and long-term follow-up of 40 patients. *Am J Med* 1980, 69:287–308.

45. Ferri C, Marzo E, Longombardo G, *et al.*: Interferon-alpha in mixed cryoglobulinemia patients—A randomized, crossover-controlled trial. *Blood* 1993, 81:1132–1136.

46. Cohen P, Tri Nguyen Q, Ferrière F, *et al.*: Treatment of mixed cryoglobulinemia with recombinant interferon alpha and adjuvant therapies. *Ann Med Intern* 1996, 147:81–86.

47. Agnello V, Chung RT, Kaplan LM: A role for hepatitis C virus infection in type II cryoglobulinemia. *N Engl J Med* 1992, 327:1490–1495.

48. Ghérardi R, Belec L, Mhiri C, *et al.*: The spectrum of vasculitis in human immunodeficiency virus-infected patients. A clinicopathologic evaluation. *Arthritis Rheum* 1993, 36:1164–1174.

49. Somer T, Finegold S: Vasculitides associated with infections, immunization and antimicrobial drugs. *Clin Infect Dis* 1995, 20:1010–1036.

50. Gisselbrecht M, Cohen P, Lortholary O, *et al.*: Human immunodeficiency virus-related vasculitis: clinical presentation and therapeutic approach on six cases. *AIDS* 1997, 11:121–123.

51. Wooten MJH: Vasculitis and lymphoproliferative diseases. *Semin Arthritis Rheum* 1996, 26:564–574.

52. Breeveld R: Vasculitis associated with connective tissue disease. *Baillere's Clin Rheumatol* 1997, 11:315–334.

53. Luqmani R, Watts R, Scott D, Bacon P: Treatment of vasculitis in rheumatoid arthritis. *Ann Médecine Interne (Paris)* 1994, 145:566–576.

54. Gross WL: New developments in the treatment of systemic vasculitis. *Curr Opin Rheumatol* 1994, 6:11–19.

55. Guillevin L, Lhote F, Gayraud M, *et al.*: Prognostic factors in polyarteritis nodosa and Churg-Strauss syndrome. A prospective study in 342 patients. *Medicine (Baltimore)* 1996, 75:17–28.

56. Guillevin L, Lhote F, Cohen P, *et al.*: Corticosteroids plus pulse cyclophosphamide and plasma exchanges versus corticosteroids plus pulse cyclophosphamide alone in the treatment of polyarteritis nodosa and Churg-Strauss syndrome patients with factors predicting poor prognosis. A prospective, randomized trial in sixty-two patients. *Arthritis Rheum* 1995, 38:1638–1645.

57. Généreau T, Lortholary O, Leclerq P, *et al.*: Treatment of systemic vasculitis with cyclophosphamide and steroids: daily oral low-dose cyclophosphamide administration after failure of a pulse intravenous high-dose regimen in four patients. *Br J Rheumatol* 1994, 33:959–962.

58. Barrier J: Treatment of giant cell arteritis. *Ann Méd Interne (Paris)* 1994, 145:533–537.

59. Hunder GSS, Allen G, *et al.*: Daily and alternate day corticosteroid regimens in treatment of giant cell arteritis. Comparison in a prospective study. *Ann Intern Med* 1975, 48:662–666.

# 5

# Spondyloarthropathies

## MUHAMMAD ASIM KHAN

Spondyloarthropathies comprise ankylosing spondylitis, reactive arthritis (including Reiter's syndrome), psoriatic and enteropathic arthritis, a form of juvenile chronic arthritis (pauciarticular late onset), and undifferentiated forms of the disease [1–7]. These diseases tend to occur more often among men who are in their late teens and early twenties and may start with features such as enthesitis (inflammatory lesions of the entheses, *ie*, sites of ligamentous or tendinous attachments to bone), dactylitis, or oligoarthritis, and in some cases may progress to sacroiliitis and spondylitis, with or without extra-articular features such as acute anterior uveitis or mucocutaneous lesions.

The HLA-B27 gene is strongly associated with susceptibility to these diseases, but the strength of the association varies markedly not only among the various spondyloarthropathies but also among various racial and ethnic groups [8,9]. Bacterial infections have long been suspected as the environmental triggers for many of these diseases. Substantial evidence strongly favors a direct role for HLA-B27 in enhancing genetic susceptibility, and additional genetic factors may also influence disease expression or severity. The disease association with HLA-B27 is currently being reinvestigated because at least 11 different natural variants of this molecule are now known that show different ethnic distributions, and some of them may also show differences in disease association. (see Figures 5-7 and 5-8); for example, HLA-B*2706 in Southeast Asians and HLA-B*2709 in Sardinian Italians seem to lack association with the spondyloarthropathies.

It may not always be possible to differentiate clearly among the various forms of spondyloarthropathies in early stages because these diseases generally share many clinical features. Moreover, the clinical spectrum is much wider than previously realized, and the clinical features typical of spondyloarthropathies may occur in different combinations so that the previously established criteria for disease classification may be inappropriate for a large subset of such patients. For example, there are now defined HLA-B27-associated clinical syndromes such as seronegative oligoarthritis or polyarthritis (mostly affecting joints of the lower extremities),

dactylitis, and enthesitis (plantar fascitis or calcaneal periostitis, Achilles tendonitis, and tenderness of tibial tubercles), even in children and in persons over age 50 years [5,10,11]. The European Spondyloarthropathy Study Group (see Figure 5-2) and Amor (see Figure 5-3) classification criteria have been developed to encompass this currently recognized wider spectrum of spondyloarthropathies [13–15].

*Ankylosing spondylitis* is a chronic systemic inflammatory disorder of undetermined etiology, usually beginning in early adulthood, primarily affecting the axial skeleton (sacroilitis being its hallmark), but it can also exhibit some extra-articular features. It is three times more common in males, and the clinical and roentgenographic features seem to evolve more slowly in females. The inflammation appears to originate in ligamentous and capsular sites of attachment to bones (enthesitis), juxta-articular ligamentous structures, and the synovium, articular cartilage, and subchondral bones of involved joints. The site of enthesitis is infiltrated by lymphocytes, plasma cells, and polymorphonuclear cells, and there is also edema and infiltration of the adjacent marrow space. A striking feature is a high frequency of axial enthesitis and synovitis that can result in fibrous and later bony ankylosis of the sacroiliac joints and the spine. The characteristic early symptom is insidious onset of chronic low back pain and stiffness, beginning usually in late adolescence or early adulthood (mean age of onset, 24 years). The pain owing to sacroiliitis is dull in character, difficult to localize, and felt somewhere deep in the gluteal region. It may be unilateral or intermittent at first; however, within a few months it generally becomes persistent and bilateral, and the lower lumbar spine area also becomes painful. Sometimes pain in the lumbar area may be the initial presentation. The symptoms typically worsen with prolonged inactivity or on waking up in the morning ("morning stiffness"), and improve with physical activity and a hot shower.

*Reactive arthritis* is defined as an aseptic inflammatory arthritis, usually asymmetric and oligoarticular, after an episode of urethritis or cervicitis or diarrhea, often with some characteristic extra-articular features, such as conjunctivitis, iritis, or mucocutaneous lesions [16,17]. It is triggered by microbial infection at a distant site usually in the gastrointestinal or genitourinary tract. The term *reactive arthritis* is often used when the identity of the triggering organism is known, and it encompasses the more restrictive term *Reiter's syndrome*, which in its complete or classic form consists of oligoarthritis and conjunctivitis following a nongonococcal urethritis or cervicitis or an episode of diarrhea. Genitourinary tract infection with *Chlamydia trachomatis* is the more commonly recognized initiator in most of the patients in the United States; enteric infections with *Shigella, Salmonella, Yersinia,* or *Campylobacter* are the more common triggers in developing parts of the world [7,17]. (see Figure 5-31). The full clinical spectrum of reactive arthritis has been broadened considerably and "incomplete" forms are observed much more commonly than the classic triad. Some patients may not demonstrate any recognized antecedent infection or may have asymptomatic triggering infection, and some forms of the undifferentiated spondyloarthropathies and juvenile arthritis may be triggered by reactive arthritis-associated bacteria. The disease is most commonly seen in young sexually active adults, mostly men, when it is triggered by *C. trachomatis.* However, reactive arthritis is underdiagnosed in women due to the frequently subclinical or asymptomatic chlamydial infection among them and the infrequent performance of pelvic examinations by physicians to look for the presence of cervicitis. Postenteritic reactive arthritis affects children and adults, including the elderly, of both genders. The joints involved are usually those of the lower limbs, with often asymmetric involvement, and the presence of any associated tenosynovitis, enthesitis, or "sausage" digits is highly suggestive of the diagnosis. A history of a preceding or associated diarrhea, urethral discharge, urinary frequency, dysuria, lower abdominal discomfort, tender enlarged prostate, circinate balanitis, conjunctivitis, mucosal lesions, onycholysis, or keratoderma blenorrhagica should suggest the possibility of reactive arthritis. Septic arthritis should be ruled out by joint aspiration, Gram stain, and culture of any accessible joint fluid.

*Enteropathic arthritis* develops in up to 20% of patients with Crohn's disease and ulcerative colitis, mostly peripheral synovitis that correlates with flare-up of bowel disease, especially in case of ulcerative colitis [1–3,18,19]. However, one-fourth have axial disease (sacroiliitis alone or with classic features of "primary" ankylosing spondylitis), which does not fluctuate with bowel disease activity. Initial treatment of arthritis is with nonsteroidal anti-inflammatory drugs, although they may aggravate bowel disease in some patients. Sulfasalazine is effective in treating inflammatory bowel disease and arthritis. Some patients may need methotrexate or other immunosuppressive drugs. Subclinical inflammatory lesions in the gut have been observed on ileocolonoscopic mucosal biopsy in many patients with spondyloarthropathy without any gastrointestinal symptoms, and these patients seem to respond better to treatment with sulfasalazine than those with normal gut histology, suggesting that sulfasalazine may have a beneficial effect on the patients with spondyloarthropathy by healing their gut inflammation [18,20]. Disease in some of the patients can later evolve into clinically obvious Crohn's disease.

*Psoriasis* is one of the most common chronic dermatoses, affecting close to 2% of the Eurocaucasoid population. It results from abnormal keratinocyte proliferation induced by T lymphocytes, but the precise cause is unknown. Psoriatic arthritis is defined as an inflammatory arthritis associated with psoriasis, but occurring in the absence of rheumatoid nodules and serum rheumatoid factor. It affects men and women equally and usually begins between 30 and 50 years of age, although it can begin in childhood [1–3,21]. The arthritis may precede the onset or diagnosis of cutaneous lesions of psoriasis in 10% to 15% of patients. Psoriatic arthritis probably occurs in 10% of the patients with psoriasis, although some studies suggest that the figure may be close to 30%. Various clinical forms of psoriatic arthritis are recognized and include distal interphalangeal joint arthritis, symmetric peripheral arthritis, asymmetric oligoarthritis, dactylitis ("sausage" digits), sacroiliitis with or without spondylitis, and arthritis mutilans. A subset of patients may show peripheral enthesitis without arthritis. The exact prevalence of each of these various forms is difficult to establish because the pattern in some patients may change with time, and some may show overlapping features.

*Juvenile spondyloarthropathy* begins before the age of 16, mostly in boys aged 9 years or older, and the common presentation is that of a seronegative oligoarthritis of the lower extremities, frequently with enthesitis, and there may be no clinically or roentgenographically identifiable involvement of the sacroiliac joints or the spine [10,22,23]. Recent epidemiologic studies suggest that this disease may be much more prevalent than previously realized. These patients may lack inflammatory back symptoms, mucocutaneous lesions, or gastrointestinal problems, and therefore they may be misclassified as having a late-onset form of pauciarticular juvenile chronic arthritis.

## THE CONCEPT OF SPONDYLOARTHROPATHY

### Disease Subgroups

1. Ankylosing Spondylitis
2. Reactive arthritis (Reiter's syndrome)
3. Enteropathic arthritis
4. Psoriatic arthritis
5. Undifferentiated spondyloarthropathy
6. Juvenile spondyloarthropathy

### All These Diseases Share Rheumatologic Features

- Sacroiliac and spinal (axial) involvement
- Enthesitis at long attachments of ligaments and tendons causing: Achilles tendonitis and plantar fasciitis, syndesmophyte formation ("bamboo spine"), sacroiliitis (due to a combination of enthesitis and synovitis), and periosteal reaction ("whiskering") at gluteal tuberosity and other parts of pelvis and other sites
- Peripheral, often asymmetric, inflammatory arthritis and dactylitis ("sausage" digits)

### Share Extra-articular Features

- Propensity to ocular inflammation (acute anterior uveitis conjunctivitis)
- Mucocutaneous lesions, variable for the subgroups
- Rare aortic incompetence or heart block
- Lack of association with rheumatoid factor and rheumatoid nodules

### Share Genetic Predisposition

- Strong association with HLA-B27 gene
- Familial clustering

**FIGURE 5-1.** The concept of spondyloarthropathy. The clinical spectrum of the rheumatologic diseases included under the term *spondyloarthropathies* consists of ankylosing spondylitis, reactive arthritis or Reiter's syndrome, spondyloarthritis associated with psoriasis and chronic inflammatory bowel diseases, and a form of juvenile chronic arthritis (pauciarticular, late-onset type) [1–6]. All forms of the spondyloarthropathies are associated with the histocompatibility antigen HLA-B27, although the strength of this association varies markedly not only among the various disease forms but also among the various ethnic and racial groups worldwide [8,9]. These diseases tend to occur more often among young men who are in their late teens and early twenties and may start with features such as enthesitis (inflammatory lesions of the entheses, ie, sites of ligamentous of tendinous attachments to bone) or dactylitis oligoarthritis, and in some cases may progress to sacroiliitis and spondylitis, with or without extra-articular features such as acute anterior uveitis or mucocutaneous lesions [4,5]. The clinical features typical of the spondyloarthropathies may occur in different combinations so that the existing classification criteria may be inappropriate for a subset of such patients. For example, there are now well-defined HLA-B27-associated clinical syndromes such as seronegative oligoarthritis or polyarthritis (mostly affecting joints of the lower extremities), dactylitis, and enthesitis (plantar fascitis or calcaneal periostitis, Achilles tendonitis, and tenderness of tibial tubercles) [5]. The overall prevalence of this form of undifferentiated spondyloarthropathy may be higher than that of reactive arthritis in some parts of the world [1,10–12].

## EUROPEAN SPONDYLOARTHROPATHY STUDY GROUP (ESSG) CRITERIA FOR SPONDYLOARTHROPATHY

| Inflammatory Spinal Pain | or | Synovitis |
|---|---|---|
| | | Asymmetric *or* Predominantly in lower limbs |

plus

### One or more of the following:

Alternate buttock pain
Sacroiliitis
Enthesopathy
Positive family history
Psoriasis
Inflammatory bowel disease
Urethritis or cervicitis or acute diarrhea occurring within 1 mo before onset of arthritis

**FIGURE 5-2.** Criteria for spondyloarthropathy. Features typical of the spondyloarthropathies may occur in various combinations, and it was recognized a few years ago that the available disease criteria are inadequate for many patients. Therefore, new classification criteria were proposed by the European Spondyloarthropathy Study Group to encompass the currently recognized wider spectrum [13]. These criteria have high degree of sensitivity and specificity, but they cannot help in identifying patients who have either an isolated peripheral arthritis, dactylitis, enthesitis, inflammatory spinal pain, acute anterior uveitis, or aortic insufficiency with heart block as the only clinical manifestation of the disease.

## AMOR CRITERIA FOR SPONDYLOARTHROPATHY

| Parameter | Scoring |
|---|---|
| A. Clinical symptoms or past history of | |
|    1. Lumbar or dorsal pain at night or morning stiffness of lumbar or dorsal pain | 1 |
|    2. Asymmetric oligoarthritis | 2 |
|    3. Buttock pain | 1 |
| | or |
|      if alternate buttock pain | 2 |
|    4. Sausage-like toe or digit | 2 |
|    5. Heel pain or other well-defined enthesiopathic pain | 2 |
|    6. Iritis | 2 |
|    7. Nongonococcal uretritis or cervicitis within 1 mo before the onset of arthritis | 1 |
|    8. Acute diarrhea within 1 mo before the onset of arthritis | 1 |
|    9. Psoriasis, balanitis, or inflammatory bowel disease (IBD) (ulcerative colitis or Crohn's disease) | 2 |
| B. Radiologic findings | |
|    10. Sacroiliitis (bilateral grade 2 or unilateral grade 3) | 2 |
| C. Genetic background | |
|    11. Presence of HLA-B27 or family history of ankylosing spondylitis, reactive arthritis, uveitis, psoriasis, or IBD | 2 |
| D. Response to treatment | |
|    12. Clear-cut improvement within 48 h after NSAID intake or rapid relapse of the pain after their discontinuation | 2 |

*A patient is considered as suffering from a spondyloarthropathy if the sum is 6.*

**FIGURE 5-3.** Amor criteria for spondyloarthropathy. The Amor's multiple entry criteria system has one advantage over the European group criteria in that the patients with undifferentiated spondyloarthropathy without arthritis or inflammatory back pain can be classified as having a form of spondyloarthropathy with the Amor citeria but not the European criteria [14]. No single item in the criteria list can contribute the 6 points needed to classify the patient as having spondyloarthropathy. Relief of pain within 24 to 48 hours after initiating treatment with a nonsteroidal anti-inflammatory drug (NSAID) or recurrence of pain within 24 to 48 hours after discontinuation of this treatment is of great clinical usefulness (2 points). For this component to be valid, the dosage of the NSAID should be large enough (ie, anti-inflammatory dose) and the dosage regimen sufficient to have appropriate therapeutic anti-inflammatory blood levels in the morning.

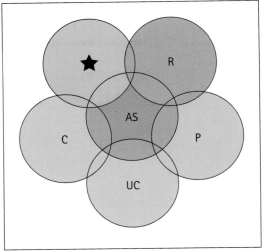

**FIGURE 5-4.** Ven diagram showing overlap among various spondyloarthropathies. The *star* denotes juvenile and undifferentiated spondyloarthropathies. The intensity of the *shaded area* indicates association with HLA-B27; the strongest association is with primary ankylosing spondylitis (represented by the nonoverlapped central part of the central circle). Note that psoriasis, ulcerative colitis, and Crohn's disease in the absence of associated spondyloarthropathy do not show any association with HLA-B27. AS—ankylosing spondylitis, p—psoriasis, UC—ulcerative colitis, C—Crohn's disease, R—reactive arthritis, including Reiter's syndrome.

## RECENT PREVELANCE STUDIES OF ANKYLOSING SPONDYLITIS (AS) AND RELATED SPONDYLOARTHROPATHIES (SPA)

| Populations | B27 Frequency (%) | Prevalence of AS (%) | | Prevalence of SpA (including AS) (%) | |
|---|---|---|---|---|---|
| | | General Population | B27(+) population | General Population | B27(+) Population |
| Eskimos (Alaska) | 40 | 0.4 | | 2.5 | |
| Eskimos (Alaska and Siberia) + Chukchi | 25–40 | | 1.6 | 2–3.4 | 4.2 |
| Saamis (Lapland) | 24 | 1.8 | 6.8 | | |
| Northern Norway | 14 | 1.4 | 6.7 | | |
| Mordovia | 16 | 0.5 | | | |
| Holland | 8 | 0.2 | 2 | | |
| Germany | 9 | 0.86 | 6.4 | 1.9 | 13.6 |

**FIGURE 5-5.** Prevalence studies. Recent studies in the native populations of Siberia (Chukchi and Eskimos) and Alaska (Inupiaq and Yupik Eskimos) that have a very high prevalence of HLA-B27 (25% to 40%) show an overall prevalence of spondyloarthropathies to vary between 2% and 3.4% [19]. The figure similarly lists the data derived from the recent epidemiologic studies in other populations as well.

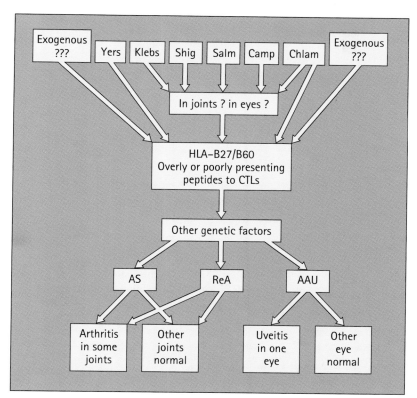

**FIGURE 5-6.** HLA-B27 as a common pathogenetic pathway. Feltkamp [25] has suggested a scheme with HLA-B27 acting as a common pathogenic pathway between several exogenous factors and the disease clinical features. HLA-B27-associated disease risk is enhanced by the presence of HLA-B60, and a great deal of research is being done to identify other genetic factors that play an important role in disease predisposition [26,29,30]. One of the reasons for the unilateral episode of acute anterior uveitis (AAU), and the often asymmetric peripheral arthritis of reactive arthritis (ReA), may be the randomness of the arrival of the exogenous antigenic inflammatory triggers at these sites. AS—ankylosing spondylitis; Camp—*Campylobacter*; Chlam—*Chlamydia*; CTL—cytotoxic T lymphocytes; Klebs—*Klebsiella*; Salm—*Salmonella*; Shig—*Shigella*; Yers—*Yersinia*. (*Adapted from* Feltcamp [25].)

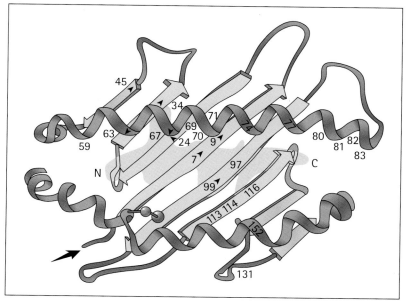

**FIGURE 5-7.** Schematic ribbon diagram of the antigen-binding cleft of the HLA-B*2705 molecule, the most common subtype of HLA-B27 in caucasoid populations. A nonameric (nine amino acid long) antigenic peptide is shown anchored bound in the antigen-binding cleft of the molecule. The view is from above, as seen from the viewpoint of a T-cell receptor. The letters *N* and *C* indicate the amino (N) and carboxy (C) termini of the bound peptide. The *arrow* indicates the amino-terminus of the alpha (heavy) chain of the HLA-B27 molecule. The floor of the antigen-binding cleft is formed by the beta strands (*broad arrows* pointing away from the amino-terminus), and the margins are formed by alpha-helices shown as *helical ribbons*. The top alpha helix and the four beta strands to the left are from the alpha-1 domain of the heavy chain and the bottom alpha helix and the four beta strands to the right are from the alpha-2 domain. The disulfide bond is shown as two *connecting spheres*. The sites of the polymorphic residues of the 12 subtypes of HLA-B27 (B*2701 to B*2712) are shown. Twelve subtypes differ from each other at one to seven residues in the antigen-binding cleft at positions 59, 69, 70, 71, 74, 77, 80, 81, 82, 83, 97, 113, 114, 116, 131, and 152. Not marked are the six side-pockets (assigned the letters a, b, c, d, e, and f) on the surface of the antigen-binding cleft. Pockets a and f are highly conserved deep pockets at the two ends of the antigen-binding cleft. The residues that form pocket b are marked by *black arrowheads* (at positions 7, 9, 24, 34, 45, 63, 67, and 99). The side chain of the second amino acid (arginine) of the bound peptide is shown anchored into pocket b. The two subtypes of HLA-B27 that are not associated with ankylosing spondylitis and related spondyloarthopathies, that is, B*2706 and B*2709, differ from the other subtypes at residues 114 and 116, primarily affecting the conformation of pocket e. (*Adapted from* Khan MA: Spondyloarthropathies: Editorial overview. *Curr Opin Rheumatol* 1994, 6:351–353. Copyright Rapid Science Publishers.)

| Residue Positions | 59 | 69 | 70 | 71 | 74 | 77 | 80 | 81 | 82 | 83 | 97 | 113 | 114 | 116 | 131 | 152 |
|---|---|---|---|---|---|---|---|---|---|---|---|---|---|---|---|---|
| Side-pockets | a | | b | | c/f | c/f | c/f | c/f | | | e/c/f | d | d/e | e/f | | e |
| B*2705 | Tyr | Ala | Lys | Ala | Asp | Asp | Thr | Leu | Leu | Arg | Asn | Tyr | His | Asp | Ser | Val |
| B*2701 | – | – | – | – | Tyr | Asn | – | Ala | – | – | – | – | – | – | – | – |
| B*2702 | – | – | – | – | – | Asn | Ile | Ala | – | – | – | – | – | – | – | – |
| B*2703 | His | – | – | – | – | – | – | – | – | – | – | – | – | – | – | – |
| B*2704 | – | – | – | – | – | Ser | – | – | – | – | – | – | – | – | – | Glu |
| B*2706 | – | – | – | – | – | Ser | – | – | – | – | – | – | Asp | Tyr | – | Glu |
| B*2707 | – | – | – | – | – | – | – | – | – | – | Ser | His | Asn | Tyr | Arg | – |
| B*2708 | – | – | – | – | – | Ser | Asn | – | Arg | Gly | – | – | – | – | – | – |
| B*2709 | – | – | – | – | – | – | – | – | – | – | – | – | – | His | – | – |
| B*2710 | – | – | – | – | – | – | – | – | – | – | – | – | – | – | – | Glu |
| B*2711 | – | – | – | – | – | Ser | – | – | – | – | Ser | His | Asn | Tyr | Arg | – |
| B*2712 | – | Thr | Asn | Thr | – | Ser | Asn | – | Arg | Gly | – | – | – | – | – | – |

**FIGURE 5-8.** Subtypes of HLA-B27. There are 12 different natural variants (subtypes) of HLA-B27 molecule [28]. These subtypes are named B*2701 to B*2711. They differ from each other by one to seven amino acids in the antigen-binding cleft of the molecule. HLA-B27*2705 is listed first in the figure because it is the major subtype, particularly in the caucasoid populations; *dashes* indicate identity with B*2705. The amino acid substitutions are shown by the conventional three-letter abbreviations for the various amino acids, along with the substitution sites and the various side pockets (a to f) affected by the substitutions. B*2705 has been split further into B*27052 and B*27053 by a single silent nucleotide substitution.

The various subtypes of HLA-B27 show different ethnic distributions, and some of them may also show differences in disease association; for example, the common subtypes in various world populations—B*2705, B*2702, B*2704, and B*2707—are clearly associated with spondyloarthropathies, whereas B*2709 in Sardinian Italians and B*2706 in Southeast Asians seem to lack such an association [28–31]. It is difficult to assess the disease association of the relatively uncommon subtypes— B*2701, B*2703, B*2708, B*2710, B*2711, and B*2712—at the population level, but occurrence of at least one case of spondyloarthropathy has been noted with all the subtypes except B*2708, B*2709, B*2711 and B*2712 [27,45]. Ala—alanine; Arg—arginine; Asn—asparagine; Asp—aspartic acid; Glu—glutamic acid; Gly—glycine; His—histidine; Ile—isoleucine; Leu—leucine; Lys—lysine; Ser—serine; Thr—threonine; Tyr—tyrosine. (*Updated and adapted from* Khan MA: Ankylosing spondylitis and heterogeneity of HLA-B27. *Semin Arthritis Rheum* 1988, 18:134.)

# Ankylosing Spondylitis

## Diagnosis and Clinical Features

### DIAGNOSTIC CRITERIA FOR ANKYLOSING SPONDYLITIS

**Rome, 1961**

**Clinical Criteria**
1. Low back pain and stiffness for more than 3 mo, not relieved by rest
2. Pain and stiffness in the thoracic region
3. Limited motion in the lumbar spine
4. Limited chest expansion
5. History or evidence of iritis or its sequelae

**Radiologic Criterion**
6. Roentgenogram showing bilateral sacroiliac changes characteristic of ankylosing spondylitis (this would exclude bilateral osteoarthritis of the sacroiliac joints)

**Definite ankylosing spondylitis if:**
1. Grade 3–4 bilateral sacroiliitis with at least one clinical criterion
2. At least four clinical criteria

**New York, 1966**

**Diagnosis**
1. Limitation of motion of the lumbar spine in all three planes: anterior flexion, lateral flexion, and extension
2. Pain at the dorsolumbar junction or in the lumbar spine
3. Limitation of chest expansion to 2.5 cm or less measured at the level of the fourth intercostal space

**Grading of Radiographs**
Normal, 0; suspicious, 1; minimal sacroiliitis, 2; moderate sacroiliitis, 3; ankylosis, 4

**Definite ankylosing spondylitis if:**
1. Grade 3–4 bilateral sacroiliitis with at least one clinical criterion
2. Grade 3–4 unilateral or grade 2 bilateral sacroiliitis with clinical criterion 1 or with both clinical criteria 2 and 3

**Probable ankylosing spondylitis**
Grade 3–4 bilateral sacroiliitis with no clinical criteria

**Modified New York, 1984**

**Criteria**
1. Low back pain at least 3 mo duration improved by exercise and not relieved by rest
2. Limitation of lumbar spine in sagittal and frontal planes
3. Chest expansion decreased relative to normal values for age and sex
4. Bilateral sacroiliitis grade 2–4
5. Unilateral sacroiliitis grade 3–4

Definite ankylosing spondylitis if unilateral grade 3 or 4, or bilateral grade 2–4 sacroiliitis and any clinical criterion

**FIGURE 5-9.** Diagnostic criteria for ankylosing spondylitis. These are the widely used diagnostic criteria for ankylosing spondylitis; they greatly depend on the radiographic evidence of sacroiliitis, which is the best nonclinical indicator of the disease presence. However, the status of the sacroiliac joints on routine pelvis radiographs may not always be easy to interpret in the early phase of the disease because of slow evolution in some patients and in adolescent patients. (*Data modified from* van der Linden [4].)

**FIGURE 5-10.** Clinical features of ankylosing spondylitis. Ankylosing spondylitis is a chronic systemic inflammatory disorder of undetermined etiology, usually beginning in early adulthood, primarily affecting the axial skeleton (sacroiliitis being its hallmark), but can also exhibit some extra-articular features. Acute anterior uveitis is the most common extra-articular feature, occurring in 25% to 30% of patients. The prevalence of the disease generally varies with the prevalence of HLA-B27 gene in the population. Studies in Eurocaucasoid populations suggest that the disease prevalence in the adult population is close to 0.2% [1,2,4]. It is three times more common in males, and the clinical anc roentgernographic features seem to evolve more slowly in females [4–32].

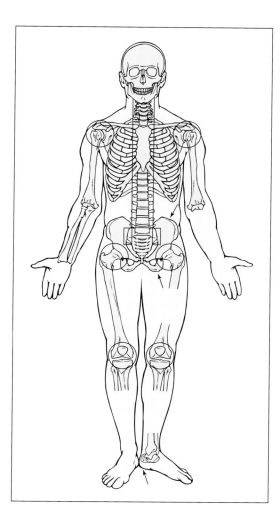

**FIGURE 5-11.** Sites of inflammation. The inflammation primarily affects the axial skeleton and appears to originate in ligamentous and capsular sites of attachment to bones (enthesitis), juxta-articular ligamentous structures, and the synovium, articular cartilage, and subchondral bones of involved joints. The site of enthesitis is infiltrated by lymphocytes, plasma cells, and polymorphonuclear cells; edema and infiltration of the adjacent marrow space are present. A striking feature is a high frequency of axial enthesitis and synovitis that can result in fibrous and later bony ankylosis of the sacroiliac joints and the spine [45].

Extra-articular or juxta-articular bony tenderness due to enthesitis at costosternal junctions, spinous processes, iliac crests, ischial tuberosities, or heels (*arrows*) may be an early feature of the disease. Stiffness and pain in the cervical spine and tenderness of the spinous processes may occur in early stages of the disease in some patients, but generally this tends to occur after some years. Back symptoms may be absent or very mild in an occasional patient, whereas others may complain only of back stiffness, fleeting muscle aches, or musculotendinous tender spots. These symptoms may be worsened on exposure to cold or dampness, and such patients may occasionally be misdiagnosed as having fibrositis (fibromyalgia). Some may have mild constitutional symptoms such as anorexia, malaise, or mild fever in early disease, and this may be more common among patients with juvenile onset, especially in developing countries [1–4]. Involvement of the costovertebral and the costotransverse joints, and occurrence of enthesitis at costosternal areas may cause chest pain that may be accentuated on coughing or sneezing. Some patients may note their inability to fully expand their chest on inspiration, but moderate to severe pulmonary restriction mostly occurs after long-standing disease.

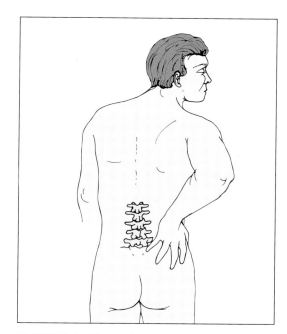

**FIGURE 5-12.** Early symptoms. The characteristic early symptom is insidious onset of chronic low back pain and stiffness, beginning usually in late adolescence or early adulthood (mean age of onset, 24 years). The pain due to sacroiliitis is dull in character, difficult to localize, and felt somewhere deep in the gluteal region. It may be unilateral or intermittent at first; however, within a few months it generally becomes persistent and bilateral, and the lower lumbar spine area also becomes painful. Sometimes pain in the lumbar area may be the initial presentation. The symptoms typically worsen with prolonged inactivity or on waking up in the morning ("morning stiffness"), and improve with physical activity and a hot shower. The back pain and stiffness may awaken some patients from sleep and some may experience considerable difficulty in getting out of bed in the morning. Others may find it necessary to wake up at night to move about or exercise for a few minutes before returning to bed. Some patients may complain of easy fatigueability, perhaps resulting, in part, from their disturbed sleep pattern.

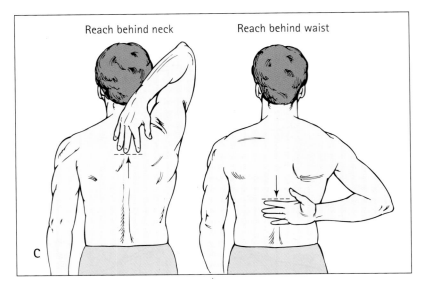

Reach behind neck          Reach behind waist

C

**FIGURE 5-14.** (*Continued*) **C,** Shoulder joint involvement is generally relatively mild, but resulting limitation of motion can easily detected by asking the patient to scratch his upper back. Normal range of shoulder motion is slower. Involvement of peripheral joints other than hips and shoulders in "primary" disease (*ie,* unassociated with psoriasis, inflammatory bowel disease, or reactive arthritis) is infrequent, rarely persistent or erosive, and tends to resolve without any residual joint deformity. Intermittent knee effusions may occasionally be the presenting manifestation of juvenile ankylosing spondylitis. Ten percent of the patients may show episodes of temporomandibular joint inflammation, which can result in limitation of jaw motion in some patients.

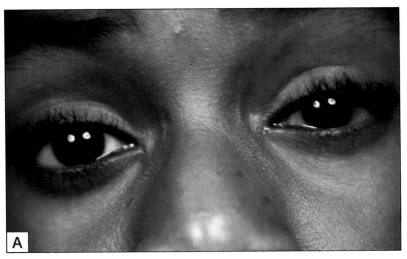

A

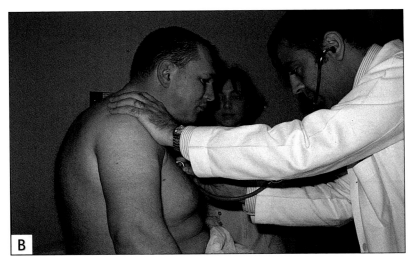

B

**FIGURE 5-15.** Uveitis. Acute anterior uveitis occurs in 25% to 30% of patients at some time in the course of their disease and is relatively more common among B27-positive than B27-negative patients [6,34,35]. **A,** The acute inflammation is typically unilateral, but it can recur in either eye. The patient presents with unilateral left ocular pain, redness, lacrimation, and photophobia evolving over a few days, which resulted in blurred vision owing to accumulation of inflammatory cells in the anterior chamber and abnormal accommodation of the ciliary muscles secondary to inflammation. There is circumcorneal congestion, and on slit-lamp examination increased numbers of white blood cells are seen in the aqueous humor of the inflamed eye. **B,** The other extra-articular manifestations are relatively uncommon and include aortitis (leading to slowly progressive aortic valve incompetency and conduction abnormalities, sometimes requiring a pacemaker), myocardial diastolic dysfunction, apical pulmonary fibrosis and cavitation, amyloidosis, and IgA nephropathy [36–42]. The marked muscle wasting seen in some patients with advanced disease results from disuse atrophy. Neurologic involvement may occur owing to fracture or dislocation, atlantoaxial subluxation, or cauda equina syndrome [1,6,43–46].

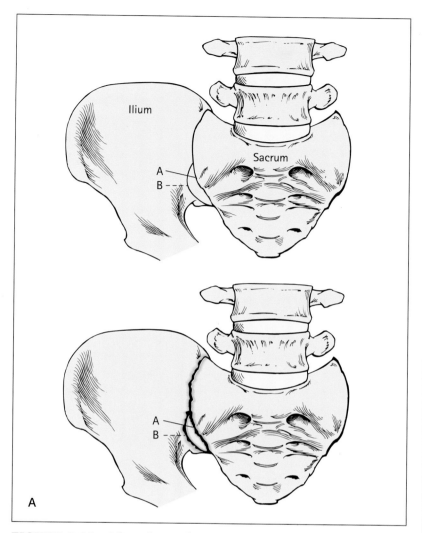

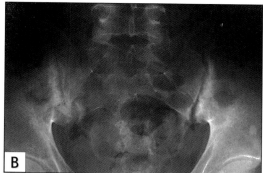

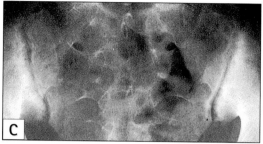

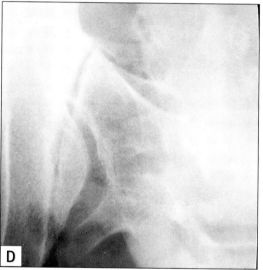

**FIGURE 5-16.** Bilateral sacroiliitis. Schematic (**A**) and anteroposterior roentgenographic views (**B** and **C**) of the pelvis show bilateral sacroiliitis in ankylosing spondylitis. There are erosions and blurring of the subchondral bone plate and reactive bone sclerosis that are more prominent on the iliac side of the joint. **D** shows a relatively mild sacroiliitis with a relatively slow evolution. The patient is a 30-year-old man with a 10-year history of disease.

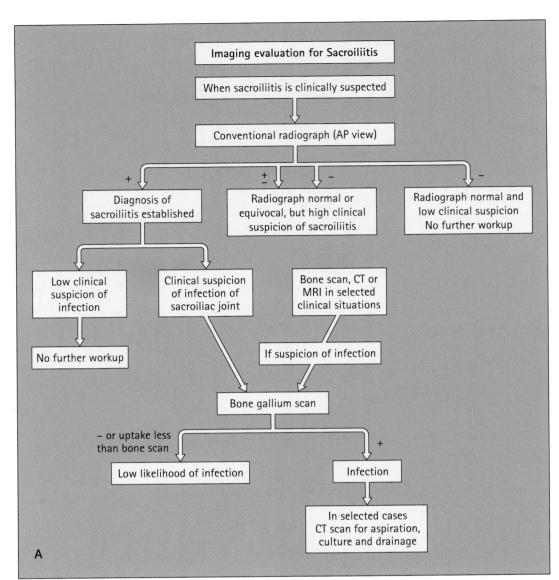

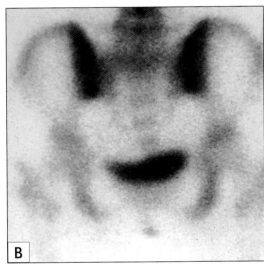

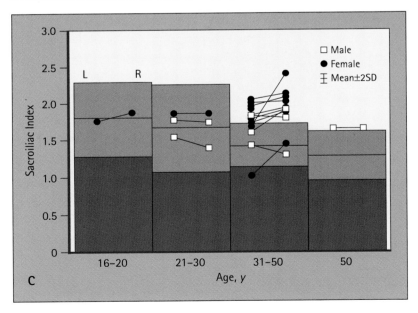

**FIGURE 5-17.** Imaging evaluation. **A**, Algorhythm for characteristic radiographic changes. Ankylosing spondylitis may sometimes evolve over many years, but changes are usually present by the time the patient seeks medical attention. They are primarily seen in the axial skeleton, especially in the sacroiliac joints. **B**, Radiographic evidence of sacroiliitis is required for definitive diagnosis and is the most consistent finding; a simple anteroposterior (AP) roentgenogram is usually sufficient for its detection, and oblique views should not be requested. In patients with early disease in whom standard roentgenography of the sacroiliac joints may be normal or show equivocal changes, quantitative bone scintigraphy may be too nonspecific to be useful [47]; computed tomography (CT) is more sensitive but equally specific when compared with conventional roentgenography. **C**, Sacroiliac index.

*(Continued on next page)*

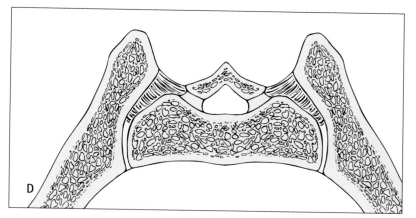

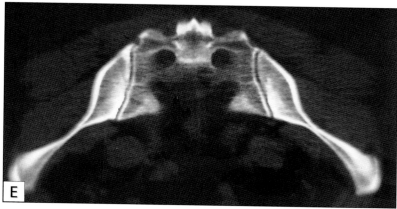

**FIGURE 5-17.** (*Continued*) **D,** Schematic horizontal cut across the sacroiliac joints at a level a little more cephalic to the CT image shown in **E**. Magnetic resonance imaging (MRI) gives excellent results and without radiation; it can show abnormalities of the periarticular bone marrow and subchondral bone but at a greater cost. These two imaging modalities, however, are rarely needed for the diagnosis of ankylosing spondylitis in most patients [48–50]. SD—standard deviation.

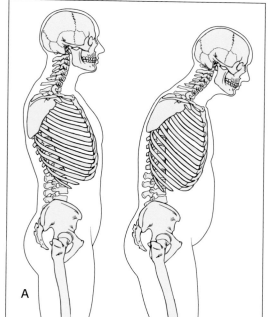

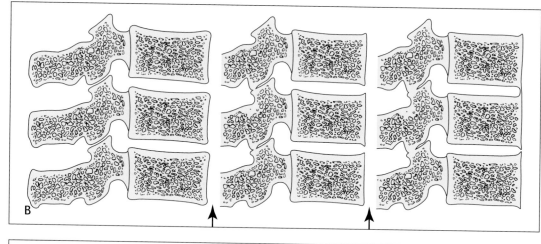

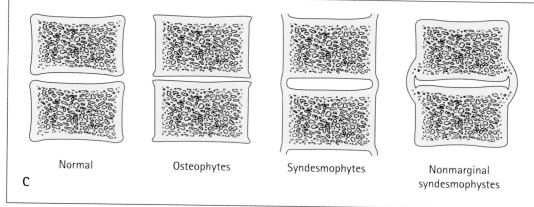

Normal     Osteophytes     Syndesmophytes     Nonmarginal syndesmophystes

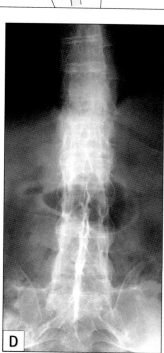

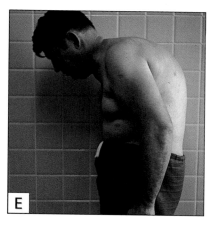

**FIGURE 5-18.** Inflammation. **A,** The inflammation of the superficial layers of the annulus fibrosus and at their sites of attachment to the corners of the vertebral bodies results in reactive bony sclerosis ("shiny corners") and subsequent bone resorption (erosions). **B** and **C,** Ultimately, this leads to "squaring" of the vertebral bodies (best visualized on lateral radiograph of the spine) and a gradual formation of intervertebral bony "bridgings" called syndesmophytes. There are often concomitant inflammatory changes in the apophyseal joints that may lead to their ankylosis, and ossification of the interspinous ligaments may also occur. **D** and **E,** This can result in complete fusion of the vertebral column ("bamboo spine") in patients with severe ankylosing spondylitis of long duration. Spinal osteoporosis, although usually seen in patients with long-standing ankylosing spondylitis, can sometimes develop in a relatively early stage of the disease.

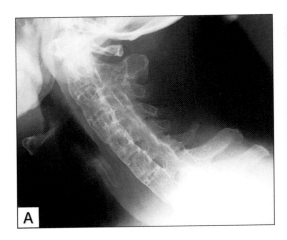

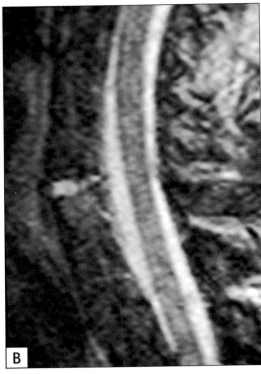

**FIGURE 5-19.** "Bamboo spine." **A**, This lateral view of the cervical spine shows a rigid and forward stooping cervical spine of a patient with severe ankylosing spondylitis for more than 35 years. The spine is completely anky-losed ("bamboo spine" due to syndesmophytes and fused facet (apophyseal) joints. Spinal osteoporosis is also present. Such patients are prone to spinal fracture. In fact, this patient had sustained lower cervical spine fracture that day and it could not be visualized on this radiograph. However, it was easily detected on a mangetic resonance imaging scan **B**.

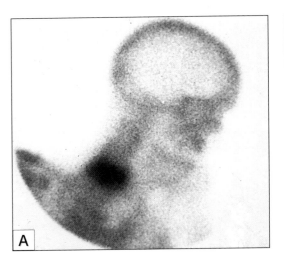

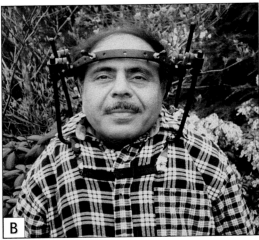

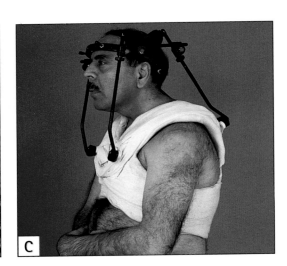

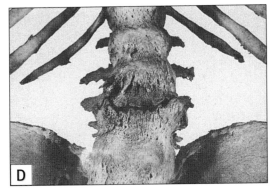

### E. IMAGING EVALUATION FOR PSEUDOARTHROSIS

Clinical evidence of cord compression

| Present | Absent |
|---|---|
| MRI | X-ray spine (including flexion view) |
| ⊖ | ⊕ |
| Bone scan | Do CT or sagittal tomography |
|   If positive, do CT or sagittal    tomography | |

**FIGURE 5-20.** Spinal fracture. **A** through **D**, Spinal fracture can follow a relatively minor trauma in patients with long-standing severe anky-losing spondylitis because the ankylosed and osteoporotic spine is prone to fractures, usually occurring in the lower cervical spine. Quadriplegia is the most dreaded complication because it has a high mortality rate. Isolate or mulitple vertebral compression fractures may also occur. The pain associated with spinal fractures may be overlooked or wrongly attributed to exacerbation of the spondylitic process and could lead to diskovertebral destruction (spinal pseudoarthrosis) [48]. **A**, Bone scan showing lower cervical spine fracture. **B** and **C**, Firm bracing needed to allow fracture to heal. **D**, Skeleton of spondylitic patient showing lumbar fracture. Imaging evaluation is necessary (**E**). The best early clinical clues to spinal fracture may be a history of acute or unexplained episode of back pain that is aggravated by movement, even in the absence of obvious physical trauma. It may sometimes be associated with localized spinal tenderness. Some patients may develop aseptic spondylodiskitis, mostly in the midthoracic spine. It is usually asymptomatic and without any physical trauma or infection and is relatively more common in the patients whose spondylitis also involves the cervical spine. CT— computed tomography; MRI—magnetic resonance imaging.

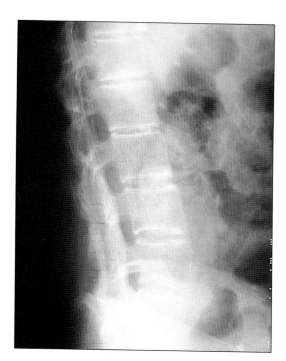

FIGURE 5-21. Reactive bony sclerosis. A lateral view of the lumbar spine of patient with anky-losing spondylitis shows reactive bony sclerosis of the corners ("shiny corners") of two adjacent vertevral bodies and bone resoption of the anterior corners of the vertebral bodies that has resulted in vertebral "squaring." Spondylodiskitis is present at the intervertebral disk between T12 and L1 vertebrae.

## Survival and Familial Aggregation

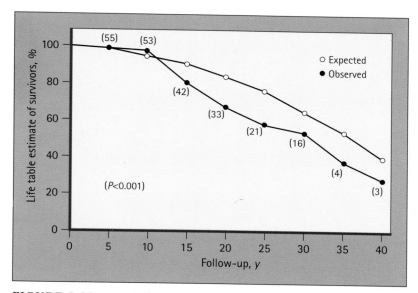

FIGURE 5-22. Survival time. Long-term survival studies indicate that severe ankylosing spondylitis may result in slight shortening of the lifespan beginning 15 years after diagnosis [63,64]. Because the average age of diag-nosis is 30 to 32 years (mean age of onset 25 and 5- to 7-year delay in diag-nosis), this means that the trend toward a slight reduction in survival starts at about age 50. Life-table estimates of percent survival as compared to what is expected are shown; the numbers in parentheses indicate the patient sample size followed in an arthritis outpatient clinic. Three patients had a maximum follow-up of up to 40 years. Because most patients with anky-losing spondylitis do not suffer from very severe disease, these data do not apply to such patients who have a normal life span.

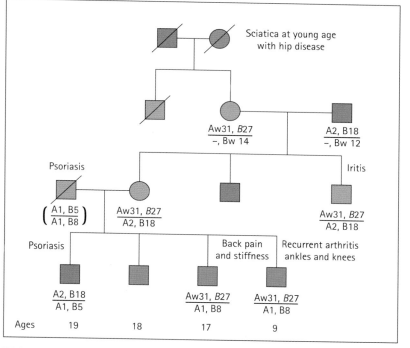

FIGURE 5-23. Family pedigree. This family shows marked familial aggregation of spondyloarthropathies. There is also presence of psoriasis in this family. Other families may show a presence of Crohn's disease or ulcerative colitis. Patients with psoriasis or inflammatory bowel disease are more likely to later develop ankylosing spondylitis than the rest of population without these diseases, and the reverse is also true, that is patients with ankylosing spondylitis are more often found to have Crohn's disease, ulcerative colitis, or psoriasis. Ileocolonoscopic studies have disclosed the presence of subclinical bowel inflammation in a large number of patients with spondyloarthropathies who had no other evidence of inflammatory bowel disease [18,19].

## COMPARISON OF CLINICAL FEATURES OF B27-POSITIVE AND B27-NEGATIVE PATIENTS WITH PRIMARY ANKYLOSING SPONDYLITIS

|  | B27(+) AS | B27(–) AS |
|---|---|---|
| Racial group | all races | Increased in non-Caucasions |
| HLA antigens | B27 | Increased B7 in blacks |
|  |  | Increased Bw16 (Bw38) in whites[†] |
|  |  | (? IBD* or psoriasis genes) |
| Age of onset | 15–40 y | 18–50 y |
| Family history | ++ | – |
| Acute anterior uveitis | ++ | + |
| Skeletal manifestations | ++ | ++ |

*IBD—inflammatory bowel disease; Some groups have reported an increased incidence of B7 cross-reacting groups of HLA antigens, but we have not been able to confirm these results.

**FIGURE 5-24.** Clinical features of HLA-B27-positive and HLA-B27-negative patients with ankylosing spondylitis. AS—ankylosing spondylitis; HLA—human leukocyte antigen; IBD—inflammatory bowel disease.

## A. HLA-B27 FREQUENCY IN PATIENTS AND NORMAL CONTROLS

| Group | Whites | | Blacks | |
|---|---|---|---|---|
|  | n | B27(+), % | n | B27(+), % |
| Control | 485 | 8 | 60 | 2 |
| Ankylosing spondylitis | 140 | 92 | 36 | 49 |
| Reiter's syndrome | 54 | 72 | 20 | 40 |

**FIGURE 5-25.** Laboratory evaluation. There are no "diagnostic" or pathognomonic laboratory tests. An elevated erythrocyte sedimentation rate and C-reactive protein are observed in 75% of patients, and a mild to moderate elevation of serum IgA concentration is also commonly present. There is no association with rheumatoid factor and antinuclear antibodies, and the synovial fluid and synovial biopsy do not show markedly distinctive features as compared with other inflammatory arthropathies. Most patients with ankylosing spondylitis (AS) can be readily diagnosed clinically on the basis of history, physical examination, and roentgenographic findings. **A**, **B**, and **C**, The presence or absence of HLA-B27 cannot definitely establish or exclude the diagnosis because the HLA-B27 as a test for the disease is neither 100% specific nor 100% sensitive. The prevalence of HLA-B27 in the general population (from which is derived the specificity of the HLA-B27 test) and the strength of its disease association (*ie*, the sensitivity of the test) also vary markedly among many ethnic and racial groups [52–54]. HLA-B27 typing cannot be used as a "routine," "diagnostic," "confirmatory," or "screening" test for AS in patients with back pain or arthritis.

(Continued on next page)

## B. PERCENT OF B27-POSITIVE PATIENTS AND NORMAL CONTROLS BY VARIOUS POPULATIONS

| Populations | Ankylosing Spondylitis | | Normal Controls | |
|---|---|---|---|---|
|  | Number of Patients | B27-positive (%) | Number of Controls | B27-positive (%) |
| Caucasoid |  |  |  |  |
| Euro-caucasoids (whites) | 2022 | 79–100 | 16,162 | 4–13 |
| Indians and Pakistanis | 130 | 83–100 | 456 | 2–8 |
| Iranians | 25 | 92 | 400 | 3 |
| Arabs | 32 | 81 | 355 | 3 |
| Jews | 31 | 81 | 456 | 3 |
| Mongoloid |  |  |  |  |
| Chinese |  |  |  |  |
| Mainland China | 196 | 89–91 | 726 | 2–7 |
| Hong Kong | 77 | 99 | 102 | 4 |
| Taiwan | 76 | 95 | 297 | 9 |
| Singapore | 29 | 97 | 238 | 7 |
| Japanese | 72 | 82 | 208 | <1 |
| Filipino | 17 | 94 | 529 | 5–8 |
| Thai | 71 | 86 | 138 | 5 |
| North American Indians |  |  |  |  |
| Haida | 17 | 100 | 222 | 50 |
| Navajo | 5 | 80 | 100 | 36 |
| Bella Colla | 3 | 100 | 129 | 25 |
| Pima | 14 | 100 | 400 | 18 |
| Zuni |  |  | 158 | 13 |
| Hopi |  |  | 100 | 9 |
| Mestizo | 239 | 69–81 | 1404 | 3–7 |
| South American Indians |  |  | 440 | 0 |
| Negroid |  |  |  |  |
| African blacks |  |  |  |  |
| Central Africans |  |  |  |  |
| Congo and Zambia |  |  | 259 | 0 |
| West Africans |  |  |  |  |
| Mali |  |  | 82 | 9.7 |
| Gambia |  |  | 702 | 2.6 |
| South Africans |  |  |  |  |
| Zimbabwe | 7 | 0 |  | <0.01 |
| South Africa | 9 | 22 | 798 | 1 |
| American Blacks | 67 | 57 | 1330 | 2–4 |

*Eskimos are not listed in the table; they have 25%–37% frequency of B27, and virtually all patients, with ankylosing spondylitis are B27 positive [4,8]. Frequency of B27 is 9% in Indonesia [64] and >25% in an isolated community in Papua, New Guinea [21].

## C. IMPORTANT ASPECTS OF THE HLA-B27 TEST

It is not a "routine" or "diagnostic" or "confirmatory" test.

Most patients with AS can be diagnosed clinically and do not need this test.

It cannot be used as a screening test for AS in the general population.

The sensitivity and specificity of the test depend on the racial and ethnic background of the patient.

The clinical usefulness of the test, like any other "imperfect" test, depends on the clinical setting in which it is performed, and requires Bayesian analysis to correctly interpret the clinical meaning of positive or negative test results.

The test can, in a similar manner, also be used as an aid to support the diagnosis of other B27-associated spondyloarthropathies besides AS.

The test does not help distinguish AS from other B27-associated spondyloarthropathies.

**FIGURE 5-25.** (*Continued*) A physician who understands the principles of probability reasoning (Bayesian analysis) can, however, use the test appropriately to support the diagnosis is positive in cases that might be less clear-cut (primarily owing to slow evolution of diagnostic radiographic sacroiliitis). HLA-B27 is associated with all the spondyloarthropathies, and differentiation between these diseases is based on the clinical findings summarized in **D**. (D *adapted from* Arnett FC, JR, Khan MA, Willkins RF: A new look at ankylosing spondylitis. *Patient Care* 1989, November 30:82–101; and Kahn [6].)

## D. CLINICAL FEATURES COMPARED

| | Disorder | | | | |
| Characteristic | Ankylosing Spondylitis | Reactive Arthritis (Reiter's Syndrome) | Juvenile Spondyloarthropathy | Psoriatic Arthropathy* | Enteropathic Arthropathy[†] |
|---|---|---|---|---|---|
| Usual age at onset | Young adult age < 40 | Young to middle age adult | Childhood onset, ages 8–18 | Young to middle age adult | Young to middle age adult |
| Sex ratio | 3× more common in males | Predominantly males | Predominantly males | Equally distributed | Equally distributed |
| Usual type of onset | Gradual | Acute | Variable | Variable | Gradual |
| Sacroiliitis or spondylitis | Virtually 100% | < 50% | < 50% | ~ 20% | < 20% |
| Symmetry of sacroiliitis | Symmetric | Asymmetric | Variable | Asymmetric | Symmetric |
| Peripheral joint involvement | ~ 25% | ~ 90% | ~ 90% | ~ 95% | 15%–20% |
| HLA-B27 (in whites) | > 90% | ~ 75% | ~ 85% | < 50%[†] | ~ 50% |
| Eye involvement[§] | 25–30% | ~ 50% | ~ 20% | ~ 20% | ~ 15% |
| Cardiac involvement | 1%–4% | 5%–10% | Rare | Rare | Rare |
| Skin, mucosal, or nail involvement | None | ~ 40% | Uncommon | Virtually 100% | Uncommon |

*About 5%–7% of patients with psoriasis develop arthritis, and psoriatic spondylitis accounts for about 5% of all patients with psoriatic arthritis.

[†]Associated with chronic inflammatory bowel disease.

[‡]B27 prevalence is higher in those with spondylitis or sacroiliitis.

[§]Predominantly conjunctivitis in reactive and psoriatic arthritis, acute anterior uveitis in the other disorders listed above.

## SALIENT PRINCIPLES OF MANAGEMENT OF ANKYLOSING SPONDYLITIS

- No cure, but most patients can be well managed with NSAIDs
- A concerned (primary) physician providing continuity of care; consultation as needed by a rheumatologist, ophthatlmologist, orthopedist, etc.
- Education of the patient about the disease to help increase compliance
- Importance of daily exercises to preserve good posture and minimize limitation of chest expansion; swimming is the best exercise; appropriate sports and recreations; sleeping on firm mattress; avoiding pillows under the head, if possible; avoidance of smoking and prevention of spinal trauma
- Supportive measures and counseling with regard to social, sexual and vocational aspects; importance of patient support groups
- Family counseling; thorough family history; physical examination of the relatives may disclose remarkable disease aggregation and many undiagnosed or misdiagnosed affected relatives in some families
- Surgical measures: arthroplasty, correction of deformity, etc.
- Early diagnosis is important, as is the early recognition and treatment of extraskeletal manifestations, such as acute anterior ureitis (iritis), and of the associated diseases or complications

**FIGURE 5-26.** Management of ankylosing spondylitis. Most patients with ankylosing spondylitis can be well managed, even though there is currently no known method to cure or prevent the disease, and there is no special diet or any specific food that has a role in its initiation or exacerbation. Aspirin seldom provides an adequate therapeutic response but other nonsteroidal anti-inflammatory drugs (NSAIDs) are more helpful and should be used in full therapeutic anti-inflammatory doses during active phase of the disease. The patients should be informed about this because otherwise they may use the drugs occasionally and for their analgesic effect only. The responses by patients differ, as do the side effects, and it is worthwhile to search out the best alternative NSAID that works for each individual.

When the disease is not being adequately controlled by NSAIDs, or for those intolerant to such drugs, sulphasalazine may be effective in those with peripheral arthritis, but it has no appreciable influence on purely axial disease and on peripheral enthesitis [55]. Because of its efficacy in inflammatory bowel disease and psoriasis, sulfasalazine may be especially useful for ankylosing spondylitis associated with those diseases. A few patients with severe ankylosing spondylitis with peripheral joint involvement unresonsive to NSAID and sulfasalazine have sometimes responded to oral methotrexate therapy [56,57]. D-Penicillamine is not effective, and antimalarial drugs and gold have not been well studied in ankylosing spondylitis. Oral corticosteroids have no therapeutic value in the long-term management of the musculoskeletal aspects of this disease because of their serious side effects, and they do not halt disease progression.

Recalcitrant enthesitis and persistent synovitis may respond to a local corticosteroid injection, and therapeutic contribution of injection into the sacroiliac joints is being evaluated [58]. There seems to be a consensus that spinal radiotherapy has no role in the modern management of patients with ankylosing spondylitis because of the high risk of leukemia and aplastic anemia. There are occaional uncontrolled reports of efficacy of low-dose external beam radiotherapy of persistent peripheral enthesitis and synovitis resistant to standard treatments. Splints, braces, and corsets are generally not helpful and are not advised. Pregnancy does not usually affect the disease symptoms, and fertility, course of pregnancy, and childbirth have been reported to be normal [31].

The patient should walk erect, keeping the spine as traight as possible, and sleep on a firm mattress using as thin a pillow as possible. Physical activity that places prolonged strain on the back muscles, such as prolonged stooping or bending, should be avoided. Regular exercises are of fundamental importance in preventing or minimizing deformity. Spinal extension exercises and deep-breathing exercises should be done routinely once or twice daily, and smoking should be avoided. Formal physical therapy is of value especially in teaching the patient the proper posture, appropriate exercises, and recreational sports, and the need for maintaining the exercise program. Group exercise sessions that include hydrotherapy in warm water are helpful. Regular swimming is considered to be one of the best exercises for these patients. Some patients have difficulty driving their car because of the impaired neck mobility, and they may find special wide-view mirrors to be helpful. Patient support groups enlist enthusiastic patient cooperation and provide information about the disease and advice about life and health insurance, jobs, working environment, wide-view mirrors, and other useful items.

Acute anterior uveitis requires prompt and vigorous treatment with dilation of the pupil and use of corticosteroid eyedrops. Systemic steroids or immunosuppressives may be needed for rare patients with severe refractory uveitis. The patient should be informed about the possibility of recurrences of acute iritis. Total hip arthroplasty gives very good results and prevents partial or total disability from severe hip disease. Vertebral wedge osteotomy may be needed for correction of severe kyphosis in some patients, although it carries a relatively high risk of paraplegia. Cardiac complications may require aortic valve replacement or pacemaker implantation. Apical pulmonary fibrosis and cavitation are not easy to manage; surgical resection may rarely be required. (*Adapted from* Khan MA, Skosey JR: Ankylosing spondylitis and related spondyloarthropathies. In: *Immunological Diseases*, edn 4. Edited by Samter M, Talmage DW, Frank MM, Austen KF, Claman HN. Boston: Little, Brown; 1988:1509–1538.)

## Presentation and Diagnosis

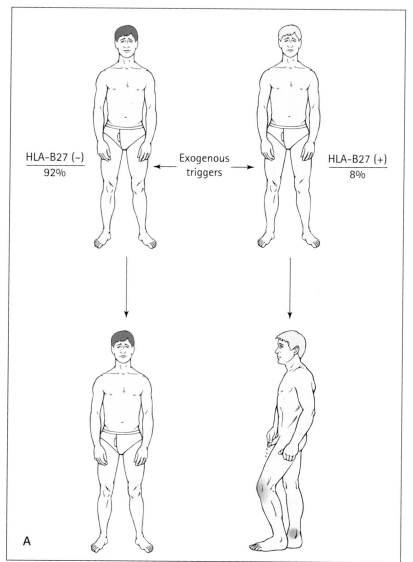

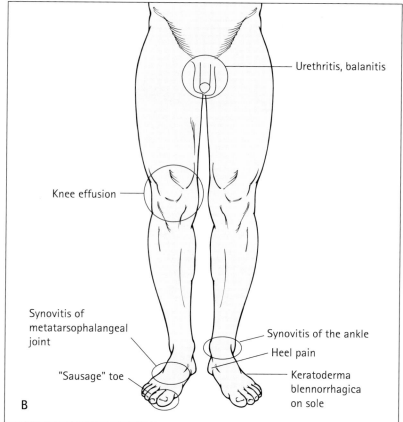

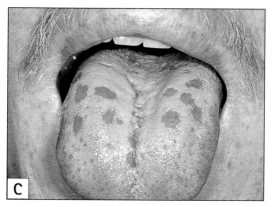

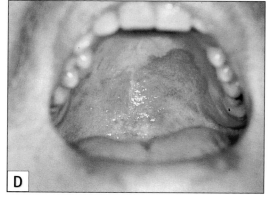

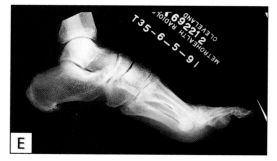

**FIGURE 5-27.** Presentation. **A** and **B**, Reactive arthritis or Reiter's syndrome usually presents with acute oligoarticular arthritis, affecting more often the joints of the lower extremities. HLA-B27 predisposes the person exposed to the exogenous triggering agent. Individuals who are HLA-B27 negative who are exposed to the agent do not develop Reiter's syndrome. The arthritis usually resolves in 3 months but can have recurrences or become chronic. The patient can show urethritis, diarrhea, balanitis or cervicitis, conjunctivitis, acute anterior uveitis, psoriasiform rashes (keratodermia, or pustular psoriasiform lesion on palms and soles), painless superficial mucosal ulcerations (**C** and **D**), onycholysis without pitting of the nails, diffuse swelling digits ("sausage" digits), Achilles tendonitis, and plantar fasciitis. **E** shows resultant erosions and periosteal "whiskering" at sites of attachment of the Achilles tendon and the plantar fascia.

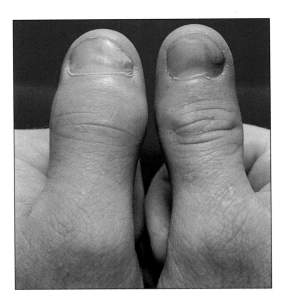

**FIGURE 5-28.** Onycholysis of thumb nail and dactylitis ("sausage"). The left thumb in a patient with reactive arthritis shows no pitting or ridging of the nail as is typical of psoriasis digit. (*From* Kahn MA, Skosey JL: Ankylosing spondylitis and related spondyloarthropathies. In: *Immunological Diseases*, edn 4. Edited by Samter M, Talmage DW, Frank MM, Austen KF, Claman HN. Boston: Little, Brown; 1988:1509–1538, with permission of the publisher.)

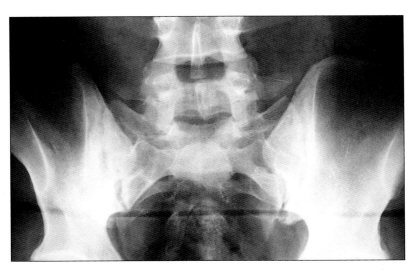

**FIGURE 5-29.** Asymmetric sacroiliitis. Anteroposterior roentgenographic view of the pelvis shows bilateral but somewhat asymmetric sacroiliitis in a patient with reactive arthritis.

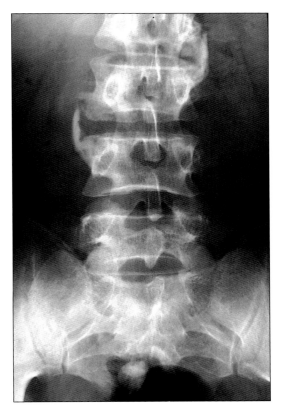

**FIGURE 5-30.** Chronic reactive arthritis. Anteroposterior roentgenographic view of the pelvis and lumbar spine in a patient with chronic reactive arthritis shows asymmetric nonmarginal syndesmophytes that originate a little distance away from the corners of the vertebrae, in contradistinction to the marginal syndesmophytes of ankylosing spondyliitis. Patients with psoriatic spondyloarthropathy are also more likely to develop similar nonmarginal syndesmophytes. Involvement of sacroiliac joints (sacoiliitis) is frequently observed and often asymmetric. There are no erosive changes of the sacroiliac joints in the patient's radiograph shown although the right-sided joint is slightly indistinct. (*From* Mustafa K, Khan MA: Recognizing and managing reactive arthritis. *J Musculoskeletal Med* 1996, 13(6):28–41, with permission of the publisher.)

## BACTERIAL INFECTIONS THAT CAN TRIGGER HLA-B27-ASSOCIATED REACTIVE ARTHRITIS

### Gastointestinal Infection

a. **Usual triggers:**
   *Shigella fexneri*
   *Salmonella enteritides* and *S. typhimurium*
   *Yersinia enterocolitica* and *Y. pseudotuberculosis*
   *Campylobacter jejuni*

b. **Unusual triggers:**
   *Shigella sonnei* and *S. dysenteriae*
   *Salmonella paratyphi*
   Bacillus Calmette-Guerin
   *Clostridium dificille*

### Urogenital infection

a. **Usual triggers:**
   *Chlamydia trachomatis*

b. **Unusual triggers:**
   ?*Ureaplasma urealyticum*

### Respiratory infection

*Chlamydia pnenumoniae*

**FIGURE 5-31.** Bacterial infections and treatment. Reactive arthritis is an aseptic inflammatory arthritis developing in an immunologically sensitized host with nonproliferating antigens thought to be present in the joint. The sensitization is usually triggered by chlamydial urethritis or cervicitis or enteric infection with *Shigella, Salmonella, Yersinia,* or *Campylobacter* in a genetically susceptible individual; HLA-B27 is the major currently known genetic risk factor. There has been a dramatic increase of reactive arthritis and related spondyloarthropathies in sub-Saharan Africa resulting from the current epidemic of human immunodeficiency virus (HIV). The link between HIV infection and increasing prevalence of reactive arthritis has been clearly demonstrated in a recent study from Lusaka, Zambia (Njobvueral, Br J Rheumatol 1997, 36:404–405). This is all the more remarkable given the almost complete absence of HLA-B27 in Bantu populations of Africa, and the fact that the HIV-associated reactive arthritis in Eurocaucasoid populations, on the other hand, retains its strong assocation with HLA-B27.

Nonsteroidal anti-inflammatory drugs (NSAIDs) form the basis of therapy, and they should be used regularly in full therapeutic anti-inflammatory dose over an extended period of time [63–65]. The patient should be advised against using the NSAIDs occasionally or only for their analgesic effect. Joint aspiration and intra-articualr corticosteroid administration of triamcinolone hexacetonide may help to obtain prompt and prolonged relief from severe or persistent synovitis, only after septic arthritis has been excluded. The differential diagnosis from septic arthritis may sometimes be difficult, and short hospitalization may be needed for patients with severe arthritis. Antibiotic treatment should be initiated if true joint infection is not excluded. Joint rest and even temporary splinting may be needed in severe cases to alleviate pain, but should be used sparingly because it may result in muscle wasting. Physical therapy is valuable during convalescence, to regain mussele strength and full range of joint motion. A comfortable pair of shoes and shoe inserts to alter weight bearing may help the patient with painful feet.

In a very severe case of acute reactive arthritis where many joints are affected and NSAIDs alone have failed, a short course of oral corticosteroids may be needed, tapering down the dose according to improvement. It is advisable to avoid prolonged low dose oral corticosteroid therapy in chronic cases because it is rarely effective. Sulphasalazine may benefit patients with chronic disease; the drug should be started with 0.5 to 1.0 g daily, which should then be gradually increased to a tolerated level of 2 to 3 g daily. Antirheumatic "disease-modifying" drugs can be tried in some patients with persistent polyarthritis. Injectable and oral gold have been used, but rheumatolagists would be more likely, in severe cases, to suggest methotrexate or azathioprine. Skin lesions are treated either with topical corticosteroids or keratinolytic agents such as salicylic acid ointment. In severe cases, retinoids or methotrexate are most commonly used. Acute anterior uveitis must be diagnosed and treated promptly to prevent synechiae and other resultant complications; the inflammation may on rare occasions affect even the posterior uveal tract.

Antibiotic treatment of the triggering infection is recommended if the presence of infection can still be identified after the onset of arthritis. For example, in *Yersinia* infections, the aim of such antibiotic therapy is rather to minimize the spread of infection within the family. However, a cautious approach should be exercised because antibiotic treatment may prolong the carrier state in some forms of enteritis, and short-term antibiotic treatment does not influence the course of postenteritic reactive arthritis. It is obvious that once the trigger has been pulled, the chain of events takes its path anyway. It is of interest that early treatment of patients with urogenital chlamydial infection in endemic areas has resulted in decreasing subsequent development of reactive arthritis and vigorous antibiotic treatment of chlamydial reinfections significantly reduced relapses of reactive arthritis. (*From* Khan [7]).

# Psoriasis

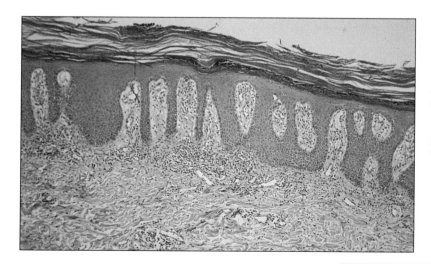

**FIGURE 5-32.** Histology. Psoriasis is a disease of abnormal keratinocyte proliferation (scale production) accompanied by inflammatory component (redness, heat, itch) induced by T cells, but the precise cause is unknow. The activated T cells in the epidermis are predominantly CD8+, whereas those in the dermis are mostly CD4+. The infiltration of CD4+ cells precedes that of CD8+ cells. The epidermal CD8+ T cells possessing receptor are stimulated by a triggering factor (as yet unknown) and produce cytokines that stimulate keratinocytes and cause inflammation. These keratinocytes produce cytokines that in turn, stimulate T cells.

## A. CLINICAL FEATURES OF PSORIATIC ARTHRITIS IN REPORTED SERIES

| Feature | Wright | Little | Roberts | Leonard | Krammer | Scarpa | Gladman |
|---------|--------|--------|---------|---------|---------|--------|---------|
| Asymmetric oligoarthritis (%) | 53 | ? | ? | 63 | 54* | 16.1 | 11† |
| Symmetric polyarthritis (%) | 31 | ? | 79 | 23 | 25* | 39 | 19‡ |
| Distal (%) | 3 | ? | 28* | 3 | ? | 7.5 | 12 |
| Back (%) | 10 | ? | 5* | 7 | 21 | 21 | 2§ |
| Mutilans (%) | ? | ? | 5* | 3 | ? | 2.3 | 16 |
| Sacroiliitis (%) | 87 | 30 | ? | 30 | ? | 16 | 27 |

*Includes patients with only distal joints involved
†14, including symmetric oligoarthritis
‡40, including asymmetric polyarthritis
§33, including peripheral joint and back involvement
*Includes more than one category.

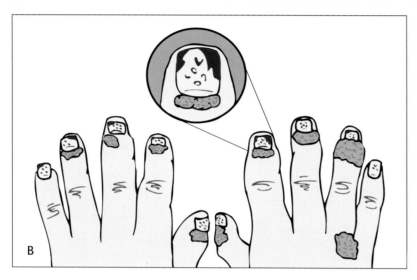

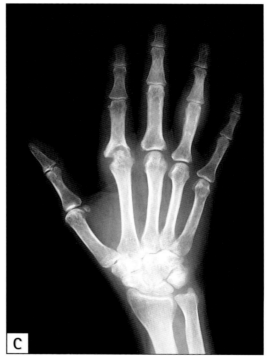

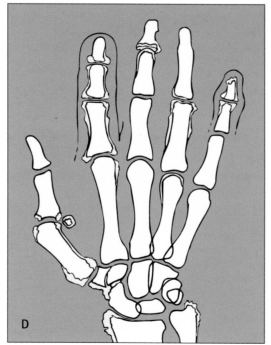

**FIGURE 5-33.** Psoriatic arthritis. Psoriatic arthritis is an inflammatory arthritis associated with psoriasis. The exact prevalence of each of its many forms has been difficult to establish (**A**); the disease pattern may change with time in an individual patient, and some patients may show overlapping features. Psoriasis and psoriatic arthritis are relatively more common in whites and are very uncommon among Africans, Chinese, and native North American Indians of unmixed ancestry. Distal interphalangeal joints are frequently affected in psoriatic arthritis (**B**). An asymmetric oligoarthritis is noted in 40% and symmetric polyarthritis in 35%; this latter subgroup has the more erosive, deforming and disabling disease (**C** and **D**). Radiographs of the involved joints as in C may show soft tissue swelling or mild erosions to severe joint destruction, and occasionally bony fusion. Sacroiliitis occurs in up to 20% of patients and 5% show predominant spondylitis.

# Miscellaneous Forms of Disease

## A. B27 ASSOCIATED "FORME FRUSTES"

Chronic enthesitis (enthesopathies)
Dactylitis ("sausage" digits)
Keratodermia (pustular psoriasis)
Aortic insufficincy with heart block
Acute anterior uveitis (acute iritis)
Symptomatic spondylitis without sacroiliitis

**FIGURE 5-34.** Undifferentiated spondyloarthropathies. **A** and **B**, The concept of spondyloarthropathies has expanded to include undifferentiated forms of the disease [5,69,70]. (B from Zeidler and coworkers [5].)

## B. SYMPTOMS AND SIGNS OF UNDIFFERENTIATED SPONDYLOARTHROPATHIES IN FAMILIES OF PATIENTS WITH ANKYLOSING SPONDYLITIS (AS)

| Symptoms and Signs | Reference | Year | Relatives, n | Relative Frequencies, % |
|---|---|---|---|---|
| Sacroiliitis without AS | Emery | 1967 | 188 | 11 |
| | Daneo | 1977 | 37 | 16 |
| | Chritiansen | 1977 | 63 | 11 |
| | Calin | 1983 | 282 | 7* |
| | LeClerco | 1984 | 261 | 9 |
| | van der Linden | 1984 | 101 | 7 |
| Inflammatory back pain | Calin | 1983 | 282 | 38 |
| | Khan | 1985 | 100 | 9† |
| Chest pain | Khan | 1985 | 86 | 15† |
| | Van der Linden | 1988 | 405 | 11† |

\* Minimal frequency, because only 70 (65%) of 107 symptomatic relatives were examined.
† Only individuals without radiographic changes.

## REPRESENTATIVE STUDIES ON THE LIKELIHOOD OF RHEUMATIC DISEASE WITH IRITIS

| Author | Conclusion |
|---|---|
| Haarr | 34% of patients with acute iritis had AS |
| Beckingsale *et al.* | 60% of patients with HLA-B27-associated iritis had significant back pain |
| Saari *et al.* | 51% of HLA-B27-associated acute anterior uveitis had rheumatic disease |
| Russell *et al.* | 63% of paitents with acute anterior uveitis had sacroiliitis by radionuclide scan |
| Stanworth and Sharp | 42% of patients with nongranulomatous anterior uveitis had AS or RS |
| Pedersen | 33% of patients with acute anterior uveitis had rheumatic disease |
| Vinje *et al.* | 35% with acute anterior uveitis had radiographic sacroiliitis |
| Linssen *et al.* | 73% of HLA-B27-positive patients with acute anterior uveitis had rheumatic disease |
| Feltkamp | 90% of patients with HLA-B27-associated acute anterior uveitis had definite or possible AS |
| Rosenbaum | 84% of patients with HLA-B27-associated acute anterior uveitis had AS, RS, or incomplete RS |

**FIGURE 5-35.** Rhematic disease with iritis. Acute anterior uveitis has a strong association with spondyloarthropathies and with HLA-B27 even in the absence of any associated spondyloarthropathy. It is also associated with Crohn's disease and ulcerative colitis, with or without associated (enteropathic) arthritis. AS—Ankylosing spondylitis; RS—Reiter's syndrome. (From Rosenbaum [34]).

# References

1. Khan MA, ed: Ankylosing spondylitis and related spondyloarthropathies. *Spine: State of the Art Reviews* Philadelphia: Hanley & Belfus; 1990:

2. Khan MA, ed: Spondyloarthropathies. *Rheum Dis Clin North Am* 1992, 18:1–276.

3. Richens J, McGill PE: The spondyloarthropathies. *Baillieres Clin Rheumatol* 1995, 9:95–109.

4. van der Linden S: Ankylosing spondylitis. In: *Textbook of Rheumatology*, edn 5. Edited by Kelly WN, Harris ED, Ruddy S, Sledge CB. Philadelphia: WB Saunders; 1996:969–982.

5. Zeidler H, Mau W, Khan MA: Undifferentiated spondyloarthropathies. *Rheum Dis Clin North Am* 1992, 18:187–202.

6. Khan MA: Ankylosing spondylitis: Clinical features. In: Rheumatology, edn 2. Edited by Klippel JH, Dieppe PA. London: Mosby-Wolfe; 1994:3.25.1–3.25.10.

7. Khan MA: Seronegative spondyloarthropathies. In: *Textbook of Clinical Rheumatology*. Edited by Feng PH, Hwee-Siew H. Singapore: National Arthritis Foundation of Singapore; 1997 (in press).

8. Khan MA: HLA-B27 and its subtypes in world populations. *Curr Opin Rheumatol* 1995, 7:263–269.

9. Carlos Lopez-Larrea, ed: *HLA-B27 in the Development of Spondyloarthropathies*. Austin, TX: Chapman & Hall (RG Landes Company); 1997.

10. Burgos-Vargos R, Vasquez-Mellado J: The early clinical recognition of juvenile-onset ankylosing spondylitis and its differentiation from juvenile rheumatoid arthritis. *Arthritis Rheum* 1995, 38:835–844.

11. Olivieri I, Padula A, Pierro A, *et al.*: Late onset undifferentiated spondyloarthropathy. *J Rheumatol* 1995, 22:899–903.

12. Uppal SS, Pande I, Singh G, *et al.*: Profile of HLA-B27-related "unclassifiable" seronegative spondyloarthropathy in females and its comparison with the profile in males. *Br J Rheumatol* 1995, 34:137–140.

13. Dougados M, van der Linden S, Juhlin R, *et al.*: The European Spondyloarthropathy Study Group preliminary criteria for the classification of spondyloarthropathies. *Arthritis Rheum* 1991, 34:1218–1227.

14. Amor B, Dougados M, Listrat V, *et al.*: Are classification criteria for spondyloarthropathy useful as diagnostic criteria? *Rev Rhum (Engl Ed)* 1995, 6:10–15.

15. Collantes-Estevez E, Cisnal del Mazo A, Muñoz-Gomariz E: Assessment of 2 systems of spondyloarthropathy diagnostic and classification criteria (Amor and ESSG) by a Spanish multicenter study. European Spondyloarthropathy Study Group. *J Rheumatol* 1995, 22:246–251.

16. Hughes RA, Keat AC: Reiter's syndrome and reactive arthritis: a current view. *Semin Arthritis Rheum* 1994, 24:190–210.

17. Kingsley G, Sieper J: Third International Workshop on Reactive Arthritis, 23–26 September 1995, Berlin, Germany. *Ann Rheum Dis* 1996, 55:564–584.

18. Mielants H, Veys EM, DeVos M, *et al.*: The evolution of spondylarthropathies in relation to gut histology. I. Clinical aspects. *J Rheumatol* 1995, 22:2266–2278.

19. Leirisalo-Repo M, Turunen U, Stenman S, *et al.*: High frequency of silent inflammatory bowel disease in spondyloarthropathy. *Arthritis Rheum* 1994, 37:23–31.

20. Wollheim FA: Enteropathic arthritis. In: *Textbook of Rheumatology*, edn 5. Edited by Kelly WN, Harris ED, Ruddy S, Sledge CB. Philadelphia: WB Saunders; 1996:1006–1014.

21. Roberton DM, Cebral DA, Malleson PN, Petty RE: Juvenile psoriatic arthritis: Followup and evaluation of diagnostic criteria. *J Rheumatol* 1996, 23:166–170.

22. Cabral DA, Oen KG, Petty RE: SEA syndrome revisited: a longterm followup of children with a syndrome of seronegative enthesopathy and arthropathy. *J Rheumatol* 1992, 19:1282–1285.

23. Cassidy JT, Petty RE. *Textbook of Pediatric Rheumatology*, edn 3. Philadelphia: WB Saunders, 1996:

24. Khan M: Worldwide overview: The epidemiology of HLA-B27 and associated spondyloarthropathies. In: *The Spondyloarthropathies*. Edited by Calin A, Taurog J. Oxford Medical Press (in press) 1998.

25. Feltkamp TE: Factors involved in the pathogenesis of HLA-B27 associated arthritis. *Scand J Rheumatol Suppl* 1995, 101:213–217.

26. Robinson WP, van der Linden SM, Khan MA, *et al.*: HLA-Bw60 increases susceptibility to ankylosing spondylitis in HLA-B27 positive individuals. *Arthritis Rheum* 1989, 32:1135–1141.

27. Feltkamp TEW, Khan MA, de Castro JAL: The pathogenetic role of HLA-B27. *Immunol Today* 1996, 7:5–7.

28. D'Amato M, Fiorillo MT, Carcassi C, *et al.*: Relevance of residue 116 of HLA-B27 in determining susceptibility to ankylosing spondylitis. *Eur J Immunol* 1995, 25:3199–3201.

29. Gonzales-Roces S, Alvarez MV, Gonzalez S, *et al.*: HLA-B27 polymorphism and ankylosing spondylitis susceptibility in world populations. *Tissue Antigens* 1997 (in press).

30. Nasution AR, Mardjuadi A, Kunmartini S, *et al.*: HLA-B27 subtypes positively and negatively associated with spondyloarthropathy. *J Rheumatol* 1997 (in press).

31. Gran JT, Husby G: Ankylosing spondylitis in women. *Semin Arthritis Rheum* 1990, 19:303–312.

32. Resnick D, Niwayama G: Ankylosing spondylitis. In: *Diagnosis of Bone and Joint Disorders*, edn 3. Edited by Resnick D. Philadelphia: WB Saunders; 1995:1008–1074.

33. Khan MA, Kushner I: Diagnosis of ankylosing spondylitis. In: *Progress in Clinical Rheumatology*, vol. 1. Edited by Cohen AS. Orlando, FL: Grune and Stratton; 1984:145–178.

34. Rosenbaum JT: Acute anterior uveitis and spondyloarthropathies. *Rheum Dis Clin North Am* 1992, 18:143–51.

35. Tay-Kearney ML, Schwam BL, Lowder C, *et al.*: Clinical features and associated systemic diseases of HLA-B27 uveitis. *Am J Ophthalmol* 1996, 121:47–56.

36. Bergfeldt L, Insulander P, Lindblom D, *et al.*: HLA-B27: an important genetic risk factor for lone aortic regurgitation and severe conduction system abnormalities. *Am J Med* 1988, 85:12–18.

37. Sun JP, Khan MA, Farhat AZ, Bahler RC: Alterations in cardiac diastolic function in patients with ankylosing spondylitis. *Int J Cardiol* 1992, 37:65–72.

38. Gould BA, Turner J, Keeling DH, *et al.*: Myocardial dysfunction in ankylosing spondylitis. *Ann Rheum Dis* 1992, 51:227–232.

39. Aranson JA, Patel AK, Rahko PS, Sundstrom WR: Transthoracic and trans-esophageal echocardiographic evaluation of the aortic root and subvalvular structures in ankylosing spondylitis. *J Rheumatol* 1996, 23:120–123.

40. Rosenow EC III, Strimlan CV, Muhm JR, *et al.*: Pleuropulmonary manifestations of ankylosing spondylitis. *Mayo Clin Proc* 1977, 52:641–649.

41. Escalante A, Weaver WJ, Beardmore TD: An estimate of the prevalence of reactive systemic amyloidosis in ankylosing spondylitis (Letter). *J Rheumatol* 1995, 22:2192–2193.

42. Bruneau C, Villiaumeocy J, Avouac B, *et al.*: Seronegative spondyloarthropathies and IgA glomerulonephritis: a report of four cases and a review of the literature. *Semin Arthritis Rheum* 1986, 15:179–184.

43. Tullous MW, Skerhut HEI, Story JL, *et al.*: Cauda equina syndrome of long-standing ankylosing spondylitis. Case report and review of the literature. *J Neurosurg* 1990, 73:441–447.

44. Tyrrell PNM, Davies AM, Evans N: Neurological disturbances in ankylosing spondylitis. *Ann Rheum Dis* 1994, 53:714–717.

45. Thomas GH, Khan MA, Bilenker RM: Spontaneous atlantoaxial subluxation as a presenting manifestation of juvenile ankylosing spondylitis. *Spine* 1982, 7:78–79.

46. Khan MA, Lai J-H, Chou C-T, *et al.*: Spinal fractures in ankylosing spondylitis. *J Musculoskeletal Med* 1993, 10:45–57.

47. Miron SD, Khan MA, Wiesen E, *et al.*: The value of quantitative sacroiliac scintigraphy in detection of sacroiliitis. *Clin Rheumatol* 1993, 2:407–414.

48. Wittram C, Whitehouse GH, Williams JW, Bucknall RC: A comparison of MR and CT in suspected sacroiliitis. *J Comput Assist Tomogr* 1996, 20:68–72.

49. Ballow M, Braun J, Hamm B, *et al.*: Early sacroiliitis in patient with spondyloarthropathy: evaluation with dynamic gadolinium-enhanced MR imaging. *Radiology* 1995, 194:529–526.

50. Blum U, Buitargo-Tellez C, Mundinger A, *et al.*: Magnetic resonance imaging (MRI) for detection of active sacroiliitis—A prospective study comparing conventional radiography, scintigraphy, and contrast enhanced MRI. *J Rheumatol* 1996, 23:2107–2115.

51. Pettersson T, Laasonen L, Leirisalo-Repo M, Tervahartiala P: Spinal pseudoarthrosis complicating ankylosing spondylitis: a report of two patients. *Br J Rheumatol* 1996, 34:1319–1323.

52. Khan MA, Khan MK: Diagnostic value of HLA-B27 testing in ankylosing spondylitis and Reiter's syndrome. *Ann Intern Med* 1982, 96:70–76.

53. Arnett FC Jr, Khan MA, Wilkens RF: Are you missing ankylosing spondylitis? *Patient Care* 1986, 20(January 30): 51–78.

54. Al-Attra HM, Al-Amiri N: HLA-B27 in healthy adults in UAE: an extremely low prevalence in Emirian Arabs. *Scand J Rheumatol* 1995, 24:225–227.

55. Khan MA: Medical and surgical treatment of spondyloarthropathies. *Curr Opin Rheumatol* 1990, 2:592–599.

56. Toivanen A, Khan MA: Therapeutic dilemma in ankylosing spondylitis and related spondylarthropathies. *Rheum Rev* 1994, 3:21–27.

57. Dougados M, Amor BP, Khan MA: Management of severe forms of spondyloarthropathies, and recent therapeutic advances. *Rheum Dis Clin North Am* 1995, 21:117–128.

58. Lehtinen A, Lerisalo-Repo M, Taavitsainen M: Persistence of enthesopathic changes in patients with spondylarthropathy during a six month follow-up. *Clin Exp Rheumatol* 1995, 13:733–736.

59. Clegg DO, Reda DJ, Weisman MH, *et al.*: Comparison of sulfasalazine and placebo in the treatment of ankylosing spondylitis: a Department of Veterans Affairs cooperative study. *Arthritis Rheum* 1996, 39:2004–2012.

60. Creemers MCW, van Riel PLCM, Franssen MJAM, *et al.*: Second line treatment in seronegative spondylarthropathies. *Semin Arthritis Rheum* 1994, 24:71–81.

61. Creemers MCW, Franssen MJAM, van de Putte LBA, *et al.*: Methotrexate in severe ankylosing spondylitis: an open study. *J Rheumatol* 1995, 22:1104–1107.

62. Braun J, Bollow M, Seyrekbasan F, *et al.*: Computed tomography guided corticoid injection of the sacroiliac joint in patients with sacroiliitis: clinical outcome and followup by dynamic magnetic resonance imaging. *J Rheumatol* 1996, 23:659–664.

63. Khan MA, Khan MK, Kushner I: Survival among patients with ankylosing spondylitis: A life-table analysis. *J Rheumatol* 1981, 8:86–90.

64. Callahan LF, Pincus T: Mortality in the rheumatic diseases. *Arthritis Care & Research* 1995, 8:229–241.

65. Toivanen A: Reactive arthritis. In: *Rheumatology*. Edited by Klippel, J, Dieppe PA. St. Louis: Mosby, 1993:4.9.1–4.9.8.

66. Khan MA, van der Linden SM: Ankylosing spondylitis and other spondyloarthropathies. *Rheum Dis Clin North Am* 1990, 16:551–579.

67. Fan PT, Yu DTY: Reiter's syndrome. In: *Textbook of Rheumatology*, edn 5. Edited by Kelly WN, Harris ED, Ruddy S, Sledge CB. Philadelphia: WB Saunders; 1996:983–997.

68. Toivanen A, Toivanen P: Reactive arthritis. *Curr Opin Rheumatol* 1996, 8:334–340.

69. Khan MA, van der Linden SM: A wider spectrum of spondyloarthropathies. *Semin Arthritis Rheum* 1990, 20:107–113.

70. Khan MA: An overview of clinical spectrum and heterogeneity of spondyloarthropathies. *Rheum Dis Clin North Am* 1992, 18:1–10.

# 6

# Disease of Bone and Connective Tissue

MICHAEL J. MARICIC and MARCIA KO

Diseases of bone and connective tissue discussed include osteo-porosis, primary and secondary hyperparathyroidism and osteoma-lacia, Paget's disease of bone, osteonecrosis and avascular necrosis, hereditary disorders of collagen metabolism, and sclerotic bone disorders.

Osteoporosis is a systemic skeletal disease characterized by low bone mass and microarchitectural deterioration of bone tissue, leading to enhanced bone fragility and consequent increase in fracture risk [1]. It has become a major medical, economic, and social health problem in the United States, with more than 1.2 million fractures attributable to osteoporosis occurring each year. This includes 600,000 vertebral crush fractures and 250,000 frac-tures of the hip [2].

After hip fracture in the elderly, there is a 12% to 20% excess mortality rate in the next year caused by complications of immobi-lization (pneumonia, pulmonary embolus). Approximately 50% of elderly patients with hip fractures never regain the same level of functional independence, and 25% require long-term institutional care. The total direct and indirect annual costs for osteoporosis exceed $12 billion.

Osteomalacia is a syndrome caused by a number of specific disorders all characterized histologically ultimately by excessive unmineralized osteoid. To understand the early biochemical, histologic, and radiologic events in osteomalacia, however, it is important to understand these events in hyperparathyroidism, because most cases of osteomalacia (those caused by calcium or vitamin D deficiency) are accompanied by secondary hyper-parathyroidism.

Paget's disease of bone is a disorder of unknown etiology with a prevalence of approximately 3% in the adult population. The heri-table disorders of collagen metabolism are of great importance to rheumatologists and orthopedists because these patients frequently present with musculolskeletal symptoms. Recent advances in molecular genetics have continued to shed light on the genetic basis for these disorders.

Disorders that result in either local or generalized osteosclerosis are relatively rare. They may be due to genetic (osteopetrosis), neoplastic (lymphoma, multiple myeloma, systemic mastocytosis), metabolic (fluorosis, hypervitaminosis A or D, renal osteodystrophy, x-linked hypophosphatemic rickets), or idiopathic (Paget's disease, sarcoidosis) causes. Two major forms of osteopetrosis have been described: an autosomal dominant form with none or few symp-toms and an autosomal recessive type that is usually fatal during infancy. The basic metabolic disorder in all types involves defective osteoclast function leading to impaired bone resorption. In the autosomal form, most patients are symptomatic although patho-logic fractures, deafness, facial palsy, carpal tunnel syndrome, and osteoarthritis may occur.

## Epidemiology and Pathogenesis

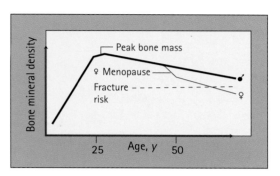

**FIGURE 6-1.** Bone density changes with age. Age related changes in bone density in both men and women are displayed. Bone density (as measured by dual energy x-ray absorptiometry) increases through childhood and adolescence, reaching its peak in the early part of the third decade of life. Bone density decreases rapidly in women immediately after menopause, owing to estrogen deficiency. As a result of this rapid loss, and because women usually have lower peak bone density than men, women are more likely to cross the theoretical "fracture risk threshold."

### RISK OF FRACTURE AFTER 50 YEARS OF AGE

| Fracture Site | Females | Males | Median Age |
|---|---|---|---|
| Proximal femur | 15.6% | 5% | 79 |
| Vertebra | 15%–32% | 5%–15% | > 70 |
| Distal radius | 15% | 2% | 66 |
| Any site | 40% | 13% | |

**FIGURE 6-2.** Lifetime risk of fracture after age 50. The lifetime risk of fracture for white men and women after age 50 is displayed. Black men and women have a substantially lower risk for all fractures. The risk of vertebral "deformities" varies depending on the criteria used to define them. Although previous studies suggested that vertebral deformities are much less common in men, recent studies suggest they may be equal. The lifetime risk of fracture for a postmenopausal woman is 40% to 50%. This includes a 1 in 6 risk of wrist fracture, a 1 in 6 risk of hip fracture, and 1 in 6 to 1 in 3 risk of vertebral fracture, depending on how this is identified and defined. The risk of hip fracture begins to rise after age 45, then rises exponentially, doubling for every 5 years of age.

### RISK FACTORS FOR OSTEOPOROSIS

Genetics

Race

Gonadal hormone deficiency

Lifelong calcium deficiency

Cigarette smoking

Excessive alcohol intake

Prolonged immobility

**FIGURE 6-3.** Risk factors for osteoporosis. Genetics accounts for 75% to 80% of the variance of bone mass and is the most important risk factor for developing osteoporosis. Whites and Asians have lower bone mass than blacks. Estrogen deficiency in women and testosterone deficiency in men lead to similar rapid bone loss. Cigarette smoking causes a lowering of bone density in both genders, in women by reducing estradiol levels and inducing earlier than normal menopause. Excessive alcohol intake (more than 1 drink a day) has been associated with reduced bone density. Although somewhat controversial, lifelong low calcium intakes have been associated with reduced bone density and increased fracture rates. An assessment of probability of the patient being osteoporotic may be made from reviewing the patient's risk factors. They are genetics (small body frame, family history of fractures), white or Asian race, estrogen deficiency, poor lifelong calcium intake, sedentary lifestyle, and excess alcohol or nicotine consumption. Multiple studies have now shown, however, that the ability to predict bone density (the best predictor of future fracture risk) from clinical risk factors is poor. The only way to know if a patient has low bone density and to assess their future risk for fracture is through the measurement of bone density.

### SECONDARY CAUSES OF OSTEOPOROSIS

| Endocrine | Neoplasm | Congenital | Miscellaneous |
|---|---|---|---|
| Hyperparathyroidism | Mulitple myeloma | Osteogenesis | Rheumatoid arthritis |
| Hyperthyroidism | Lymphoma | Homocystinuria | Gastrectomy |
| Cushing's syndrome | Mastocytosis | Gaucher's disease | Cirrhosis |
| Hypopituitarism | | | Renal failure |
| Hyperprolactinemia | | | Malabsorption (sprue) |

**FIGURE 6-4.** Secondary causes of osteoporosis. Disorders causing bone loss need to be excluded with a complete history, physical examination, routine laboratory tests such as a complete blood count, serum creatinine, calcium, phosphorus, and alkaline phosphatase. If abnormal, a secondary cause may be present. Because more than 100 disorders can lead to osteoporosis, secondary causes other than postmenopausal estrogen deficiency that need to be recognized include the endocrinopathies (hyperthyroidism, hyperparathyroidism, hypercortisolism, and premature sex hormone deficiencies), neoplastic diseases such as myeloma and lymphoma, and drug-induced causes (corticosteroids, heparin). A Z score (age-matched bone density) greater than 2 standard deviations below normal may also heighten suspicion of a secondary cause of osteoporosis and lead to further testing. (*See* Figs. 6-15 and 6-16 for an explanation of the Z score.)

## SECONDARY CAUSES OF OSTEOPOROSIS: DRUGS

Glucocorticoids
Excessive thyroid replacement
Anticonvulsants
Heparin
Methotrexate, cyclosporin A

**FIGURE 6-5.** Drugs as a secondary cause of osteoporosis. Bone loss with glucocorticoid usage is dose and duration dependent. Many studies suggest the greatest percentage of bone loss occurs within the first 6 months. Excessive thyroid replacement, as evidenced by a low thyroid-stimulating hormone assay, accelerates bone loss, even in clinically euthyroid individuals. Anticonvulsants such as phenytoin and phenobarbitol may lead to accelerated degradation of 25-hydroxyvitamin D. Long-term heparin use has been associated with severe osteoporosis in certain indivuduals. Methotexate and cyclosporin A have adverse effects on bone turnover in animal models, but their effects in humans are less clear.

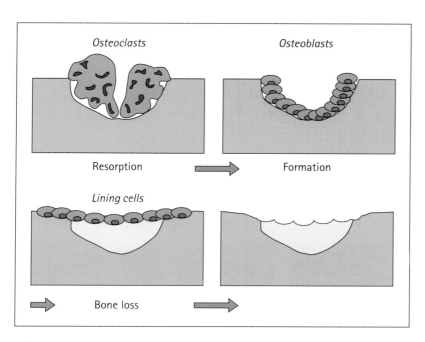

Osteoclasts — Osteoblasts

Resorption — Formation

Lining cells

Bone loss

**FIGURE 6-6.** Bone remodeling unit in osteoporosis. Bone remodeling normally occurs throughout the body in discrete packets called bone remodeling units. Trabecular bone, which accounts for 20% of the total bone mass, accounts for 80% of the turnover, due to its greater surface area. Eighty percent of bone mass is cortical bone, but this accounts for only 20% of total turnover. The normal remodeling unit in humans takes approximately 80 days. Bone is removed by osteoclasts. Osteoblasts lay down osteoid, which is then mineralized. In the patient with osteoporosis, the amount of new bone laid down is less than that removed.

## BIOCHEMICAL MARKERS OF BONE METABOLISM

| Bone Formation | Bone Resorption |
|---|---|
| Serum alkaline phosphatase | Urinary hydroxyproline |
| Serum bone-specific alkaline phosphatase | Urinary N-telopeptides |
| Serum osteocalcin | Urinary deoxypyridinoline |
| Serum type I collagen extension peptides | Serum tartrate-resistant acid Phosphatase |

**FIGURE 6-7.** Biochemical markers of bone metabolism. Biochemical markers of bone metabolism reflect bone turnover and are important in understanding pathophysiolgic states and studies of pharmacologic agents. Their use in following individual patients is currently an area of great interest. The serum bone-specific alkaline phosphatase and urinary collagen cross-links such as N-telopeptides and deoxypyridinoline appear to have the greatest sensitivity and specificity for following formation and resorption, respectively.

## Clinical and Radiologic Features

## CLINICAL FEATURES OF OSTEOPOROSIS

May be asymptomatic
Height loss
Dorsal kyphosis
Back pain
Restrictive lung disease
Protuberant abdomen with early satiety

**FIGURE 6-8.** Clinical features of osteoporosis. Patients with osteoporosis may have no warning signs until the first fracture occurs. Gradual height loss and dorsal kyphosis may result from microfractures or complete fractures of vertebral bodies. Acute back pain is caused by stretching of the periosteum, whereas chronic back pain derives from paraspinal muscles and other local soft tissues. Progressive thoracic kyphosis with encroachment of the ribs onto the pelvic brim may decrease the space available for abdominal contents and lead to gastrointestinal symptoms such as nausea and early satiety.

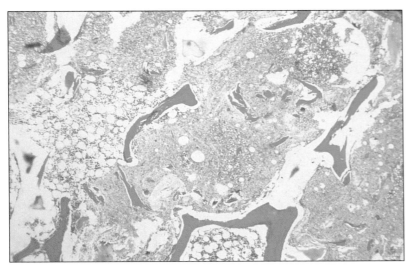

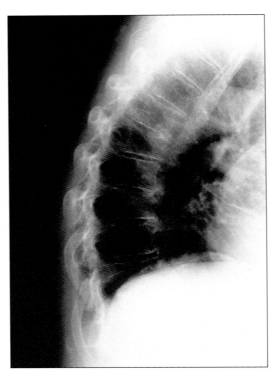

**FIGURE 6-10.**
Dorsal kyphosis and
osteopenia. Diffuse
osteopenia is present
in the thoracic spine.
In most vertebrae, no
trabeculae are visible.
In the upper verte-
brae, only vertical
striations are visible
because the hori-
zontal striations are
usually the first to
disappear. Although
no definite fractures
are seen, dorsal
kyphosis is present
due to anterior
wedging of multiple
vertebrae.

**FIGURE 6-9.** Histopathology of osteoporosis. This hematoxylin and
eosin-stained slide displays decreased bone mass from thinning of the
trabeculae and loss of microarchitectural connectivity, the two cardinal
features of osteoporosis. Both of these qualities lead to increased fragility
of bone and a subsequent increase in fracture risk. There is also an
increased number of fat cells seen among the marrow elements,
a common finding as trabecular bone volume decreases with age.

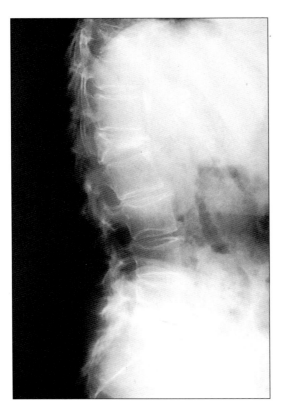

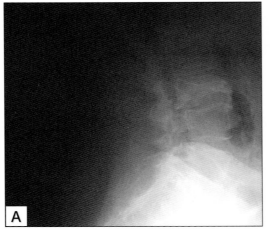

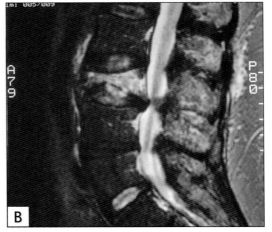

**FIGURE 6-12.** Burst fracture of L2. **A**, The L2 vertebral body displays fragmentation and
a through-and-through fracture. Burst fractures account for 1.5% of all spinal fractures and are
usually caused by a combination of axial loading with flexion. Posterior disruption or displacement
of the posterior vertebral margin, as seen in this radiograph, in association with an acute neurologic deficit (seen in about 40% of patients) are important clues to differentiate burst from usual
compression fractures. **B**, This magnetic resonance image from the same patient reveals cord
compression at the level of L2 caused by a retropulsed fragment and accompanying edema.
Because normal vertebral fractures involve only the anterior body, they do not result in acute
neurologic signs and symptoms. Radicular or cord symptoms or signs should alert the clinician
to the possibility of a burst fracture, especially in the patient with secondary osteoporosis. Burst
fractures often occur in the setting of secondary osteoporosis such as from glucocorticoid use or
multiple myeloma, but may also occur in postmenopausal osteoporosis, as in this patient.

**FIGURE 6-11.** Crush fracture, lumbar
vertebra. Diffuse osteopenia and a crush
fracture of L1 are present. Central end-plate
deformities of L3 and L4 are also present.

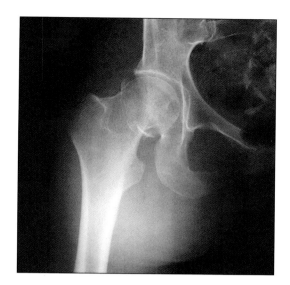

**FIGURE 6-13.** Femoral neck fracture. Hip fractures are usually classified as femoral neck (between the base of the femoral neck and intertrochanteric line), intertrochanteric (between the greater and lesser trochanters), or subtrochanteric. Femoral neck and intertrochanteric fractures account for over 90% of the hip fractures, occurring in roughly equal proportions. Femoral neck fractures are intracapsular fractures. The blood supply to the femoral head is frequently disrupted, which can lead to an increased frequency of complications (non-union and avascular necrosis).

## Bone Mineral Density Measurement

### COMPARISON OF AVAILABLE BONE DENSITY TECHNIQUES

| Site | DXA | QCT | pDXA | RA |
|------|-----|-----|------|-----|
| Precision | 1%–2% | 2%–4% | 1%–2% | 1%–2% |
| Accuracy | 3%–5% | 5%–15% | 2%–5% | 5% |
| Radiation dose (uSv) | 1–2 | 50 | <1 | 5 |

*Note: Annual background radiation equals approximately 2000 μSv*

**FIGURE 6-14.** Comparison of bone density tests. Dual energy x-ray absorptiometry (DXA) is currently considered the gold standard for measuring bone density because of its high precision and accuracy, low radiation, and ability to measure central sites such as the hip and spine [3]. Quantitative computed tomography (QCT) scans are able to discriminate trabecular bone better than the other techniques, which may be helpful in certain research applications. The radiation dose, however, is much higher than with other techniques. Peripheral techniques such as peripheral DXA (pDXA) and radiographic absorptiometry (RA) are highly precise and accurate. Their major limitation is their inability to measure central sites such as the hip and spine.

Bone mineral density as assessed by DXA has been able to predict the relative risk for future fracture of the hip and other bones. Large epidemiologic studies [4] have shown that for each 1 standard deviation (SD; approximately 10%) below a mean peak normal bone mass (T score on Hologic densitometer or young adult Z score on the Lunar), the risk of future spinal fracture is increased approximately twofold. The predictive value for low hip density is slightly higher at about 2.6-fold for each 1 SD decrease. When combined with a history of prevalent fracture after the menopause (which by itself increases future fracture risk) there is a synergistic increase in future fracture risk. The major value of obtaining bone mineral density in patients is to determine whether the patient has osteopenia significant enough to result in a nontraumatic fracture, to assess the relative risk of future fracture, and to follow response to treatment.

### WHO CRITERIA FOR OSTEOPOROSIS

| Diagnosis | T–Score |
|-----------|---------|
| Normal | ≥–1.0 SD |
| Osteopenia | –1.0 to –2.5 SD |
| Osteoporosis | ≤–2.5 SD |
| Severe osteoporosis | ≤–2.5 SD (with fragility fractures) |

**FIGURE 6-15.** Criteria for the diagnosis of osteoporosis. In 1993, a World Health Organization (WHO) consensus conference established criteria for the densitometric diagnosis of osteoporosis in postmenopausal women. A T score (comparison to peak normal mean bone density) above or better than -1 standard deviation (SD) is considered normal. A T score of worse than or below -2.5 SD represents osteoporosis. The intermediate category (between -1.0 and -2.5 SD) is labeled osteopenia, or low bone mass.

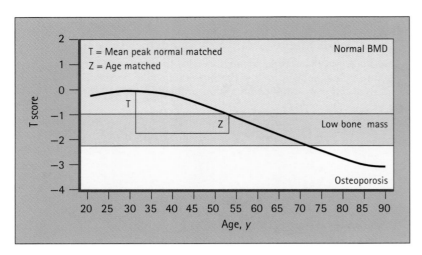

**FIGURE 6-16.** Bone density interpretation. Z scores are comparisons of the patient's bone density to sex-, race-, and age-matched controls. T scores are comparisons of the patient's bone density to subjects with mean peak normal bone density, matched for race and sex. T scores, rather than Z scores, are used for the densitometric diagnosis of osteoporosis. Using Z scores would imply that the prevalence of osteoporosis does not increase with age, which is incorrect. As seen here, approximately 50% of women aged 75 have osteoporosis, with the prevalence increasing with advancing age. BMD—bone mineral density.

## INDICATIONS FOR BONE DENSITY MEASUREMENT

1. In estrogen-deficient women, to make decisions about therapy
2. In patients with vertebral abnormalities or roentgenographic osteopenia, to establish a diagnosis of osteoporosis
3. In patients receiving long-term glucocorticoid therapy, to diagnose low bone mass to adjust therapy
4. In patients with primary asymptomatic hyperparathyroidism, to diagnose low bone mass to identify those at risk of severe skeletal disease who may be candidates for surgical intervention
5. To monitor response to treatment

**FIGURE 6-17.** Indications for bone density measurement. In general, bone density measurement should be performed only when it will influence therapeutic decisions. The results of bone density measurement have been shown to influence patient acceptance of hormone replacement therapy, and this would be the most common indication for its use. Dual energy x-ray absorptiometry (DXA) may also be extremely useful in the patient beginning long-term glucocorticoid use to categorize the patient's present risk of fracture and to aid in the tapering of glucocoritcoids or the use of prophylacitc agents. When using DXA to monitor response to treatment, because of the precision error of the test, only decreases of more than 5% should be considered significant for the purpose of changing treatment.

## Treatment

## NONPHARMACOLOGIC MANAGEMENT OF OSTEOPOROSIS

1. Patient education
2. Avoid smoking, excessive alcohol intake
3. Fall prevention intervention
4. Physical therapy
   a. Weight-bearing exercise
   b. Exercise to strengthen paraspinal muscles
   c. Balance and lower extremity strengthening

**FIGURE 6-18.** Nonpharmacologic management of osteoporosis. Management of osteoporosis begins with patient education. Risk factor reduction such as avoidance of nicotine and alcohol are mandatory. Fall prevention includes avoiding drugs that may cause sedation or hypotension, checking the patient for proper vision and hearing, and avoiding obstacles in the home that may cause falls. Physical therapy should be given to all patients, even those who have not yet sustained a fracture.

## PHARMACOLOGIC THERAPIES FOR OSTEOPOROSIS

Calcium
Vitamin D
Hormone replacement therapy
Calcitonin nasal spray
Bisphosphonates
SERMS

**FIGURE 6-19.** Pharmacologic therapies for osteoporosis. Medical treatment for osteoporosis should always begin with vitamin D (400 to 800 IU/d) and calcium (1000 mg/d) for premenopausal women and women on hormone replacement therapy (HRT), and 1500 mg/d for estrogen-deficient women and older men. HRT is currently the standard for prevention and treatment because of its global health benefits. Calcitonin nasal spray (200 IU/d) and alendronate (5 mg/d for prevention or 10 mg/d for treatment) are useful alternatives in women who cannot or will not take HRT, and bisphosphonates other than alendronate are likely to be soon approved. Selective estrogen replacement modulators (SERMS) may play a significant role in osteoporosis in the near future.

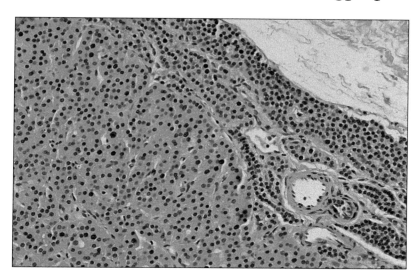

**FIGURE 6-20.** Parathyroid gland adenoma. Parathyroid adenomas are almost always solitary and usually located in the inferior glands. They are predominantly composed of chief cells that appear normal except for some variation in cell and nuclear size. In contrast to the normal gland, there is little or no stromal fat, and there is a rim of compressed normal parathyroid tissue compressed under a distinct capsule.

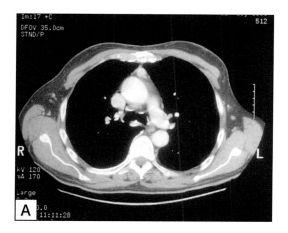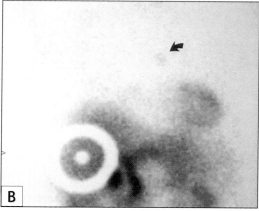

**FIGURE 6-21.** Parathyroid gland. **A**, a left inferior parathyroid adenoma seen as a left-sided retrosternal mass on the magnetic resonance image scan and **B**, an increased area of uptake (*arrow*) in the lower left area of the neck on sestimibi scan.

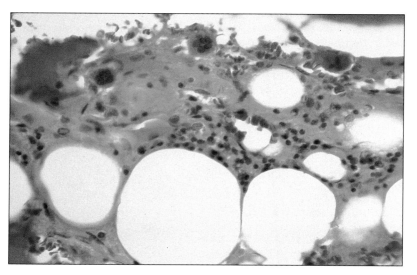

**FIGURE 6-22.** Hyperparathyroidism—osteoclasts. Three multinuclear osteoclasts are seen under but not immediately adjacent to bone. Underneath them is a large collection of fibrovascular tissue and fat. In hyperparathyroidism, cortical bone is much more severely affected than cancellous bone. Primary hyperparathyroidism is a fairly common disorder, with a prevalence of about 30/100,000. Although it has been most commonly diagnosed in the asymptomatic stage by chemistry screening in the recent past, changes in Medicare procedures for ordering these screens may result in patients presenting with more far advanced clinical disease in the future. These clinical manifestations would include osteopenia, renal stones, abdominal pain and mental status changes including depression [5].

## RADIOLOGIC FEATURES OF HYPERPARATHYROIDISM

Subperiosteal resorption
Endocortical scalloping
Thinning of cortical bone
Increased cortical porosity
Osteopenia

**FIGURE 6-23.** Radiologic features of hyper-parathyroidism. In both primary and secondary hyperparathyroidism, cortical bone is usually more commonly and severely affected than trabecular bone. Subperiosteal cortical resorption is virtually pathognomonic of hyper-parathyroidism. Intracortical resorption along Volkman's and haversian canals may cause both cortical thinning and porosity. Trabecular bone is also affected and may lead to diffuse osteopenia due to thinning and disappearance of trabeculae.

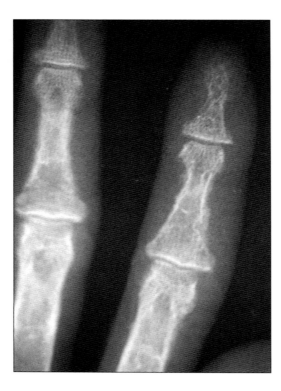

**FIGURE 6-24.** Hyperparathyroidism. Diffuse osteopenia, intracortical thinning, and subperiosteal resorption of the ulnar and radial aspects of the index middle phalanx are seen.

## Causes of Osteomalacia

### CAUSES OF OSTEOMALACIA

#### Calcium or Vitamin D Deficiency
Dietary
Gastrectomy
Small intestinal malabsorption (sprue)
Hepatobiliary disorders

#### Increased 25–hydroxyvitamin D Degradation
Anticonvulsants

#### Defective 1,25–dihydroxyvitamin D Synthesis or Action
Renal failure
Vitamin D-resistant rickets

#### Hypophosphatemia
Tumor-induced
X-linked hypophosphatemic rickets
Fanconi syndrome (partial or complete)

#### Mineralization inhibitor
Etidronate
Fluoride
Aluminum

#### Miscellaneous
Systemic acidosis
Hypophosphatasia

**FIGURE 6-25.** Causes of osteomalacia. Osteomalacia is a syndrome rather than a disease and as such demands a search for the primary etiology [6]. Insufficient dietary intake is not uncommon among the elderly, especially in nursing homes. Malabsorptive disorders such as sprue may be subtle and require a 24-hour urinary calcium determination to document malabsorption. Anticonvulsants such as phenobarbital and dilantin may cause osteomalacia in some but not all patients taking these medications because of increased hepatic degradation of 25-hydroxyvitamin D.

Hypophosphatemia may result from defective renal resorption of phosphorus or from oncogenous osteomalacia, which is usually also manifested by an inhibition of the conversion of 25-hydroxy into 1,25 dihydroxyvitamin D. Osteomalacia from inhibition of mineralization by etidronate, fluoride, or aluminum is rare, but should be searched for in the absence of more obvious etiologies.

Patients with osteomalacia often present with nonspecific bone pain due to insufficiency fractures especially in the areas of the ribs, pubis, or lesser trochanters. An elevated alkaline phosphatase level is an important clue that one may be dealing with osteomalacia rather than osteoporosis.

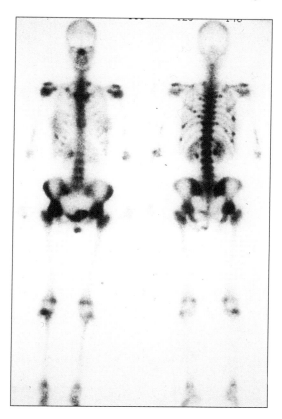

**FIGURE 6-26.**
Technetium bone scan. This technetium bone scan is remarkable for the presence of bilateral intense uptake in both trochanteric regions (representing insufficiency fractures or Looser's lines) and bilateral symmetric uptake in the ribs (pseudofractures). These rib fractures are usually spontaneous, and their presence should suggest osteomalacia rather than osteoporosis.

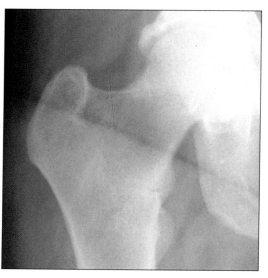

**FIGURE 6-27.** Looser's line. A Looser's line is seen as a horizontal lucency in the middle of the lesser trochanter. Looser's line represents insufficiency fractures through unmineralized osteoid in patients with osteomalacia.

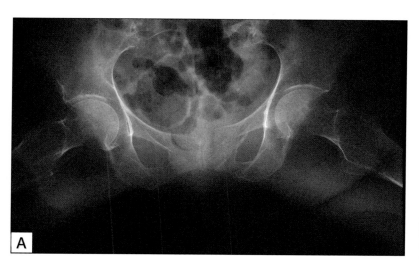
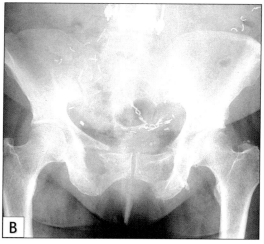

**FIGURE 6-28.** Pubic insufficiency fractures. **A,** A pubic insufficiency fracture is seen as a disruption of the cortex through the left pubic ramus. The patient was an elderly, homebound woman who was vitamin D insufficient. These fractures present with groin pain on weight bearing and may be confused clinically with intra-articular disease. **B,** Through-and-through fractures of both superior and inferior pubic rami are seen. This patient had received continuous daily etidronate for Paget's disease and developed severe osteomalacia. She had prolonged bilateral groin pain, with prior radiographs demonstrating nondisplaced pubic insufficiency fractures before they eventually became displaced.

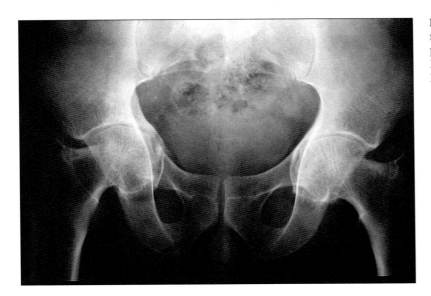

**FIGURE 6-29.** Protrusio acetabuli. Protrusio acetabuli is caused by medial or axial migration through the softened acetabular roofs in this patient with osteomalacia. Protrusion may be seen in osteomalacia, Paget's disease, or in inflammatory arthritides affecting the hip joint. Protrusio is not seen in osteoporosis.

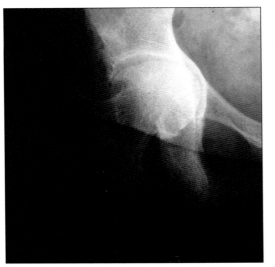

**FIGURE 6-30.** Osteomalacia simulating avascular necrosis. Flattening and collapse of the lateral portion of the femoral head may be due to insufficiency fractures from osteomalacia, as in this patient with severe renal tubular acidosis. Recognition of this appearance and the pathophysiologic basis of this collapse is important to differentiate it from avascular necrosis.

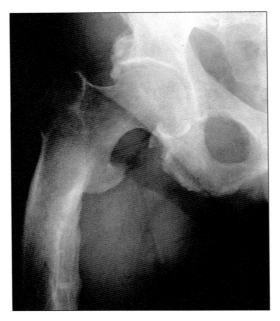

**FIGURE 6-31.** X-linked hypophosphatemic rickets. The typical radiographic features of this disease are demonstrated. There is bowing of the femoral shaft with healed insufficiency fractures on the concave surface of the midshaft. Ossification of entheses and sclerosis of the sacroilliac joints are present and may mimic ankylosing spondylitis.

# Paget's Disease of Bone

## *Histopathology*

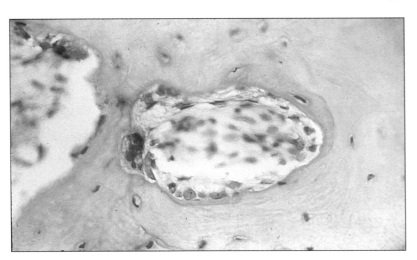

**FIGURE 6-32.** Giant osteoclast. An enlarged, multinucleated osteoclast is seen on this hemotoxylin and eosin-stained photomicrograph of bone. The osteoclasts are not only increased in size, but in numbers and activity as well. The osteoclast is believed to be the cell responsible for initiating the increased bone turnover seen in Paget's disease. The predominant current theory of the etiology of Paget's disease is a chronic viral infection leading to an increase in osteoclast number, size, and activity. Areas of intense osteolyisis are accompanied by a compensatory increase in osteoblastic bone formation. The bone formed is mechanically abnormal, however, leading to complications such as fracture and premature osteoarthritis in weight-bearing bones.

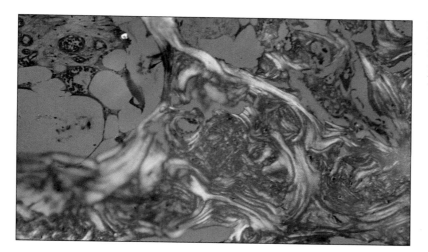

**FIGURE 6-33.** Woven bone in polarized light. Because of the greatly increased turnover of bone, the collagen fibrils are unable to achieve a normal lamellar pattern of adult bone. Instead, the fibrils are arranged in a haphazard fashion. With proper treatment, normalization of the lamellar pattern should ensue.

## Clinical Features and Complications

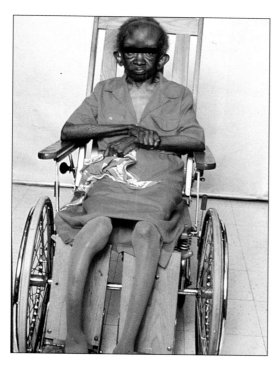

**FIGURE 6-34.** Clinical features. This patient displays many of the classic features of Paget's disease including severe bowing of the right lower leg, frontal bossing, and deafness as manifested by her hearing aid.

## Radiographic Features

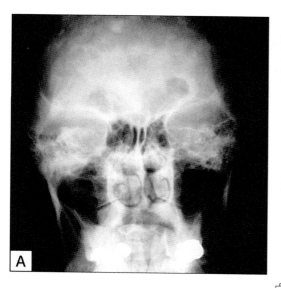

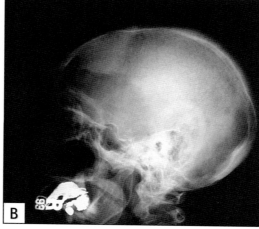

**FIGURE 6-35.** Skull radiographs. **A**, A typical mosaic pattern of areas of increased sclerosis and lucency is seen. The most common sites of involvement are the spine, pelvis, skull, and long bones of the lower extremities. Spinal complications include radiculopathies and direct cord compression secondary to enlargement of the neighboring bone. Skull involvement may lead to deafness from pagetic involvement of the ossicles or compresion of the eighth cranial nerve. **B**, In osteoporosis circumscripta, a well-demarcated zone of lucency in the frontal area is seen. This area would be intensely active on technetium bone scan.

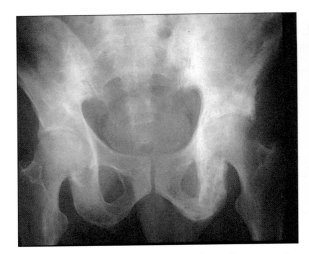

**FIGURE 6-36.** Pelvis radiograph. Diffuse pagetic involvement of the left hemipelvis is manifested by areas of mixed sclerosis and lucency. There is also pagetic involvement of the right hemipelvis near the right sacroiliac joint. Paget's disease also tends to enlarge affected bones, as seen in the greater size of the left compared with the right hemipelvis.

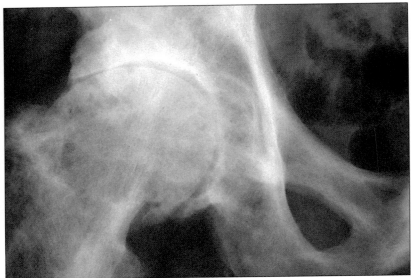

**FIGURE 6-37.** Hip joint radiograph. Symmetric joint space narrowing caused by Paget's disease is seen. Paget's disease may cause premature osteoarthritis when it affects weight-bearing joints. Such involvement is an indication for treatment, even if the patient is asymptomatic.

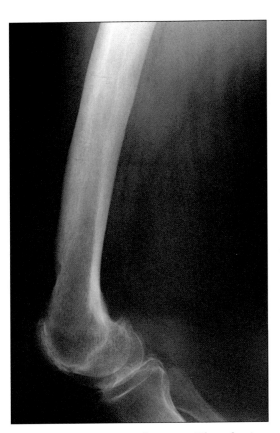

**FIGURE 6-38.** Stress fractures. Three horizontal insufficiency fractures are seen on the outer convex surface of the distal femur. The presence of these fractures is an indication for treatment, even if the patient is asymptomatic, because they may progress to complete fractures.

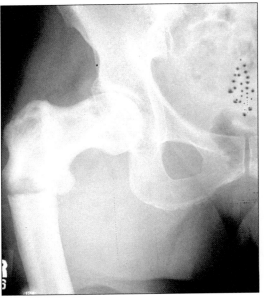

**FIGURE 6-39.** Pathologic fracture. A complete, horizontal subtrochanteric fracture through sclerotic pagetic bone is seen. This patient had no prior knowledge that she had Paget's disease before the fracture.

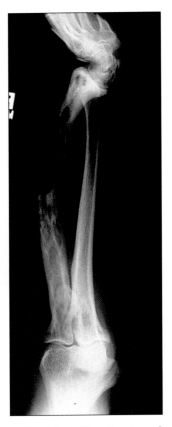

**FIGURE 6-40.** Bowing of radius. Bowing and deformity of non–weight-bearing bones such as the radius may occur in Paget's disease. The radiographic features of Paget's disease showing mixed sclerosis and lucency are present in the radius.

## INDICATIONS FOR TREATMENT OF PAGET'S DISEASE

Elevated alkaline phosphatase two times normal
Pain in an area of pagetic involvement
Skeletal deformity due to Paget's disease
Prevention of premature osteoarthritis when near joint
Osteolytic lesions of lower extremities
Hearing loss due to Paget's disease
Radiculopathy and cord compression due to Paget's disease
Hypercalcemia or high-output congestive heart failure (rare)

**FIGURE 6-41.** Indications for treatment. A common fallacy is that most patients with Paget's disease are asymptomatic and do not require treatment. In fact, most patients do have symptoms related to their pagetic involvement when carefully questioned. In those who do not, often they have other indications for treatment such as the prevention of hearing loss or premature osteoarthritis when Paget's disease involves the skull or weight-bearing joints, respectively.

## TREATMENT OF PAGET'S DISEASE

Injectable calcitonin

Etidronate

Alendronate

Tiludronate

Pamidronate (intravenous)

**FIGURE 6-42.** Treatment. With currently available therapies, the goal of treatment of Paget's disease is now normalization rather than a decrease of the alkaline phosphatase level [7]. Injectable calcitonin in doses of 50 to 100 units every day to three times a week is effective, but often inconvenient for many patients. Side effects include nausea and flushing (each about 20%). Etidronate, 400 mg/d for 6 months, followed by a rest period of not less than 3 months, is effective in many patients, and well tolerated orally. It does have the potential to induce osteomalacia if continued without pause. The oral bisphosphonates, alendronate (40 mg/d) and tiludronate (400 mg/d), should also be stopped for a rest period after 6 and 3 months, respectively. They do not cause osteomalacia, but they do have the potential to cause esophagitis if not taken correctly. Intravenous pamidronate is thought by many to be the drug of choice because of its increased potency and ease of administration (30 to 90 mg intravenously given for 1 to 3 days and repeated as necessary every 3 to 12 months).

# Osteonecrosis and Avascular Necrosis

## *Etiology and Staging*

## ETIOLOGIES OF AVASCULAR NECROSIS

**Traumatic**

Intracapsular femoral neck fracture
Hip dislocation

**Nontraumatic**

Glucocorticoids
Gaucher's disease
Sickle cell disease
Caisson's disease

## STAGING OF ISCHEMIC NECROSIS OF THE FEMORAL HEAD

| Stage | Findings |
|---|---|
| 0 | Suspected necrosis but no clinical findings and normal radiographs and bone scan |
| I | Clinical findings, normal radiographs, and abnormal bone scan |
| II | Osteopenia, cystic areas, and bone sclerosis on radiographs |
| III | Crescent sign and subchondral collapse without flattening of the femoral head on radiographs |
| IV | Flattening of the femoral head and normal joint space on radiographs |
| V | Joint space narrowing and acetabular abnormalities on radiographs |

**FIGURE 6-43.** Etiology of avascular necrosis. Although intertrochanteric hip fractures may sometimes lead to avascular necrosis, it is much more common with intracapsular femoral neck fractures. In addition to the nontraumatic etiologies listed here, others that are less well established include alcoholism, disorders of fat metabolism, systemic lupus erythematosus, and diabetes mellitus.

**FIGURE 6-44.** Staging of avascular necrosis. This is one of the staging systems for the progression of avascular necrosis. Staging systems are necessary for epidemiologic studies and to be able to compare the results of different treatments.

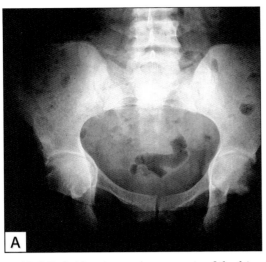

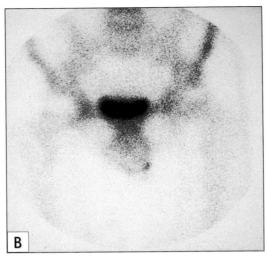

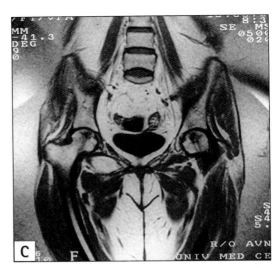

**FIGURE 6-45.** Avascular necrosis of the hip. **A**, The right hip displays flattening of the femoral head, consistent with stage IV avascular necrosis. **B**, A technetium bone scan displays decreased uptake in the right femoral head compared with the left. The decreased uptake is due the decreased blood flow in the acute stage of the disease. **C**, Magnetic resonance imaging reveals areas of decreased uptake on a T1-weighted scan, representing decreased blood flow to the femoral heads.

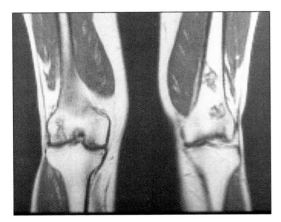

**FIGURE 6-46.** Bone infarcts in the femur. Multiple areas of decreased uptake on a T1-weighted magnetic resonance imaging scan in the distal femurs represent bone infarcts. This patient was taking high-dose glucocorticoids and developed sudden pain above both knees. Initial radiographs were normal.

# Disorders of Collagen Metabolism

## *Ehler-Danlos Syndrome*

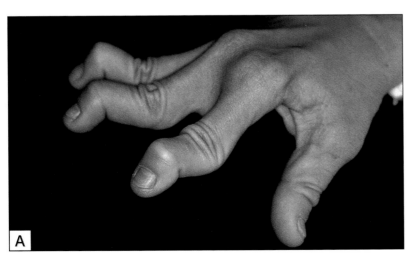

**FIGURE 6-47.** Joint hypermobility. Ehler-Danlos syndromes are disorders with wide phenotypic variability and genetic heterogeneity. Nine types have now been idenified based on genetic and phenotypic differences; however, a great deal of phenotypic variability is still seen within types. Type III (benign hypermobile joint syndrome) is the type most frequently encountered by clinicians. Patients present with complaints related to joint hypermobility. Blue-tinged sclerae, hyperextensible skin, varicosities, spontaneous pneumothorax, and mitral valve prolapse are among the extraskeletal manifestations. **A**, Spontaneous swan-necking of the fingers is shown. Swan-neck deformities are caused by laxity of ligaments and other soft tissue and are reversible in this disorder.

*(Continued on next page)*

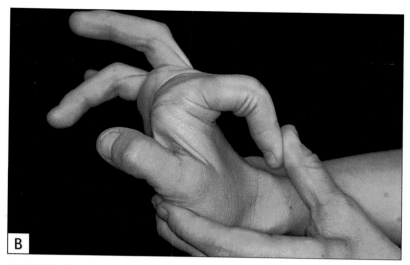

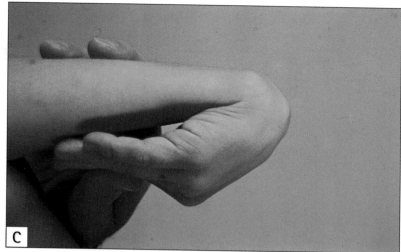

**FIGURE 6-47.** (*Continued*) **B**, Severe hyperextension of the metacarpophalangeal joint is displayed. **C**, Hyperflexion of the wrist is displayed.

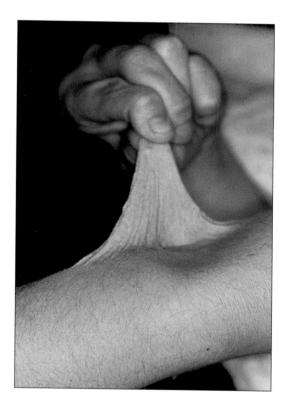

**FIGURE 6-48.** Hyperextensible skin. The skin is hyperextensible in Ehler-Danlos syndrome owing to the laxity of the collagen. Thin "cigarette-paper" scars may be another clue to the presence of this syndrome.

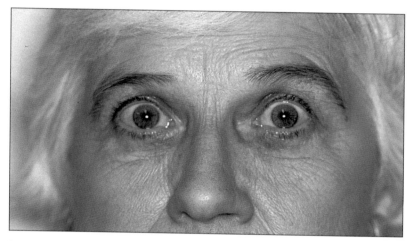

**FIGURE 6-49.** Blue sclerae. Blue-tinged sclerae are present. Blue sclerae may also be seen in osteogenesis imperfecta, which is a syndrome characterized by variable modes of inheritance, with a prevalence of at least 1 in 20,000. Abnormalities of type I collagen have been described. Type I osteogenesis imperfecta is the mildest form clinically and is characterized by autosomal dominant inheritance with variable penetrance. Type IV is also autosomal dominant, but skeletal fragility is usually more severe than in type I. Types II and III are autosomal recessive and clinically the most severe forms. Increased susceptibility to fractures, bowing of bones, premature hearing loss, and blue sclerae are among the clinical features.

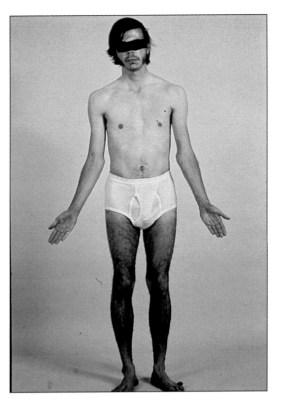

**FIGURE 6-50.** Clinical features. Many of the typical features of Marfan's syndrome are seen in this patient, including arm length greater than height, increased lower to upper extremity ratio, pectus excavatum, and pes planus. Marfan's syndrome is characterized by autosomal dominant inheritance and has a prevalence of 1 in 20,000. A disorder of fibrillin, a glycoprotein abundant in the aortic media, skin, and ciliary zones, has recently been implicated as the most likely cause of this disorder. Musculoskeletal features include limbs disproportionately long for trunk size (dolichostenomelia), arachnodactyly, pectus excavatum or carinatum, scoliosis, pes planus, and joint hypermobility. Serious extraskeletal features include dilation of the aortic root (leading to aortic dissection) and upward subluxation of the lens.

## Sclerotic Bone Disorders

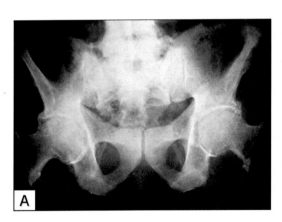

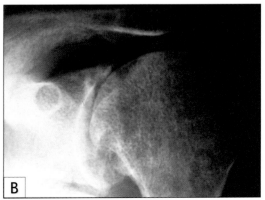

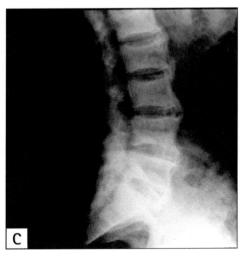

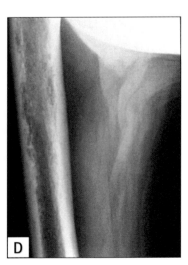

**FIGURE 6-51.** Fluorosis. Many of the typical radiographic features of fluorosis are displayed. Osteosclerosis is a typical feature and is present in the spine and sacrum (**A**), and in the glenoid fossa (**B**). The lateral spine (**C**) displays ossification of anterior longitudinal ligament. Ossification of entheses is a typical finding. The long bone (**D**) shows severe endocortical scalloping and intracortical porosity, features of hyperparathyroidism. Secondary hyperparathyroidism often accompanies fluorosis because of the rapid increase in osteoid formation and demand for calcium. Flouride may cause osteosclerosis after chronic ingestion. Diffuse bone pain (often from insufficiency fractures), joint stiffness, and a brownish mottling of the teeth are often seen clinically. Osteosclerosis, mainly of cancellous bone, and a tendency for ossification of entheses are seen on radiographs.

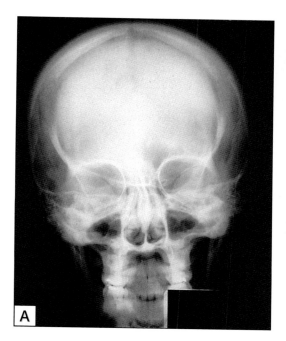

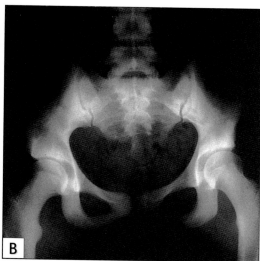

**FIGURE 6-52.** Osteosclerosis of the skull (**A**) and pelvis (**B**). Osteosclerosis is a genetic disorder caused by a failure of osteoclasts to differentiate from their normal hematopoetic precursors. As a result, bone cannot be resorbed, and severe thickening ensues.

# References

1. Kanis JA, Melton LJ, Christiansen C, Johnston CC, *et al.*: Perspective: the diagnosis of osteoporosis. *J Bone Min Res* 1994, 8:1137–1141.

2. Melton LJ III, Chrishchilles EA, Cooper C, Lane AW, *et al.*: How many women have osteoporosis? *J Bone Miner Res* 1992, 7(9):1005–1010.

3. Miller PD, Bonnick SL, Rosen CJ, *et al.*: Clinical utility of bone mass measurement in adults: consensus of an international panel. *Sem Arthritis Rheum* 1996, 25:361–372.

4. Ross PF, Davis JW, Epstein RS, Wasnich RD: Pre-existing fractures and bone mass predict vertebral fracture incidence in women. *Ann Intern Med* 1991, 114:919–923.

5. Silverberg SJ: Diagnosis, natural history, and treatment of primary hyperparathyroidism. *Cancer Treat Res* 1997, 89:163–181.

6. Francis RM, Selby PL: Osteomalacia. *Baillieres Clin Endocrinol Metab* 1997, 11(1):145–163.

7. Delmas PD, Meunier PJ: The management of Paget's disease of bone. *N Engl J Med* 1997, 336:558–566.

# 7

# Infectious Arthritis

## LEONARD SIGAL

Patterns, both spatial and temporal, and clinical associations are often the evidence that suggests and confirms specific diagnoses in rheumatology. This is certainly true in differentiating among the various infectious arthritides, where little about the examination of the affected joint is unique or pathognomonic. Among coincident physical findings, cutaneous lesions are often the clues that suggest the correct diagnosis. Radiographic patterns of abnormalities also can provide useful hints, but such changes may be significantly delayed, rendering them irrelevant to the diagnostic process.

Infectious arthritis can occur in a normal joint, but prosthetic or previously inflamed and damaged or surgically "invaded" joints are predisposed to infection. The infection may spread from an adjacent osteomyelitis, a local penetrating wound (or needle puncture), or bacteremia (hematogenous spread from a primary focus, *eg*, sinusitis, pneumonia, gastrointestinal or genitourinary infections, intravenous drugs, bed sores, sepsis, prior colonoscopy or cystoscopy). Immunologically compromised patients, such as those with underlying neoplasm, alcoholism, diabetes mellitus, malnutrition, or chemotherapeutic agents, develop septic arthritis more often than do immunocompetent individuals.

The clinical presentation can differ markedly depending on age. Neonates and small children may present with a systemic sepsis syndrome and minimal local symptoms, whereas older children may have local complaints and signs. Adults often present with severe local pain and fever.

Thus, it is often only by considering the entire clinical syndrome and the demographic and surrounding societal milieu that clinicians can render a correct judgment about diagnosis, therapy, and prognosis.

## BACTERIAL ARTHRITIS: WHICH ORGANISM TO SUSPECT?

| Organism | Age, (y) | | | |
|---|---|---|---|---|
| | < 2 | 2–15 | 16– 50 | >50 |
| Staphylococcus | 40% | 50% | 15% | 75% |
| Streptococcus | 25% | 35% | 5% | 10% |
| Haemophilus | 30% | 2% | — | — |
| Gonococcus | — | 5% | 75% | — |
| Gram-negative | 3% | 5% | 5% | 10% |

**FIGURE 7-1.** Bacterial arthritis. The demographics of the patient, especially age, can help to predict the organism causing septic arthritis. Nongonococcal infectious arthritis is usually monoarticular, most often affecting the large joints. Pain, often followed by swelling, is relatively abrupt in onset. Local signs of inflammation are usually present,

although constitutional complaints can overshadow local features. Any delay in diagnosis and effective treatment can increase the likelihood and severity of joint damage, especially if the infection is with a virulent organism. First and foremost in the evaluation of such patients is analysis of the synovial fluid: culture, Gram stain (positive in 50%–75% of cases), cell count (10,000–30,000 cells/mm$^3$ early in the septic process; 50,000–100,000 cell/mm$^3$ later, usually with neutrophil predominance), glucose and protein determinations, and examination for intracellular crystals. The only contraindication to this rule is surrounding or overlying soft tissue infection; it is usually unwise to penetrate an area of cellulitis to tap a joint. Because cellulitis and bursitis do not penetrate an intact joint capsule, differentiating between these and septic arthritis is crucial (see Figure 7-3). Blood cultures may be positive in up to 50% of patients with nongonococcal septic arthritis. Radiographs are normal in the earliest stages of septic arthritis, although they may be useful to rule out trauma and act as a baseline. Bone scans are positive 4 to 7 days after the onset of infection, but they are not specific and so are not especially useful except for sacroiliac joint infections, where the diagnosis may be obscure.

## COMPARISON OF GONOCOCCAL ARTHRITIS AND OTHER BACTERIAL ARTHRITIDES

| Gonococcal Dermatitis or Arthritis Syndrome | Nongonococcal bacterial arthritis |
|---|---|
| Usually young healthy adults | Often elderly, very young, debilitated, immune compromised, intravenous drug users |
| Initial migratory polyarthralgia | Polyarthralgia uncommon |
| Tenosynovitis in majority (66%) | Tenosynovitis rare |
| Dermatologic lesions common (33%–50%) | Dermatologic lesions rare |
| Polyarthritis in about 30% | Monoarthritis in > 85% |
| Oligoarthritis in about 30% | |
| Monoarthritis in about 40% | |
| Blood cultures positive in <10% | Blood cultures positive in about 50% |
| Synovial fluid culture positive in 25% | Synovial fluid culture positive in 90% |
| Usually rapid response, 2–4 d | Slow response, pain may last 10 d |

**FIGURE 7-2.** Comparison of gonococcal arthritis and other bacterial arthritides. Gonococcal arthritis presents in a demographic group different from the typical, and with a distinct clinical syndrome and associated findings more frequently than does nongonococcal bacterial arthritis.

## DIFFERENTIAL DIAGNOSIS OF SEPTIC ARTHRITIS

1. Periarthritis (periarticular inflammatory disease), eg, cellulitis, bursitis
2. Osteomyelitis
3. Trauma; disruption of internal structures, eg, menisceal or ligamentous tear; fracture
4. Crystal-induced inflammation, eg, monosodium urate (gout), calcium pyrophosphate dihydrate ("pseudogout")
5. Intra-articular hemorrhage: hemophilia or other bleeding disorders, hemorrhage may follow inapparent or otherwise trivial trauma
6. Viral—often polyarticular; often with a rash
7. Tuberculosis—chronic, monoarthritis, insidious onset, minimal inflammatory changes (see section on mycobacteria)
8. Presentation of chronic rheumatologic disease, eg, reactive, psoriatic, or, rheumatoid arthritis

**FIGURE 7-3.** Differential diagnosis of septic arthritis. When evaluating a patient with a painful and inflamed joint, where septic arthritis is a consideration, the processes listed would be included within the differential diagnosis. Spinal septic arthritis (septic diskitis) should be suspected in patients with chronic unrelenting back pain, fever, and marked local spine tenderness. Children with septic diskitis may present with no local pain, but refuse to walk. The thoracolumbar region is most commonly affected. The infection usually crosses the disk space on imaging studies, a finding that differentiates septic diskitis from malignancy.

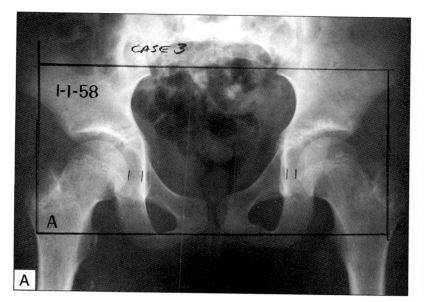

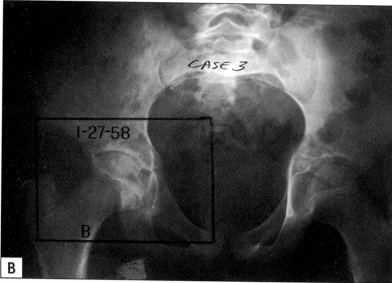

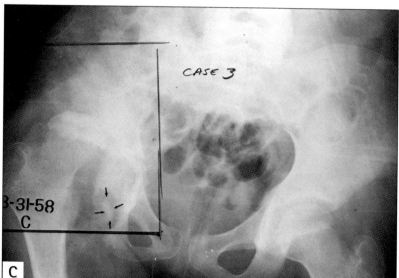

**FIGURE 7-4.** Progressive changes in a septic hip (*Staphylococcus aureus*). **A**, Note increased distance between the femoral epiphysis and acetabulum on the right compared with the left due to increased volume of synovial fluid. **B**, Four weeks later, there is frank destruction of bone and cartilage. The process now involves the proximal femur, the ilium, and the ischium. **C**, At 3 months after onset, additional destruction has caused dislocation of the hip with resultant avascular necrosis of the femoral head. A sequestrum is noted in the ischium (*arrows*). (*Courtesy of* American College of Radiology teaching collection. Used with permission.)

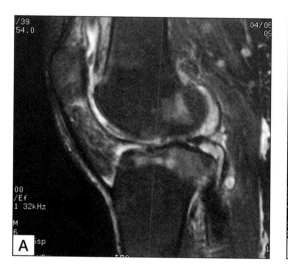

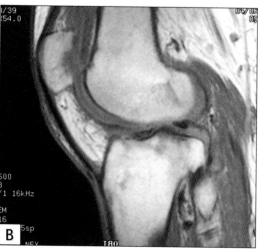

**FIGURE 7-5.** Changes of septic arthritis on magnetic resonance imaging (MRI). This MRI of the right knee was performed with a 1.5 Tesla magnet. Images include axial, sagittal, and coronal proton density and fast spin echo T2-weighted images. No joint effusion is seen, although there is a focal fluid collection superficial to the medial collateral ligament. Synovial proliferation with internal debris is seen. **A**, Osseous structures demonstrate edema on both sides of the joint (most notable in the posterior aspect of the lateral tibial condyle), compatible with septic arthritis. Focal loculation of fluid seen between the tibial spines appears to be eroding bone and may represent focal erosion related to the septic arthritis. **B**, Similar changes as in *A* also increased signal intensity within the posterior horn of the medial meniscus, extending to the inferior articular surface, represents a complex tear. (*Courtesy of* Robert Epstein, MD.)

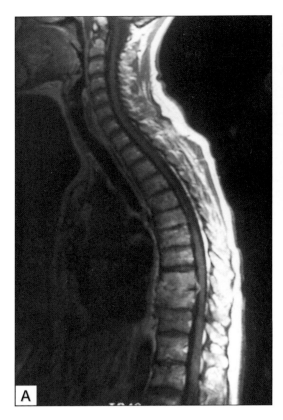

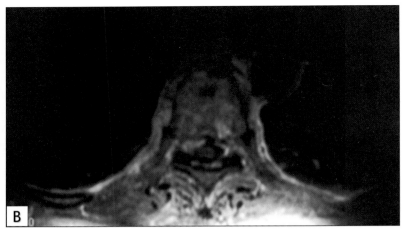

**FIGURE 7-6.** Findings characteristic of infectious spondylitis. Magnetic resonance image of the thoracic spine was performed on a 1.5 Tesla unit. T1-weighted and proton density and T2-weighted images of the cervical and thoracic spine are in the sagittal orientation. T1-weighted images were also obtained after administration of intravenous gadolinium. **A,** The thoracic spine disk demonstrates destructive changes with heterogeneous signal on T1-weighted image and patchy increase signal intensity on T2-weighted image. **B,** Associated end plates also demonstrate increased signal intensity on T2-weighted images. Soft tissue extends circumferentially in the paraspinal region with a right posterior epidural component. Thus, this process extends both anteriorly and posteriorly to the vertebral body disk complex. The disk demonstrates enhancement in patchy fashion after administration of contrast material. The soft tissue paraspinal component demonstrated profuse enhancement in a smooth circumferential fashion wrapping around the vertebral body. (*Courtesy of* Robert Epstein, MD.)

# Viral Arthritides

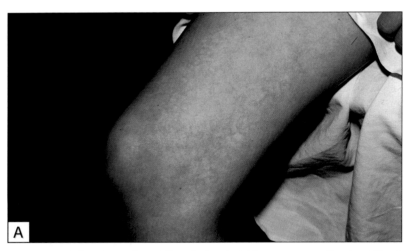

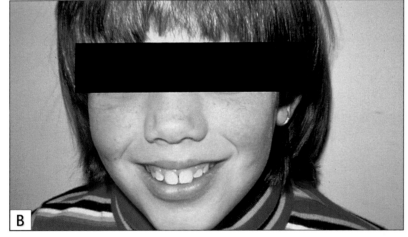

**FIGURE 7-7.** Parvovirus. The viral arthritides are generally short-lived (usually less than 6 weeks duration) and often affect females. The arthritides are often asymmetric, although bilateral symmetry can occur. The American College of Rheumatology criteria for the diagnosis of rheumatoid arthritis requires a duration of disease sufficiently long to make viral etiology unlikely [1].

Parvovirus is a small single stranded DNA virus that grows in rapidly proliferating cells, such as activated lymphocytes and erythroid precursors. The most common features of parvovirus infection are a nonspecific febrile illness and erythema infectiosum (also known as fifth disease or "slap cheek fever"). Other clinical features of parvovirus infection include aplastic anemia in sickle cell disease and other chronic hemolytic anemias and hydrops fetalis.

Arthritis occurs in up to 5% of children infected with parvovirus; arthralgias occur in about 8%. Parvovirus in adults can cause acute and occasionally persistent arthritis. About 50% of adults with infection experience arthritis (60% of women and 30% of men); arthralgias occur in 80% of adults.

Pain and stiffness can be short-lived (median duration 10 days), but a symmetrical polyarthropathy may persist for longer and may recur. The small joints of the hands, wrists, elbows, hips, knees, and feet are each involved in over 50% of cases.

A common historical feature in patients with parvovirus-induced arthritis is exposure to children with a recent febrile illness (fifth disease); affected women may have young children of their own or work with children as teachers, health care providers, or day care workers. Parvovirus should be suspected with such a history. Over half the normal adult population has measurable serum IgG antibodies to parvovirus, suggesting prior exposure. Detection of IgM, produced only in early disease, is a marker of recent infection and therefore strong evidence in favor of parvovirus being the cause of recent-onset arthritis.

**A,** Maculopapular erythematous rash is present on the legs of a patient with parvovirus infection. **B,** "Slap cheeks" are seen on the face of this child with acute parvovirus infection. (*A courtesy of* Paul Honig, MD; *B courtesy of* SYNTEX. Used with permission.)

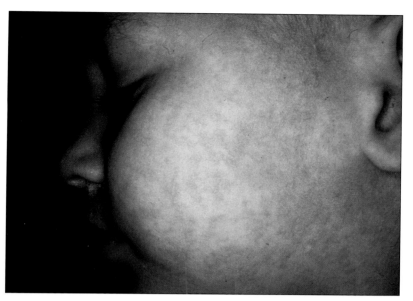

**FIGURE 7-8.** Facial rash of rubella in a child. This member of the Togavirus family is a spherical virus containing single-stranded RNA. Infection can be manifest as a mild febrile illness with a maculopapular erythematous rash and lymphadenopathy. The rash usually starts on the face and extends to the trunk and extremities, sparing the palms and soles. Rubella arthritis usually occurs in women between ages 20 and 40 (women outnumber men by 5–8:1) in a bilaterally symmetric distribution, affecting the small joints of the hands, knees, wrists, ankles, and elbows, in descending order of frequency. The onset of the arthritis is rapid, usually occurring with the rash, although the arthritis may occur up to 6 days before or 6 days after the onset of the rash. Although rubella arthritis may last up to a year, it usually resolves within 2 weeks. Use of the RA 27/3 rubella vaccine has been associated with arthritis in about 15% of female recipients, starting 1 to 4 weeks after vaccination. Unlike natural infection, vaccine-associated arthritis has been reported to recur. (*Courtesy of* Bill Witmer, MD.)

# Mycobacteria

## *Mycobacterium Tuberculosis*

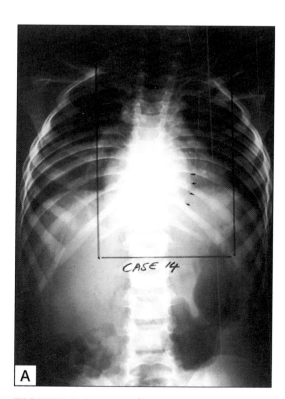

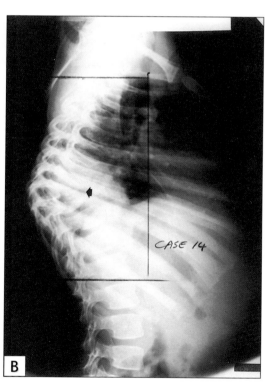

Tuberculous spondylitis starts as a subchondral infection, with spread to the vertebral body and joint space. The infection can extend along the axis of the spine to affect other vertebral bodies. The lower thoracic and the upper lumbar spine account for more than 75% of cases, with involvement of the sacral or cervical spine rare. Local signs of inflammation are usually absent. Patients may complain of pain worsened by movement, developing slowly over many months, but fever, malaise, and weight loss are rare. In late disease, patients may first present with spine deformity and even neurologic dysfunction from spinal cord compression. The first change on radiography is erosion of the anterior part of the vertebral body; subsequently symmetric end plate erosion and narrowing of the intervertebral disk space may occur. Bone destruction can cause wedging, vertebral collapse, and deformity in more advanced infection. Paraspinal abscess develops in up to 65% of patients, although this is uncommon in the lumbar spine. Especially in disease of short duration, computerized tomography and magnetic resonance imaging may be useful in documenting changes not seen on routine radiographs.

**FIGURE 7-9.** Pott's disease. Current estimates are that 15% of all new cases of tuberculosis in the United States will present with other than pulmonary disease; of these 10% will present with disease of the joints or bones. The best known articuloskeletal manifestation of tuberculosis is Pott's disease (tuberculous spondylitis), accounting for 50% of cases (peripheral arthritis occurs in about one-third and osteomyelitis/dactylitis, tenosynovitis/bursitis, and Poncet's disease in the remainder).

Spread from the primary site of infection to bones or joints occurs via hematogenous, lymphatic, or contiguous routes. The most common identified primary site is still the lungs, although only about 30% of patients have radiographic evidence of pulmonary tuberculosis at presentation. In about 20% of patients, the genitourinary tract is the original site of infection; no initiating site is found in the remaining 50% of patients.

**A**, PA and **B** lateral radiographs. These A—P and lateral radiographs are of tuberculous osteomyelitis of the spine with a paravertebral abscess in a child. Collapse of the 8th, 9th, and 10th thoracic vertebral bodies has caused a gibbous deformity. Note the sparing of the posterior vertebral elements. Lateral and anterior extension of the large paravertebral abscess is seen. (*Courtesy of* American College of Radiology.)

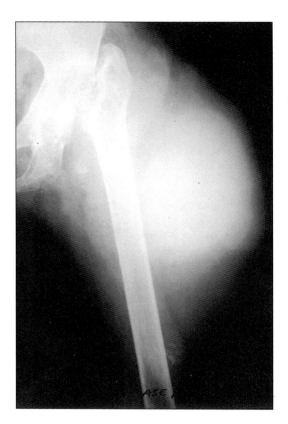

**FIGURE 7-10.** Tuberculous arthritis. Tuberculous arthritis affects the weight-bearing joints, usually the knee or hip. A monoarthritis in about 90% of cases, it affects the metaphysis, synovium, and capsule and may extend into nearby extra-articular structures. The arthritis is usually insidious, with little local inflammation, and causes minimal if any constitutional symptoms. Marked swelling of the joint is due to synovial hypertrophy and effusion and may overshadow pain. The diagnosis may be long delayed due to the paucity of symptoms as well as the fact that most physicians do not consider tuberculosis as part of the differential diagnosis of arthritis. Infection may be more virulent or multifocal in patients who are immunosuppressed or malnourished.

There may be significant bony destruction despite the minimal symptoms. Early in infection soft tissue swelling and periarticular osteopenia occur. After several weeks there may be haziness of the subchondral bone surface and poorly delineated marginal erosions. Joint space narrowing and joint destruction are late changes, occurring only after several months of untreated infection. Synovial fluid reveals 10,000 to 20,000 white cells/mm$^3$. Synovial biopsy shows changes strongly suggesting tuberculosis in the overwhelming majority of cases, with caseating granulomata and multinucleated giant cells. The diagnosis can usually be confirmed by culture of synovial tissue or fluid, the latter much less likely to grow the organism than the former.

This radiograph shows tuberculosis of the hip with extensive destruction of the femoral head and neck and little reactive bone sclerosis. Protrusio acetabuli, due to bone resorption, is present. Loculated collections of exudate are found within a large cold abscess in the thigh. (*Courtesy of American College of Radiology.*)

# Gonococcal Arthritis

## *Disseminated Gonococcal Infection Syndrome*

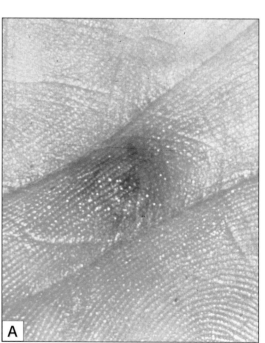

A

**FIGURE 7-11.** Cutaneous lesions of disseminated gonococcal (*Neisseria gonorrhea*) infection. There are over one million cases of gonococcal infection in the United States per year and 1% to 3% of these will disseminate. In disseminated cases, the female to male ratio is between 2 and 4:1. Gonococcal arthritis is most common in women between the ages of 15 and 30 years. The onset of gonococcal arthritis is within 1 week of menses in about two-thirds of affected women. Although recurrent, severe, difficult to treat, familial cases of disseminated gonococcal infection may be due to terminal complement component deficiencies. These account for only about 5% of all cases. Disease in children should suggest sexual abuse. Gonococcal arthritis is increasingly common in homosexual men.

The primary focus of infection is usually the genitourinary tract, but it may be the pharynx or anus. Dissemination can lead to perihepatitis (Curtis-FitzHugh syndrome, thought to be due to spread by direct continuity from the fallopian tube, although it has occurred in women with prior tubal ligations), hepatitis, meningitis, endocarditis, myocarditis, and other distant foci of infection.

The incidence of uncomplicated gonococcal urogenital infection varies with the population studied: 1.6% in private family planning clinics to 19% in venereal disease clinics, with the greatest risk being among young nonwhite single females and those of lower socioeconomic status. If gonococcus is grown or suspected, testing for syphilis, chlamydia, and human immunodeficiency virus infection should also be performed. Gonococcus can be cultured from many women and men with no urogenital symptoms.

(*Continued on next page*)

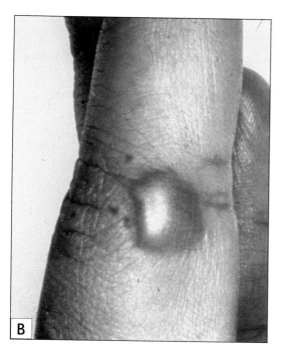

**FIGURE 7-11.** (*Continued*) Disseminated gonococcal infection can be associated with musculoskeletal problems (*see also* Figure 7-2). Gonococcal arthritis usuallly presents with migratory or diffuse arthralgias and low-grade fever. In the following few days mono- or oligoarthritis may occur, mainly affecting large joints, especially the knee, wrist, and ankle. During this phase, blood cultures are rarely positive. Synovial fluid cultures are positive in only about one-third of patients, although the yield from the genital tract may be up to 75%. In some patients the first feature may be an isolated mono- or oligoarthritis in an otherwise well person. Monoarthritis occurs in about one-third of cases and migratory polyarthritis, tenosynovitis, and ultimately mono- or oligoarthritis constitutes the remaining two-thirds of affected individuals.

During the bacteremic phase of disseminated gonococcal infection cutaneous lesions occur. Although occasionally difficult to find, these lesions may be invaluable in suggesting the correct diagnosis. Painless macular, papular, vesicular, pustular, or necrotic skin lesions, especially affecting the distal limbs, may be found early in the bacteremic phase, commonly in association with tenosynovitis and fever. Occasionally, the organism is found in a pustule, seen by Gram stain or in culture. Blood cultures may be positive in up to 40% of these patients.

A pustule with central necrosis **A** and a bullous lesion **B** are shown. (*Courtesy of* American College of Rheumatology. Used with permission.)

## Disseminated Meningococcal Infection

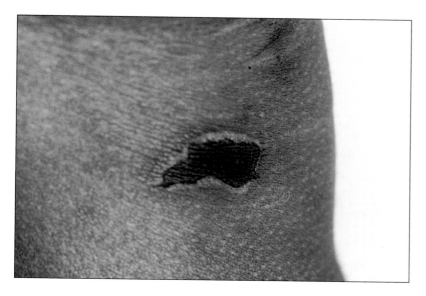

**FIGURE 7-12.** Cutaneous lesions of disseminated meningococcal infection. A syndrome similar to that of disseminated gonococcal infection, complete with similar skin lesions, can be seen in disseminated infection with *Neisseria meningitidis*. A necrotic lesion due to disseminated meningococcal infection is seen. (*Courtesy of* Paul Honig, MD.)

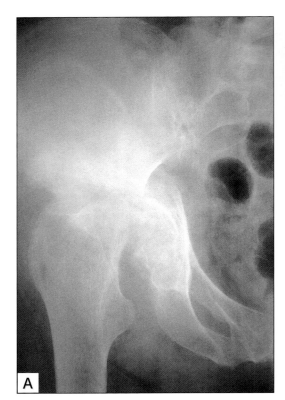

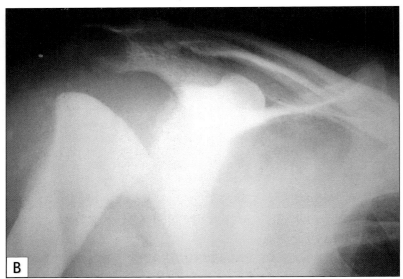

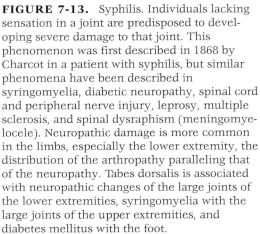

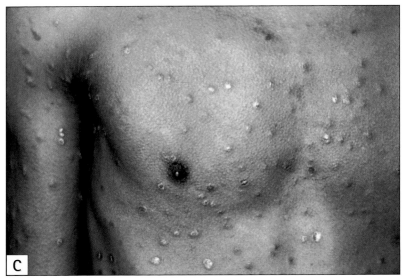

**FIGURE 7-13.** Syphilis. Individuals lacking sensation in a joint are predisposed to developing severe damage to that joint. This phenomenon was first described in 1868 by Charcot in a patient with syphilis, but similar phenomena have been described in syringomyelia, diabetic neuropathy, spinal cord and peripheral nerve injury, leprosy, multiple sclerosis, and spinal dysraphism (meningomyelocele). Neuropathic damage is more common in the limbs, especially the lower extremity, the distribution of the arthropathy paralleling that of the neuropathy. Tabes dorsalis is associated with neuropathic changes of the large joints of the lower extremities, syringomyelia with the large joints of the upper extremities, and diabetes mellitus with the foot.

The diagnosis of neuropathic joint can be made with confidence in the patient with severe joint destruction with minimal symptoms and surprisingly normal joint movement. There may be confusion with osteonecrosis, severe osteoarthritis, postseptic changes, or the arthritis mutilans of psoriasis, but a careful history and neurologic evaluation suggest the correct cause of the arthropathy. Neuropathic changes in the hip usually include bone loss or destruction, with complete absence of the femoral head. In the shoulder, resorption of the head of the humerus and the glenoidal cavity may occur, resulting in apparent increase of joint space. Bone debris may be found in and near the joint space. There is often new bone formation in neuropathic knees with bony sclerosis at weight-bearing areas and development of multiple osteophytes.

The cause of the neuropathic changes is still debated, with the leading theories being mechanical and trophic. According to the mechanical theory, the joint is subjected to repetitive trauma without the normal muscular protection afforded to a joint with normal sensation. By the trophic theory, the normal maintenance of the joint depends on autonomic nervous input; in the absence of this signal these mechanisms break down and inexorable destruction ensues.

**A** and **B**, Luetic neuropathic hip and shoulder are shown. Profound changes in the acetabulum and femoral head are seen. Occasionally, femoral neck fracture occurs. In some patients, loss of acetabular integrity leads to protrusion of the remnant of the femoral head into the pelvis. Destruction of the acromion is seen in the shoulder along with severe remodeling of the humeral head. **C**, Cutaneous lesions of secondary lesions of syphilis are seen on the torso. (*A and B courtesy of* Charlene Varnis, MD; *C courtesy of* Bill Witmer, MD.)

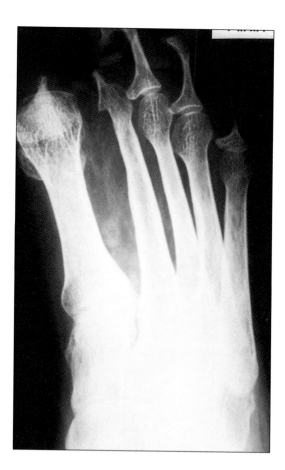

**FIGURE 7-14.** Neural leprosy. There are two types of leprosy: lepromatous that causes skin changes but bone changes in only 5% of cases and neural in which nearly two-thirds of patients have bone changes. The infection of nerve by *Mycobacteria leprae* causes neuropathic changes with resorption that starts with joints most subject to repetitive trauma, the distal phalanges of the hands and feet. "Pencil-in-cup" deformities can occur, probably from concentric atrophy and resorption. Patients with neural leprosy are predisposed to developing cellulitis and osteomyelitis due to local seeding through unappreciated ulcers and wounds. Damage to the feet of a patient with neural leprosy is shown. (*Courtesy of* American College of Radiology. Used with permission.)

# Lyme Disease

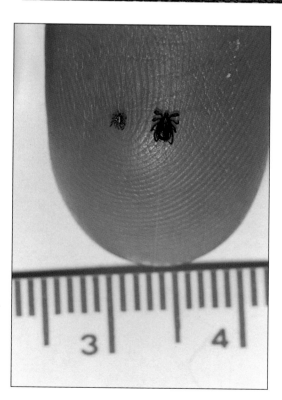

**FIGURE 7-15.** *Ixodes scapularis* ticks. Nymph and adult specimens are shown on a normal finger, with a background scale drawn in centimeters, for comparison. The etiologic agent of Lyme disease, *Borrelia burgdorferi*, was isolated from Ixodid ticks captured on Long Island and then grown from patient samples. Lyme disease is spread by the bite of infected Ixodid ticks: *I. scapularis* in the northeastern, southeastern, and midwestern United States (in the northeast previously called *Ixodid dammini*, but now known to be identical with *I. scapularis*); *Ixodid pacificus* in California and Oregon; *Ixodid ricinus* in Europe; and *Ixodid persulcatus* in Asia. Ixodid ticks have a four-stage life cycle. The egg mass is laid in the leaf clutter at the base of the forest. Larvae hatch from the mass and, in the northeastern and midwestern regions, feed in the summer and fall, typically from *Peromyscus leucopus*, the white-footed field mouse, although other animals will do, as well. Fewer than 1% of eggs are infected with *B. burgdorferi*; the spirochete is obtained with the initial blood meal. White-footed field mice maintain a persistent, although apparently asymptomatic, spirochetemia throughout their lives. Once the larval tick feeds, it falls off and after molting, it emerges in the early spring as a nymph. The nymph typically waits on a leaf of grass or low-lying shrub until something warm and exhaling carbon dioxide happens along; it will then grasp its potential host. The most common host of the nymph is a mouse, but other mammals, including dogs, cows, horses, and humans, and birds, can also provide the blood meal. Once fed, the nymphs molt. Adults appear in the fall and winter, typically taking their blood meal from white-tailed deer (*Odocolieus virginianus*) or other large mammals.

The percentage of nymphs infected with the spirochete is only half that of adult ticks. Nonetheless, 90% or more of cases of Lyme disease are spread by nymphs because adults are less abundant, larger (found and removed more quickly and easily), and active at a time when fewer people are outside. The tick takes 24 hours or longer to attach. During that time *B. burgdorferi* lies dormant on the inner aspect of the tick's midgut. As the blood meal reaches the midgut, spirochetes proliferate and escape the gut, ultimately reaching the tick's salivary glands, where the excess water of the blood meal is passed back into the host along with the spirochete.

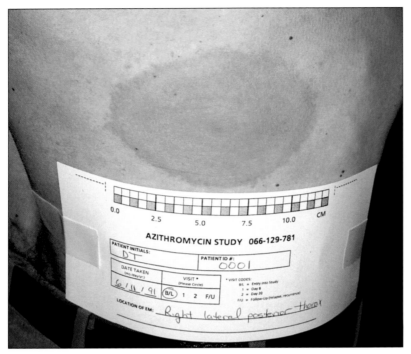

**FIGURE 7-16.** Single erythema migrans. The hallmark of early localized Lyme disease, and the only pathognomonic finding, is erythema migrans. The rash occurs at the site of the tick bite (recalled by only about 30% of patients) a mean of 7 to 10 days (range, 1–30 days) after the bite; most erythema migrans rashes are noted in the spring, summer, and early fall, as expected from the time nymphs are looking for their blood meal. Erythema migrans consists of an erythema expanding to a large circular or annular lesion, starting as a papule or macule, often with central clearing. It is typically found in the inguina, axilla, midriff, or behind the knee, the most common sites for tick bites. The rash is usually asymptomatic, but it may burn or itch and may be associated with a virus-like illness. The lesion may persist for 4 weeks before fading spontaneously.

The differential diagnosis of erythema migrans should include cellulitis, fixed drug eruption, tinea, plant dermatitis, granuloma annulare, and urticaria.

A transient erythema may develop at the site of a tick bite, within hours of the bite. Probably due to a reaction to components of the tick's saliva, this resolves within a day or two and should not be confused with erythema migrans. The bite of a spider (*eg*, brown recluse spider) is found on exposed skin and causes a painful and rapidly expanding lesions that may undergo central necrosis.

An example of single erythema migrans is shown on the back with the appearance of a "bull's eye." The lesion occurred at the site of a tick bite and slowly spread over the course of a few days.

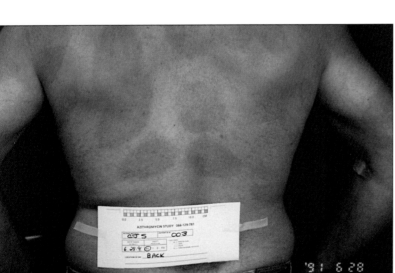

**FIGURE 7-17.** Multiple lesions of erythema migrans. Spirochetemia occurs relatively quickly after the onset of the erythema migrans lesion, probably within days. Dissemination to the heart, brain, and cranial and peripheral nerves is the cause of early disseminated disease, developing weeks to months after the infected tick bite. Spread to multiple areas of the skin causes multiple erythematous lesions, probably in about 10% of all patients with Lyme disease. The secondary erythemas are less likely to undergo central clearing. In addition to erythema migrans, individuals with early Lyme disease may develop arthralgia, myalgia, lymphadenopathy, and other symptoms of a virus-like illness, such as malaise, headache, fever, and chills.

This patient had multiple erythema migrans lesions. Spirochetemia caused dissemination of the infection. These asymptomatic lesions expanded over the course of a few days. Central clearing is seen in most of these lesions, although the absence of such central clearing in secondary lesions is common.

## CLINICAL MANIFESTATIONS OF LYME DISEASE

Early localized: occurring a few days to a month after the tick bite

Erythema migrans (in up to 90% of patients; multiple in 10% of patients with erythema migrans)*
Fatigue, malaise, lethargy
Headache
Myalgia or arthralgias
Regional or generalized lymphadenopathy

Early disseminated disease[†]: occurring days to 10 months after the tick bite

Carditis—approximately 8%–10% of untreated patients
  Conduction defects
  Mild cardiomyopathy or myopericarditis
Neurologic disease—approximately 10%–12% of untreated patients
  Cranial neuropathy (most often facial, can be bilateral)
  Lymphocytic meningitis
  Encephalitis
  Peripheral neuropathy or radiculoneuropathy
  Myelitis
Musculoskeletal—approximately 50% of untreated patients
  Migratory polyarthritis or polyarthralgias
  Fibromyalgia
Other
  Skin: Lymphadenosis benigna cutis (lymphocytoma, erythema nodosum)
  Lymphadenopathy: regional or generalized
  Eye: Conjunctivitis, iritis, choroiditis, vitritis, retinitis
  Liver: Liver function test abnormalities, hepatitis
  Kidney: Microhematuria, proteinuria

Late/chronic disease[†]: occurring months to years after the tick bite

Musculoskeletal—approximately 50% of untreated patients develop migratory polyarthritis
approximately 10% of untreated patients develop chronic monoarthritis, usually knee
  Fibromyalgia
Neurologic disease—chronic, often subtle, encephalopathy, encephalomyelitis, or peripheral
  neuropathy; ataxia, dementia, sleep disorder
Cutaneous—acrodermatitis chronica atrophicans; morphea or localized scleroderma-like lesions,
  possibly B cell lymphoma, in Europe.

---

*These figures represent more recent estimates; previously it was thought that 50% to 70% of all patients
had erythema migrans either by history or at presentation to the doctor and that up to 50% of patients with
erythema migran had multiple lesions.
[†]May occur in the absence of any prior features of Lyme disease.

**FIGURE 7-18.** Clinical manifestations of Lyme disease. Lyme disease has been described in Europe, Asia, and North America. In the United States the number of cases has been increasing and the geographic distribution has expanded. The highest focal prevalence of Lyme disease in the United States continues to be in southern New England, the Middle Atlantic states, Wisconsin, Minnesota, and California. The clinical features of Lyme disease are now well described, although there are some differences between the disease in North America and Europe, for instance, more neurologic disease in Europe and possibly more arthritis in the United States. The pathogenic *Borrelia burgdorferi* are grouped as *B. burgdorferi* sensu lato. Within this classification are the *B. burgdorferi* sensu stricto (found in North America, Europe, and Asia), and *Borrelia garinii* and *Borrelia afzelii* (found only in Europe and Asia). *B. burgdorferi* sensu stricto cause the vast majority of Lyme arthritis cases in Europe and Asia and, of course, all of the Lyme arthritis cases in North America. (*From* Sigal [2].)

## EPIDEMIOLOGIC CRITERIA FOR LYME DISEASE

Presence of erythema migrans
Cases with at least one late manifestation and laboratory confirmation of infection. The late
  manifestations include any of the following when an alternate explanation is not found:
Musculoskeletal system: Recurrent brief attacks of objective joint swelling in one or a few
  joints, sometimes followed by chronic arthritis in one or a few joints. Manifestations not
  considered as criteria for diagnosis include chronic progressive arthritis not preceded by brief
  attacks and chronic symmetric polyarthritis. Additionally, arthralgias, myalgias, or
  fibromyalgia syndromes alone are not accepted as criteria for musculoskeletal involvement.
Nervous system: Lymphocytic meningitis, cranial neuritis, particularly facial palsy (may be
  bilateral), radiculoneuropathy or rarely, encephalomyelitis alone or in combination.
  Encephalomyelitis must be confirmed by showing antibody production against *Borelia
  burgdorferi* in the cerebrospinal fluid (CSF), demonstrated by a higher titer of antibody in CSF
  than in serum. Headache, fatigue, paresthesias, or mild stiff neck alone are not accepted as
  criteria for neurologic involvement.
Cardiovascular: Acute onset, high grade (second or third degree) atrioventricular conduction
  defects that resolve in days to weeks and are sometimes associated with myocarditis.
  Palpitations, bradycardia, bundle branch block, or myocarditis alone are not accepted as
  criteria for cardiovascular involvement.

**FIGURE 7-19.**
Epidemiologic criteria for Lyme disease from the Centers for Disease Control and Prevention. Lyme disease is a reportable disease in all 50 states and has been reported from at least 46 states thus far. In most of the nonendemic states, cases are imported by people who traveled from their nonendemic homes to endemic work or vacation sites, were bitten by a tick, and then returned home before they began experiencing the clincial syndrome of Lyme disease. Thus, a travel history may be crucial in some cases.

These criteria, however, are for use in defining cases for report. They are useful as rigorous epidemiologic criteria; they were not designed for use as diagnostic criteria. The fact that a patient does not "satisfy" these criteria should not dissuade the clinician from making the diagnosis of Lyme disease. (*From* Wharton and coworkers [3].)

| CRITERIA FOR POSITIVE WESTERN BLOT (IMMUNOBLOT) ANALYSIS IN THE SEROLOGIC CONFIRMATION OF INFECTION WITH BORRELIA BURGDORFERI (LYME DISEASE) | | |
| --- | --- | --- |
| Duration of Disease | Isotype Tested | Bands to be Considered |
| First few weeks of infection | IgM | Two of the following: ospC (23), 39, 41 |
| After first weeks of infection | IgG | Five of the following: 18, 21, 28, 30, 39, 41, 45, 58, 66, 93 |

**FIGURE 7-20.** Criteria for positive Western blot (immunoblot) analysis in the serologic confirmation of infection with *Borrelia burgdorferi* (Lyme disease). The alternate criteria for IgM reactivity were proposed by the Centers for Disease Control and Prevention. IgM criteria should not be used in the confirmation of purported infection of more than a few weeks' duration. (*Criteria derived from* Dressler and coworkers [4].)

# References

1. Adapted from Arnet FC, Edworthy SM, Bloch DA, *et al*: The American Rheumatism Association 1987 revised criteria for the classification of rheumatoid arthritis. *Arthritis Rheum* 31:315-324, 1988.
2. Sigal LH (editor): Reports of the National Clinical Conference on Lyme Disease. *Am J Med* 1995, 98:1S-91S.
3. Wharton M, Chorba, TL, Vogt RL, *et al*.: Case definitions for public heatlh surveillance. *MMWR* 1990, 39:RR-13, 19–21.
4. Dressler F, Whalen JA, Reinhardt BN, Steere AC. Western blotting in the serodiagnosis of Lyme disease. *J Infect Dis* 1993, 167:392–400.

# Suggested Bibliography

Brancos MA, Peris P, Miro JM, *et al*.: Septic arthritis in heroin addicts. *Semin Arthritis Rheum* 1991, 21:81–87.

Goldenberg DL: Infectious arthritis complicating rheumatoid arthritis and other chronic rheumatic conditions. *Arthritis Rheum* 1989, 32:496–502.

Grosskopf I, Ben David A, Charach G, *et al*.: Bone and joint tuberculosis—a 120 year review. *Israel J Med Sci* 1994, 30:278–283.

Hsu V, Patella SJ, Sigal LH: "Chronic Lyme disease" as the incorrect diagnosis in patients with fibromyalgia. *Arthritis Rheum* 1993, 36:1493–1500.

Pinals RS: Polyarthritis and fever. *N Engl J Med* 1994, 330:796-774.

Cucurull E, Espinoza LR: Gonococcal arthritis. *Rheum Dis Clin North Am* 1998, 24:305-322.

Dillon M, Nourse C, Dowling F, *et al*.: Primary meningococcal arthritis. *Pediatr Infect Dis J* 1997, 16:331-332.

Ytterberg SR: Viral arthritis [review]. *Curr Opin Rheumatol* 1999, 11:275-280.

Phillips PE: Viral arthritis [review]. *Curr Opin Rheumatol* 1997, 9:337-344.

Barth WF: Office evaluation of the patient with musculoskeletal complaints [review]. *Am J Med* 1997, 102:3S-10S.

Saraux A, Taelman H, Blanche P, *et al*.: HIV infection as a risk factor for septic arthritis. *Br J Rheumatol* 1997, 36:333-337.

Naides SJ: Parvovirus B19 infection. *Rheum Dis Clin North Am* 1993, 19:457–475.

Resnick D: Neuropathic osteoarthropathy. In *Bone and Joint Imaging*, edn 2. Edited by D. Resnick. Philadelphia: WB Saunders; 1996:930–940.

Sigal LH: Lyme disease. In *Primer on the Rheumatic Disease*, edn 11. Edited by JH Klippel, CM Weyand, RL Wortmann. Atlanta: Arthritis Foundation; 1997:204–207.

Steere AC, Schoen RT, Taylor E: The clinical evolution of Lyme arthritis. *Ann Intern Med* 1987, 107:725–731.

Wise CM, Morris CR, Wasilauskas BL, Salzer WL: Gonococcal arthritis in an era of increasing penicillin resistance: presentations and outcomes in 41 recent cases (1985-1991). *Arch Intern Med* 1994, 154:2690–2695.

Yagupsky P, Dagan R, Howard C, *et al*.: Epidemiology, etiology, and clinical features of septic arthritis in children under the age of 24 months. *Arch Pediatr Adolesc Med* 1995, 32:496–502.

# 8

# Arthritis and Systemic Disease

## KENNETH T. CALAMIA, MARC D. COHEN, and DAVID M. MENKE

Muscoloskeletal symptoms occur in numerous systemic diseases. These symptoms are often the reason the patient initially seeks medical attention. An understanding and appreciation of these manifestations can correct diagnosis in a timely fashion.

Amyloidosis is characteristically the deposition of a fibrillar protein, which may affect many different organs. AA amyloidosis may occur as a complication of several inflammatory diseases, particularly rheumatoid arthritis and juvenile chronic polyarthritis and is most frequently associated with renal involvement. Amyloidosis should be considered in patients with rheumatoid arthritis and proteinuria or renal failure. AL amyloidosis has more varied clinical manifestations, which include an arthropathy. The joints most frequently affected are the shoulders, knees, wrists, and metacarpophalangeal joints. Typical findings in such patients are the "shoulder pad" sign and carpal tunnel syndrome. Confirmation of amyloid deposition may be obtained with a subcutaneous fat aspirate, which is positive in about 80% of cases, or by a more direct biopsy of involved tissues such as a renal or myocardial biopsy. Hemodialysis patients may develop an arthropathy owing to deposition of $\beta_2$ microgobulin amyloid particles. This may develop in more than 50% of patients after 5 years of dialysis.

Musculoskeletal symptoms may accompany hematologic disorders. In sickle cell disease, the occlusion of small blood vessels by sickled erythrocytes and necrosis of bone marrow are the causes of many of the complications including painful crises, dactylitis, and osteonecrosis. The painful crisis of sickle cell disease occurs most commonly in the juxta-articular areas of the long bones, but it may also occur in the back and ribs. Osteonecrosis of the femoral head occurs commonly in patients with sickle cell disease, and may occur in other joints, particularly the shoulder. Osteomyelitis should be considered if painful symptoms last longer than 1 to 2 weeks. There is an increased incidence of salmonella osteomyelitis in sickle cell disease. In hemophilia, synovitis and chronic effusions result from repeated intra-articular bleeding. Later, permanent bony changes may be seen.

Hemochromatosis often presents with musculoskeletal symptoms. The occurrence of osteoarthritis involving the second and third metacarpophalangeal occurs commonly and is an important clue to the diagnosis of hemochromatosis. Multiple other joints may be affected as well. Radiographs often demonstrate cystic lesions in association with joint space narrowing, sclerosis, and osteophytosis. There is also an increased incidence of calcium pyrophosphate dihydrate deposition disease in patients with hemochromatosis. Testing for hemochromatosis should be accomplished when the disease is suspected. All first-degree relatives of those with confirmed disease should undergo screening studies. Because of the frequency of heterozygotes in the population, screening has been suggested in all individuals over the age of 20 years. At present, liver biopsy is necessary for the diagnosis of hemochromatosis.

Hypertrophic osteoarthropathy is characterized by clubbing, periostosis, and noninflammatory effusions. For uncertain reasons, patients with malignant lung tumors often manifest hypertrophic osteoarthropathy as a painful arthropathy that may occur in advance of clubbing. A number of other secondary causes have been recognized and include specific pulmonary diseases, congenital heart disease, infective endocarditis, and a variety of other conditions.

Primary bone, cartilage, or synovial tumors may present with musculoskeletal pain or as mass lesions. Recognizing malignant lesions is critically important so that appropriate early treatment can be given. Studies with computed tomography or magnetic resonance imaging may be helpful in diagnosis but may be misleading, and biopsy is imperative.

Endocrinologic abnormalities have been associated with a myriad of musculoskeletal manifestations. Acromegaly is caused by overproduction of growth hormone, usually secondary to a pituitary tumor. This may result in enlargement of the hands and feet, thickening and darkening of the skin, and enlargement of the tongue and internal organs. Patients with acromegaly may have pain in the lower spine and a peripheral arthropathy associated with secondary degenerative changes involving multiple joints. There may be compression neuropathy from bony overgrowth. Carpal tunnel syndrome also is a common manifestation. Thyroid acropachy includes painless soft tissue swelling in fingers and toes, clubbing, periostitis, and pretibial myxedema. It is rare and may occur long after treatment of hyperthyroidism. Hypothyroidism has been associated with chronic tenosynovitis, carpal tunnel syndrome, and pseudogout. Diabetes mellitus is associated with several different types of bone and joint alterations. These include osteoporosis, hyperostosis, osteoarthritis, lytic bone changes defined as diabetic osteoarthropathy, cheiroarthropathy, Dupuytren's contractures, and periarthritis of the shoulders. Neuropathic arthropathy may occur in diabetes, usually involving the foot.

The acute polyarthritis of sarcoidosis commonly involves the knees and ankles and is often accompanied by hilar lymphadenopathy and erythema nodosum. A chronic form of polyarthritis is associated with sarcoidosis involving other organs. In addition to the chronic arthritis is dactylitis and bone lesions are found, most often in the hands and feet. These cystic lesions may also occur in the skull, nasal bones, vertebrae, and ribs.

Juvenile and adult forms of Gaucher's disease are associated with organomegaly and bone abnormalities attributable to medullary infiltration by Gaucher cells. The bone changes may result in episodic pain or even fractures. The infiltration causes the contours of long bones and

vertebral bodies to expand. Osteonecrosis may result from ischemia in infiltrated bone.

Multicentric reticulohistiocytosis affects skin and joints by an accumulation of lipid-laden histiocytes. This produces a symmetric polyarthritis, which may precede the skin lesions. Distal interphalangeal joint involvement is common, but other small and large peripheral joints and the cervical spine may be affected. Cutaneous nodules form over the dorsum of the hands and may resemble rheumatoid nodules. There may also be striking resorption of subchondral bone resulting in "arthritis multilans."

Wilson's disease is an inherited disorder characterized by accumulation of copper in various body tissues. Osteopenia may develop in the hands, feet, and spine. Bony changes often manifest as an indistinctness of the subchondral bone with focal areas of radiodensity at the joint margins. Subchondral cysts have also been associated with Wilson's disease. Small ossicles about affected joints may also occur.

Awareness of the musculoskeletal manifestations of systemic diseases often provides important clues that enable the physician to make a more timely diagnosis and initiate appropriate treatment.

# Amyloidosis

## CLASSIFICATION OF AMYLOID AND AMYLOIDOSIS

| Amyloid protein | Protein precursor | Clinical diagnosis |
|---|---|---|
| AA | apoSAA | Reactive (secondary) amyloidosis |
| | | Familial Mediterranean fever |
| | | Familial amyloid nephropathy with urticaria and deafness (Muckle-Wells' syndrome) |
| AL | κ, λ, eg, κIII | Idiopathic (primary) amyloidosis, associated with myeloma or macroglobulinemia |
| AH | IgG 1 (γ1) | |
| ATTR | Transthyretin | Familial amyloid polyneuropathy, Portuguese |
| | | Pamilial amyloid cardiomyopathy, Danish |
| | | Systemic senile amyloidosis |
| AApoAI | apoAI | Familial amyloid polyneuropathy, Iowa |
| Agel | Gelsolin | Familial amyloidosis, Finnish |
| Acys | Cystatin C | Hereditary cerebral hemorrhage with amyloidosis, Icelandic |
| Aβ | β protein precursor | Alzheimer's disease |
| | | Down syndrome |
| | | Hereditary cerebral hemorrhage with amyloidosis, Dutch |
| Aβ2M | β2-microglobulin | Associated with chronic dialysis |
| Ascr | Scrapie protein precursor | Creutzfeldt-Jakob disease, etc. |
| | 33–35′ cellular form | Gerstmann-Straüssler-Scheinker syndrome |
| Acal | (Pro)calcitonin | In medullary carcinomas of the thyroid |
| AANF | Atrial natriuretic factor | Isolated atrial amyloid |
| AIAPP | Islet amyloid polypeptide | In islets of Langerhans |
| | | Diabetes type II, insulinoma |

**FIGURE 8-1.** Classification of amyloid and amyloidosis. This classification is based on fibrillar proteins with known primary structure. These proteins are derived from protein precursors in the serum. The clinical diagnoses associated with each amyloid protein are listed. Dominant organ involvement in familial amyloid syndromes distinguishes neuro-pathic, nephropathic, and cardiopathic forms [1]. AA—amyloid A protein; apo—apolipoprotein; H—immunoglobulin heavy chain; L—immunoglobulin light chain; SAA—serum amyloid A protein. (*Adapted from* WHO-IUIS Nomenclature Subcommittee[2].)

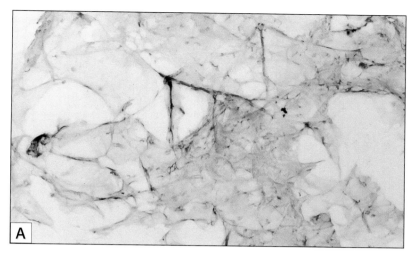

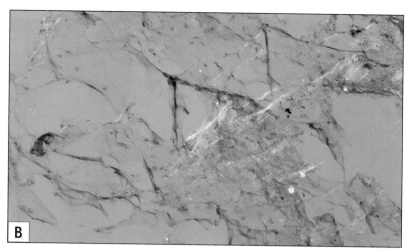

**FIGURE 8-2.** Abdominal fat aspirate in primary (AL) amyloidosis. **A**, Perivascular deposits of amyloid (Congo red positive) are identified in aspirated subcutaneous adipose tissue (X100). **B**, Polarized light microscopy shows greenish yellow amyloid deposits with scattered admixed talc particles as an artifact (X100). Abdominal fat aspiration is a sensitive, inexpensive, and convenient procedure for establishing the diagnosis of systemic amyloidosis.

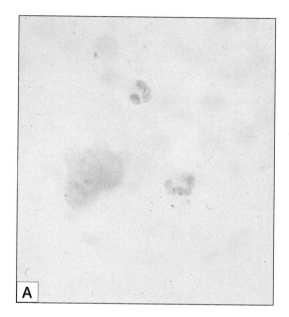

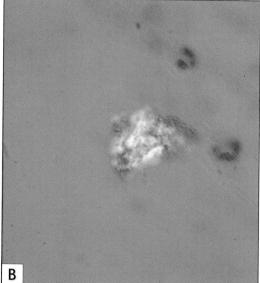

**FIGURE 8-3.** Synovial fluid analysis in amyloid arthropathy. Synovial fluid analysis may often yield diagnostic findings in patients with amyloid arthropathy. The slide shows synovial fluid from a shoulder of a 64-year-old patient with primary amyloidosis. The sample of synovial fluid was prepared in a cytocentrifuge and stained with Congo red. **A**, Synovial fluid elements were examined with light microscopy. **B**, Polarized light microscopy reveals apple-green birefringence, which is diagnostic of amyloid [3]. (*Courtesy of* Gene G. Hunder, MD.)

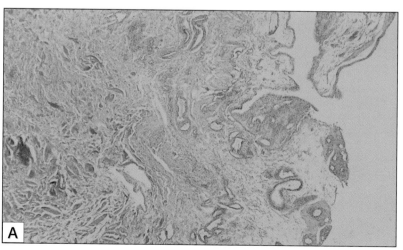

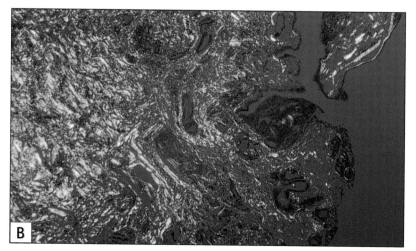

**FIGURE 8-4.** Flexor tendon synovium in $Ab_2M$ amyloidosis. **A**, Amyloid deposition (Congo red positive) and fibrosis are identified in subsynovial soft tissues (Congo red, X20). **B**, Polarized light microscopy stained with Congo red shows yellow-green birefringence of amyloid and white birefringence of collagen (Congo red, X20). (Because collagen will sometimes show Congo red positivity depending on the pH of the staining technique, the color of birefringence is essential for confirmation of amyloid deposition.) Immunohistologic stains for $beta_2$ microglobulin may be used to establish that the amyloid deposition is related to dialysis.

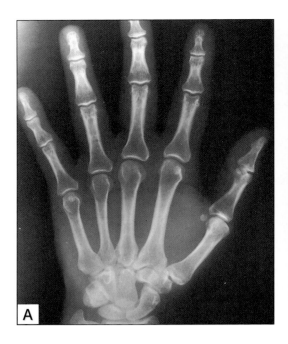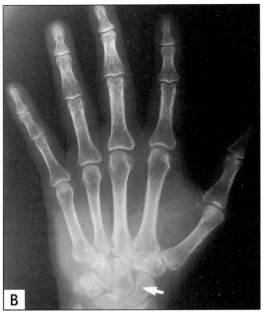

**FIGURE 8-5.** Cystic bone disease of A $\beta_2$M amyloidosis. **A**, This radiograph is from a patient on dialysis for 6 years. **B**, This radiograph shows two cystic lesions of the carpus of the same patient (*arrow*) after 14 years on dialysis. Manifestations of A $\beta_2$M amyloidosis in patients on chronic dialysis include carpal tunnel syndrome, intraosseous cysts, shoulder arthropathy, a destructive spondyloarthropathy, pseudotumors, and an erosive arthritis. (*Courtesy of* James T. McCarthy, MD.)

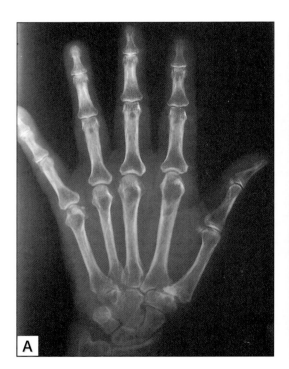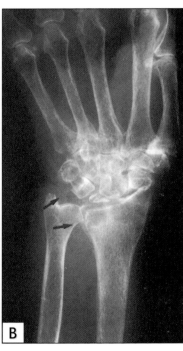

**FIGURE 8-6.** Erosive cystic arthritis of A $\beta_2$M amyloidosis. **A**, Radiograph taken at the start of hemodialysis. **B**, Radiograph taken after 9 years of hemodialysis. The *arrows* in the figure point to areas of cystic destruction of the wrist resulting from A $\beta_2$M amyloidosis. (*Courtesy of* James T. McCarthy, MD.)

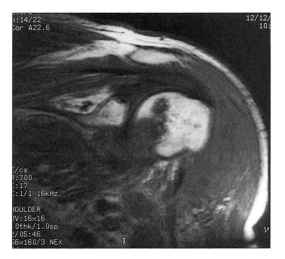

**FIGURE 8-7.** Magnetic resonance image of cystic lesion of shoulder in A $\beta_2$M amyloidosis. The patient was a 47-year-old man on chronic hemodialysis who complained of shoulder pain. The T1-weighted scan reveals a large low-intensity erosion with prominent synovium bulging from the lesion. (*Courtesy of* Thomas H. Berquist, MD.)

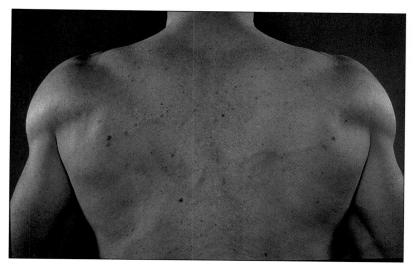

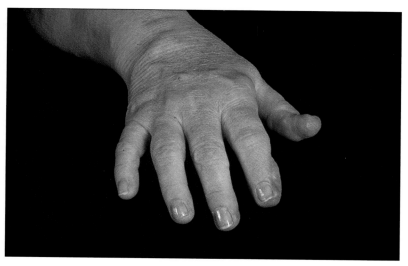

**FIGURE 8-8.** "Shoulder pad" sign in primary (AL) amyloidosis. Shoulder enlargement occurs as a consequence of amyloid deposition in synovial and periarticular tissues and may be found in AL, AA (secondary), and A $\beta_2$M amyloidosis. (*Courtesy of* Robert A. Kyle, MD.)

**FIGURE 8-9.** Arthropathy and infiltrative skin lesions of primary (AL) amyloidosis. The arthropathy of AL amyloidosis may mimic rheumatoid arthritis but is usually nonerosive. Symmetric involvement of fingers, wrists, and shoulders may occur. Skin lesions in AL are common and may be polymorphic. Localized cutaneous amyloidosis may occur in some patients. (*Courtesy of* Robert A. Kyle, MD.)

# Hemophilic Arthropathy

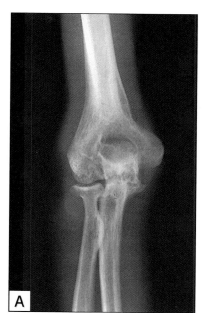

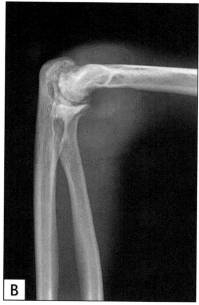

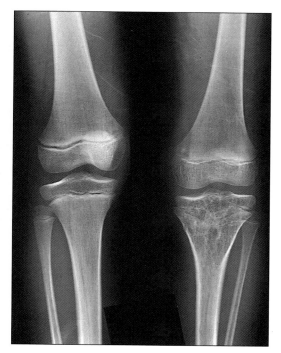

**FIGURE 8-10.** Hemophilic arthropathy, elbow. **A**, A-P, and **B**, lateral views are shown. The patient presented with acute and chronic pain in the right elbow. A large radiodense particular effusion is present, consistent with hemarthrosis. Erosive and degenerative changes are present at the articular surface. Pressure erosions are seen at the anterior and medical aspect of the distal humerus. (*Courtesy of* Thomas H. Berquist, MD.)

**FIGURE 8-11.** Radiograph of the knees of an 18-year-old man with hemophilia and a history of multiple hemarthroses. Repeated hemarthroses lead to synovitis with synovial hypertrophy and fibrosis, which contribute to articular cartilage destruction. Erosive changes resembling those in rheumatoid arthritis may be seen radiographically in chronic hemophilic arthritis. Synovial soft tissues may have increased density due to hemosiderin deposition. Advanced arthropathy resembles osteoarthritis but on knee films there may be characteristic widening of the intercondylar notch and squaring of the patella (not shown).

As seen on the left knee in this film, synovitis and increased blood flow to the joint may lead to epiphyseal overgrowth and limb length discrepancy. Postsurgical changes are present at the upper tibial epiphysis. (*Courtesy of* Thomas H. Berquist, MD.)

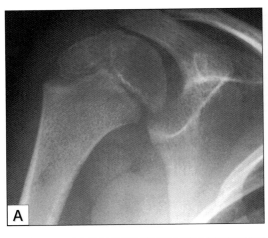

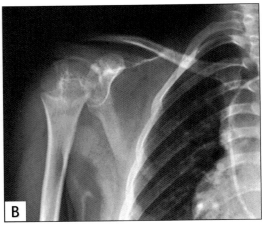

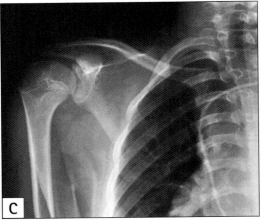

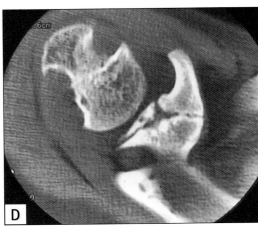

**FIGURE 8-12.** Hemophilic arthropathy, shoulder. The radiograph in (**A**) was taken after a history of multiple hemarthroses in a 12-year-old boy with hemophilia. The other films (**B** and **C**) were taken 6 years later, showing progression of the lesion. A computed tomography scan at that time (**D**) showed large erosive defects in the humeral head. (*Courtesy of* Thomas H. Berquist, MD.)

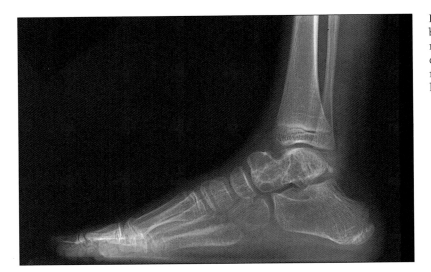

**FIGURE 8-13.** Hemophilic pseudotumor, talus. The talus has multiple benign cystic lucencies, likely owing to previous intraosseous hemorrhage in a patient with hemophilia. There is deformity and enlargement of the anterior superior aspect of the talus representing a pseudotumor, resulting from new bone formation after intraosseous and subperiosteal hemorrhage. (*Courtesy of* Thomas H. Berquist, MD.)

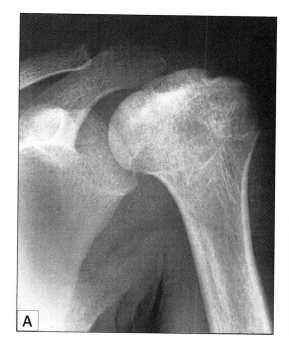

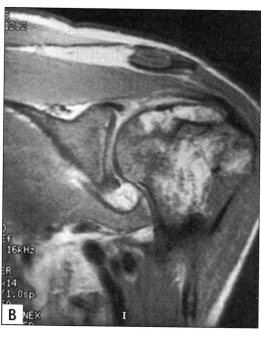

**FIGURE 8-14.** Avascular necrosis of the shoulder in sickle cell disease. **A**, x-ray and **B**, MRI of left shoulder. The most common arthropathy in patients with sickle cell anemia is related to avascular necrosis of subchondral bone. Hip and shoulder involvement are most common [4]. (*Courtesy of* Thomas H. Berquist, MD.)

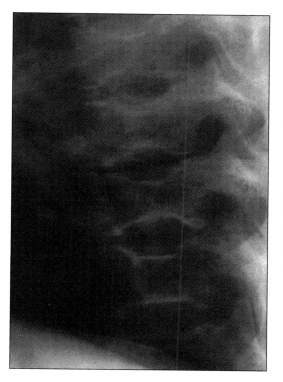

**FIGURE 8-15.** "H vertebrae" in sickle cell disease. The radiograph shows the spine of an 18-year-old woman who had experienced multiple painful crises of sickle cell disease since age 2. The superior and inferior central region of the vertebral end plates are depressed and thickened. This deformity is thought to occur as a result of ischemia during vertebral bone growth. The central vertebral body receives its nutrition from small arteries that traverse metabolically active marrow. Sickling may be more likely in these vessels as compared to the short perforating periosteal vessels that supply the periphery of the verte-brae. This abnormality is characteristic of sickle cell diseases, but similar findings have been reported in patients with thalassemia, homo-cystinuria, and Gaucher's disease [5]. (*Courtesy of* Thomas H. Berquist, MD.)

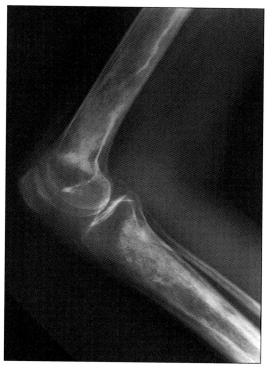

**FIGURE 8-16.** Bone infarcts in sickle cell disease. Radiographs of the knees show cortical thickening and patchy increased density due to bone infarction with repair. Skeletal complica-tions may be more common in mixed sickle cell disease. This patient had sickle-thal disease. (*Courtesy of* Thomas H. Berquist, MD.)

# Myeloproliferative Disorders

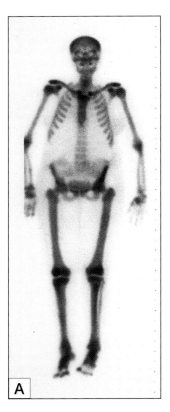
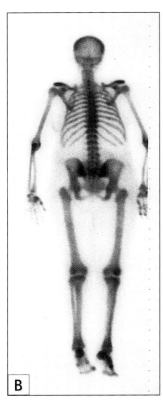

**FIGURE 8-17.** Polycythemia vera and myelofibrosis. The bone scan from an elderly woman with these conditions shows diffusely increased uptake throughout the skeleton with relatively little activity in the kidneys, **A**, anterior, and **B**, posterior. This is a "superscan" pattern that may be seen with diffuse metastatic disease, metabolic bone disease such as that with hyperparathyroidism or hyperthyroidism, or with diffuse bone marrow disorders such as myelofibrosis. (*Courtesy of* Thomas H. Berquist, MD.)

# Hemochromatosis

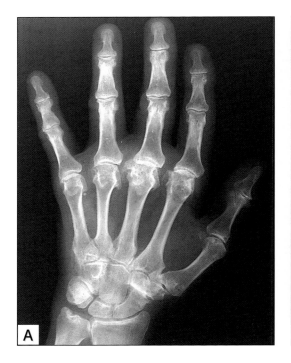
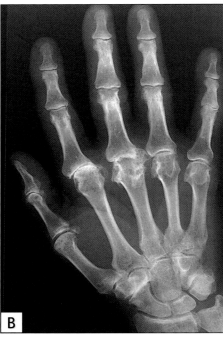

**FIGURE 8-18.** Arthropathy associated with hemochromatosis. **A** and **B**, In hemochromatosis, degenerative changes at metacaropophalangeal joints are common. Beak-type osteophytes in this location are distinctive. Chondrocalcinosis of the wrist is also present. (*Courtesy of* William W. Ginsburg, MD.)

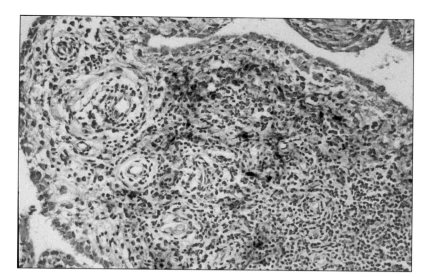

**FIGURE 8-19.** Synovial hemosiderosis. Lymphocytic synovitis with subsynovial iron deposition (*blue*) is seen in a patient with hemochromatosis (Prussian blue, X100). Lymphocytic inflammation with iron deposition in subsynovial soft tissue is not specific for hemochromatosis and is more commonly seen after trauma or previous surgical intervention.

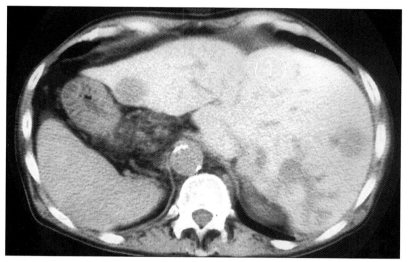

**FIGURE 8-20.** Computed tomography (CT) scan of the liver in hemochromatosis. The scan is from a 65-year-old man with known hemochromatosis. The serum ferritin level was 2660 ng/mL and the α-fetoprotein level was 6324 ng/mL. The scan reveals diffusely increased density (increased attenuation) of the hepatic parenchyma on this noncontract study. Note that the liver is more dense than the spleen. The differential diagnosis of increased liver attenuation on CT scan includes hemochromatosis, glycogen storage diseases, and the use of thoratrast (contrast agent) or mineral-containing therapeutic agents such as gold, amiodarone, or cisplatin. The scan also shows several low-density masses in the liver, which proved to be hepatoma on biopsy.

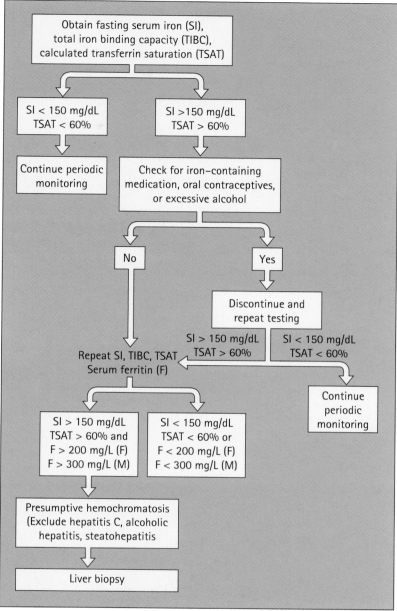

**FIGURE 8-21.** Algorhythm for suspected hemochromatosis. Laboratory evaluation for the diagnosis of homozygous hemochromatosis.

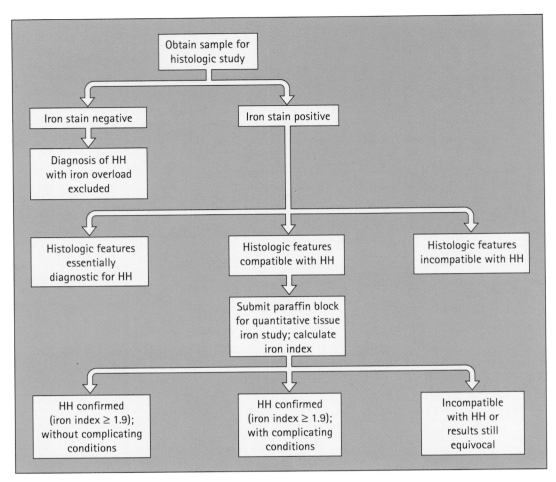

**FIGURE 8-22.** Diagnostic algorithm for liver biopsy specimens in suspected homozygous hemochromatosis (HH). The diagnosis of HH can be made when the typical histopathologic features are present on liver biopsy specimens. When the findings are equivocal, determinations of quantitative hepatic iron concentration and hepatic iron index (HII) usually allow the distinction of HH from other types of iron overload. A baseline quantitative tissue iron may also be desirable for monitoring treatment of confirmed cases.

A hepatic iron concentration of more than 10,000 mg/g dry weight is diagnostic for HH. The HII relates hepatic iron concentration to age [6]. HII equals tissue iron in mg/g dry weight divided by [55.8 X age]. (*Adapted from* Ludwig and coworkers [7].)

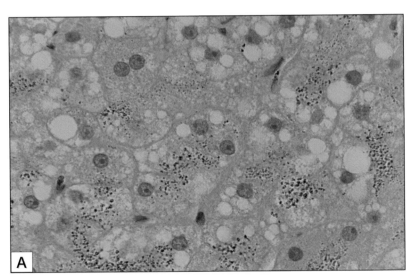

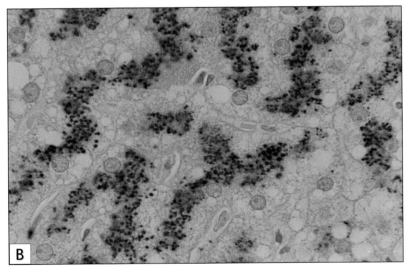

**FIGURE 8-23.** Hemochromatosis, liver biopsy. **A**, Hepatocellular iron deposition is identified as granular brown cytoplasmic pigment (hematoxylin and eosin, X400) and **B** confirmed to be iron by iron staining (Prussian blue, X400). Iron deposition in hepatocytes establishes the diagnosis of hepatic hemosiderosis. Hemochromatosis is diagnosed if hepatic hemosiderosis is identified with histologic evidence of liver damage or markedly elevated quantitative iron indices. Iron staining must be done because the brown granular pigment in hepatocytes resembles lipofuscin in hematoxylin and eosin stains.

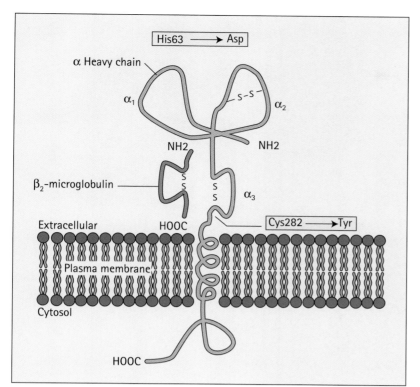

**FIGURE 8-24.** Hypothetical model of the HLA-H protein. The model is based on its homology with major histocompatibility complex (MHC) class I molecules. The HLA-H protein is a single polypeptide with three extracellular domains that would be analogous to the $\alpha_1$, $\alpha_2$, and $\alpha_3$ domains of other MHC class I proteins. In contrast to other members of the MHC class I family, the $\alpha_1$ and $\alpha_2$ domains in the HLA-H protein are nonpolymorphic. $\beta_2$-microglobulin is a separate protein and may interact with the HLA-H gene product in a noncovalent manner in the $\alpha_3$ homologous region. Additionally, the HLA-H protein contains a membrane-spanning region and a short cytoplasmic tail. The approximate locations of Cys282Tyr and His63Asp are indicated. Mutations in genes coding for these regions are thought to inactivate this protein, resulting in abnormal iron metabolism. HOOC–carboxylr group; NH$_2$–amino group. (*From* Feder and coworkers [8].)

# Hypertrophic Osteoarthropathy

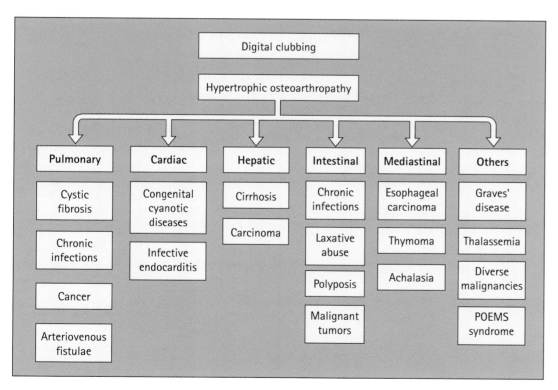

**FIGURE 8-25.** Classification of hypertrophic osteoarthropathy. POEMS—polyneuropathy, organomegaly, endocrinopathy, M protein, skin changes. (*Adapted from* Martinez-Lavin [9].)

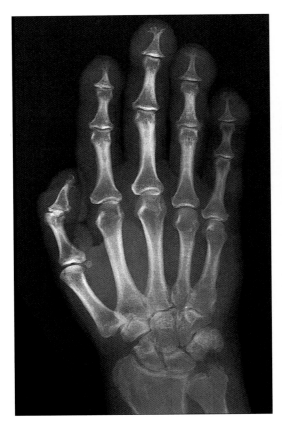

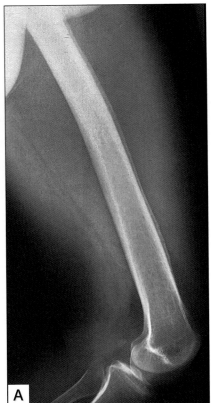

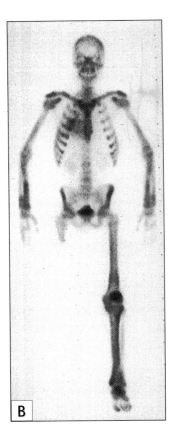

**FIGURE 8-26.** Pachydermoperiostitis. The radiograph is of the hand of a 56-year-old man who developed enlargement of the distal fingers and toes as a small child. In adolescence he developed thickening of the skin of the hands and feet. Several family members were similarly affected. The radiograph reveals soft tissue prominence of the digits with bullous distal enlargement. Acro-osteolysis is prominent. Irregular periosteal new bone formation is present in the distal long bones of the extremities, seen here as irregular enlargement of the distal radius and ulna. (*Courtesy of* Thomas H. Berquist, MD.)

**FIGURE 8-27.** Hypertrophic osteoarthropathy secondary to pulmonary metastatic osteogenic sarcoma. The 20-year-old patient presented with cough and chest pain 7 years after right above-the-knee amputation for osteogenic sarcoma of the distal femur. **A,** Plain film of left femur revealed extensive, smooth, lamellated periosteal new bone formation, consistent with hypertrophic osteoarthropathy. **B,** The bone scan on the left shows mild, irregular increased uptake involving the left femur and tibia as well as the distal humeri and radii. The right lung uptake reflects the metastatic involvement. A chest radiograph revealed a large mass in the right midlung (not shown). (*Courtesy of* Thomas H. Berquist, MD.)

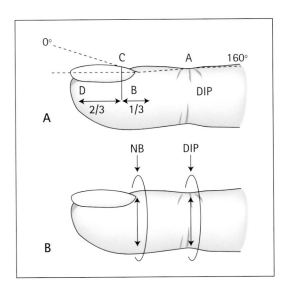

**FIGURE 8-28.** Measurement of clubbing of the fingers. **A,** Clubbing may be recognized clinically by the loss of the normal 15° to 20° angle (*CBD*) of the proximal nail as it penetrates the nail fold. Measurement of the profile (*ABC*) and hyponychial (*ABD*) angles is used to identify and quantitate digital clubbing [10]. Precise measurements of the angles can be facilitated by using an overhead projector to cast a magnified shadow from which an outline can be made [11]. Both profile and hyponychial angles are increased in clubbing of the digits, but the latter may be more characteristic of the condition. The mean hyponychial angle of right index normal subjects was found to be 180.1 ± 4.2° and in clinically clubbed patients the mean was approximately 195° [10].

Other techniques have also been used to determine the presence of clubbing or to monitor improvement after treatment. **B,** A "digital index" can be determined by measuring the perimeter of the digit at the distal interphalangeal (DIP) joint and at the nailbed (NB). A NB to DIP ratio is calculated for each joint. If the sum of these is greater than 10, clubbing is present [12].

Measurement of the dorsoventral thickness at these two sites using a caliper establishes the presence of clubbing if the NB thickness is greater [13]. (A *adapted from* Bentley and coworkers [10]; B *adapted from* Vazquez-Abad and coworkers [12].)

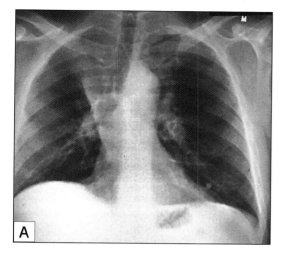

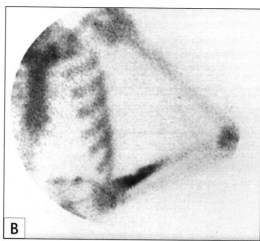

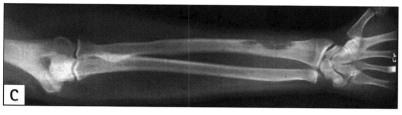

**FIGURE 8-29.** Squamous cell carcinoma of the lung metastatic to distal radius. This 64-year old male smoker presented with pain in the wrist and distal forearm of several weeks' duration. On examination there was tenderness and slight swelling of the distal radius. **A**, Chest radiograph showed consolidation and loss of volume in the right upper lobe and bronchoscopy with biopsy revealed squamous cell carcinoma. **B**, The bone scan was positive in the distal radius. **C**, Radiograph of the forearm showed a destructive lytic lesion. The differential diagnosis of the radius lesion would include a primary bone malignancy, myeloma, vascular tumor, or metastasis. The case demonstrates that a malignancy, metastatic to the joint or to periarticular structures, may mimic an arthropathy. (*Courtesy of* Thomas H. Berquist, MD.)

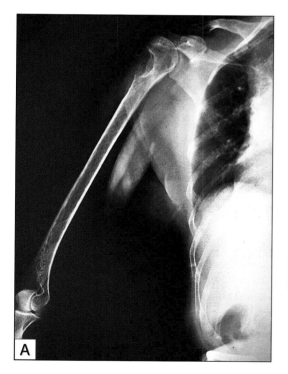

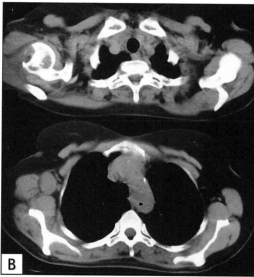

**FIGURE 8-30.** Grade IV diffuse large cell lymphoma involving the right shoulder. A 51-year-old man presented with chronic right shoulder pain. **A**, Shoulder radiograph revealed an eccentric lytic lesion in the lateral metaphysis with cortical destruction. **B**, Computed tomography scan of the chest showed cortical destruction in the proximal right humerus (*upper*), a 2-cm soft tissue mass in the right axilla (*lower*), and retroperitoneal adenopathy (not shown). Biopsy confirmed a diffuse large cell lymphoma. Lymphoma of bone usually occurs as a result of hematogenous dissemination (stage IV), but may arise as a primary tumor in bone. (*Courtesy of* Thomas H. Berquist, MD.)

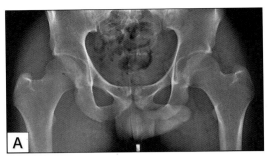

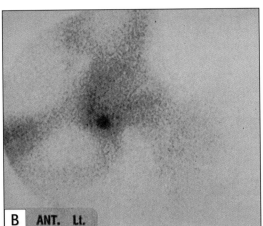

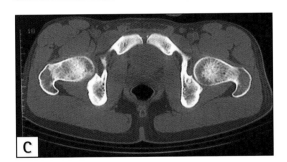

**FIGURE 8-31.**
Osteoid osteoma.
**A**, Radiograph, **B**, bone scan, and **C**, a computed tomography (CT) scan from an 18-year-old man with pain in the left groin for a duration of 1 year. The pelvis films are negative, but bone scan reveals a focus of intense uptake in the inferior left acetabular region. The CT scan shows an 8-mm nidus with a surrounding lucent rim, typical of an osteoid osteoma. (*Courtesy of* Thomas H. Berquist, MD.)

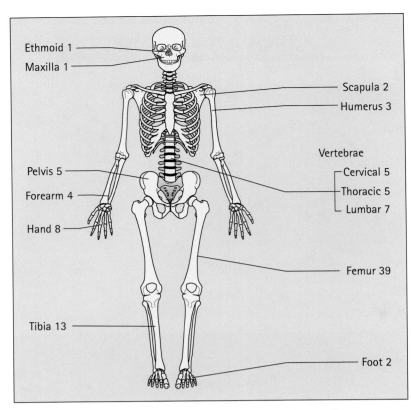

**FIGURE 8-32.** Sites of involvement in 95 cases of osteoid osteoma [14]. In 5 patients in this series, a monoarthritis was present. When osteoid osteoma occurs in or near a joint, swelling and proliferative synovitis may occur [15]. (*Adapted from* Cohen [14].)

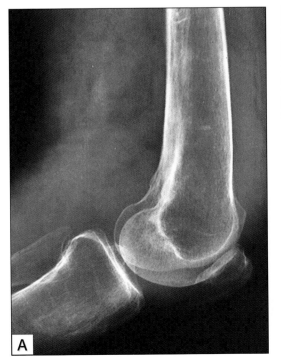

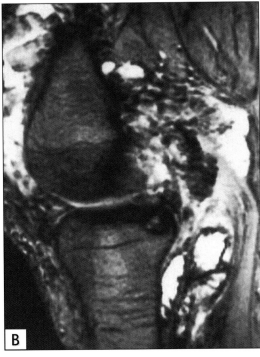

**FIGURE 8-33.** Pigmented villonodular synovitis. The radiograph is from a 72-year-old woman with pain and limited knee flexion for 1 year. **A**, Radiograph of knee, lateral view. Fluid or synovitis is seen in the suprapatellar recess and in the posterior aspect of the knee. **B**, MRI of knee. A T2-weighted sagittal magnetic resonance image demonstrates an extensive multilobulated mass of low signal intensity involving the synovium, which proved to be pigmented villonodular synovitis. (*Courtesy of* Thomas H. Berquist, MD.)

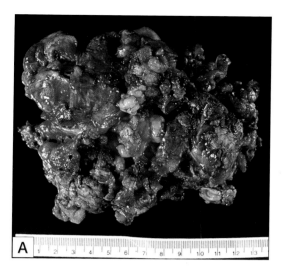

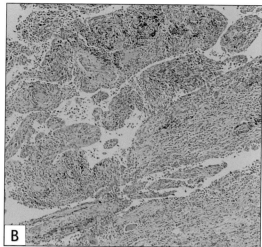

**FIGURE 8-34.** Pigmented villonodular synovitis. **A**, Gross specimen photograph shows reddish brown shaggy tumor of the right posterior knee. This tumor was one of many forming diffuse multinodular masses involving the entire synovial surface and adjacent soft tissue. Erosion of joint surfaces was also present. **B**, In the microscopic sections, proliferating fronds of synovium thickened by inflammatory or giant cell (*arrow*) infiltrates and pigment deposition can be seen (hematoxylin and eosin, X40). The pigment is typically Prussian blue positive (iron). Additional microscopic sections of these tumors may show areas of necrosis, xanthomatous histiocytic proliferation, and dense fibrosis. Although local invasion of adjacent soft tissue is common, cytologic atypia of proliferating cells with atypical mitosis are not identified.

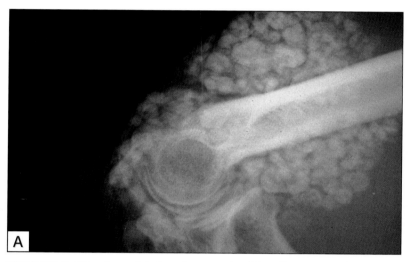

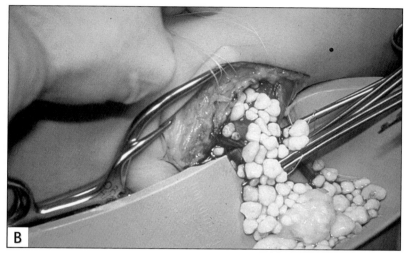

**FIGURE 8-35.** Synovial chondromatosis of the elbow. **A**, Radiograph of the elbow. **B**, operative photograph. 34-year-old man with synovial chondromatosis. The patient presented with an enlarging mass over 10 years with little pain. The joint was filled with numerous ossified loose bodies, removed at the time of surgery. The synovium at this point had become inactive, no longer forming metaplastic cartilage nodules, making complete synovectomy unnecessary. (*Courtesy of* K. Krishnan Unni, MD.)

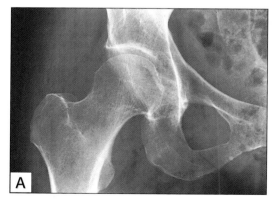

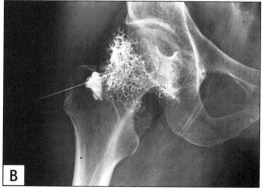

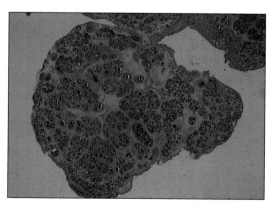

**FIGURE 8-36.** Synovial chondromatosis, **A**, Radiograph. **B**, Arthrogram. Radiographic studies in synovial chondromatosis may be normal if the metaplastic cartilage nodules do not become calcified. Affected joints may show findings of (secondary) osteoarthritis. In cases with nondiagnostic radiographs, clinical suspicion and additional imaging studies can lead to a diagnosis. Tomograms may be helpful if faint calcifications are visible. A magnetic resonance image or arthrogram may be diagnostic. (*Courtesy of* Thomas H. Berquist, MD.)

**FIGURE 8-37.** Synovial chondromatosis, microscopic view. Metaplastic nodules of cartilage are present in synovial villi (hematoxylin and eosin, X15.6). These cartilaginous nodules may detach to form free-floating cartilaginous bodies and become calcified or ossified.

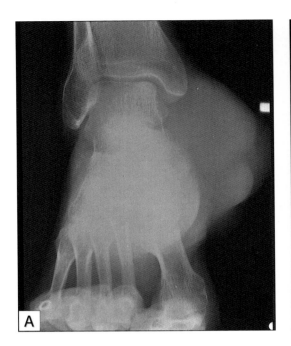

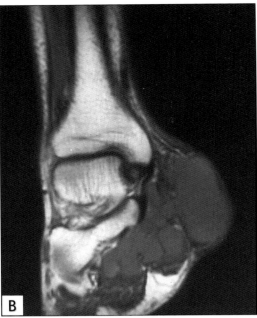

**FIGURE 8-38.** Synovial sarcoma. A 57-year-old man presented with a painless, slowly enlarging mass of the right ankle. **A**, Radiographs revealed a large lobulated mass medial to the right ankle and hindfoot. **B**, Magnetic resonance imaging (MRI) of the ankle showed a large multilocular mass of homogenous density. The consistency of the mass is that of a thick fluid, but a synovial sarcoma could not be excluded. A biopsy revealed synovial sarcoma and a below-the-knee amputation was performed. Synovial sarcomas are generally found in young adults, most often in the lower extremity. MRI is often useful in distinguishing benign from malignant soft tissue tumors but may be misleading [16,17]. (*Courtesy of* Thomas H. Berquist, MD.)

## Arthropathies with Endocrine Disorders

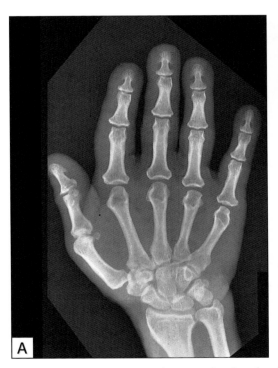

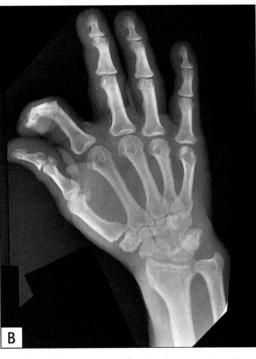

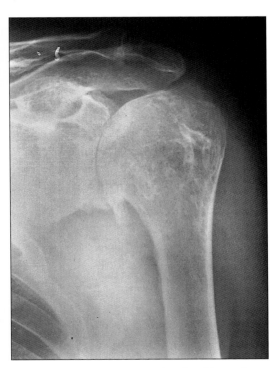

**FIGURE 8-39.** Acromegaly. **A**, and **B**, hand radiographs. Joint space widening is present owing to stimulation of cartilage growth by excess growth hormone. An increase in soft tissue density and spadelike deformity of the distal tufts is also seen. (*Courtesy of* Thomas H. Berquist, MD.)

**FIGURE 8-40.** Acromegaly, shoulder radiograph. Degenerative arthritis is common in chronic acromegaly. Growth hormone excess may lead to cartilage and osteophyte overgrowth but cartilage may wear prematurely. (*Courtesy of* Thomas H. Berquist, MD.)

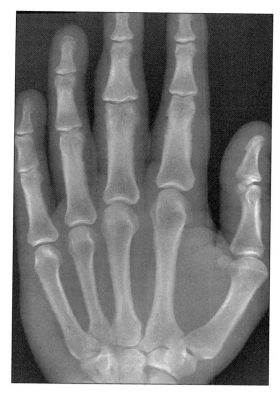

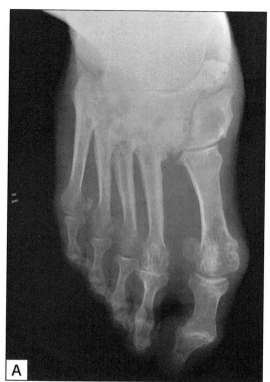

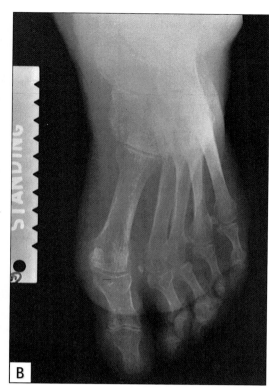

**FIGURE 8-41.** Thyroid acropachy. The radiograph is from a 34-year-old man with a history of Graves' disease and swelling of the extremities. The films show fluffy periostitis, diaphyseal enlargement, and soft tissue swelling in several regions. Clinically, clubbing of the digits may be present and acro-osteolysis may be seen radiographically. The syndrome usually occurs after treatment of Graves' disease and is often associated with exophthalmos and pretibial myxedema [18]. (*Courtesy of* Thomas H. Berquist, MD.)

**FIGURE 8-42.** Charcot arthropathy in diabetes mellitus. **A**, Right foot. **B**, Left foot. Radiographs are from a 70-year-old man with long-standing diabetes and neuropathy. Articular destruction and new bone formation is seen in the right midfoot. Separation of the first and second metatarsals on the right results from the destructive midfoot process.

# Miscellaneous Diseases with Arthritis

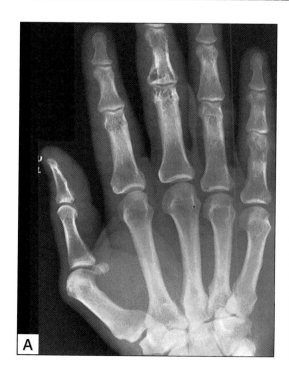

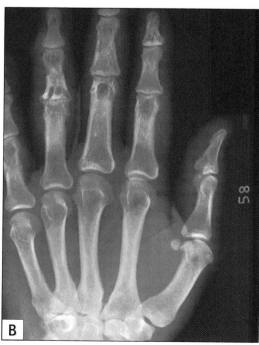

**FIGURE 8-43.** Osseous lesions in chronic sarcoidosis. **A**, and **B**, Hand radiographs. Chronic sarcoid arthritis is characterized by a persistent or remitting polyarthritis, often with dactylitis. Cutaneous lesions are often present. Synovial biopsy reveals characteristic granulomas. Although generally nonerosive, the association with osseous lesions may lead to destructive, often cystic, bony changes [19]. (*Courtesy of* Thomas H. Berquist, MD.)

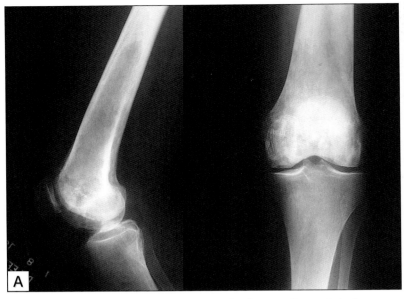

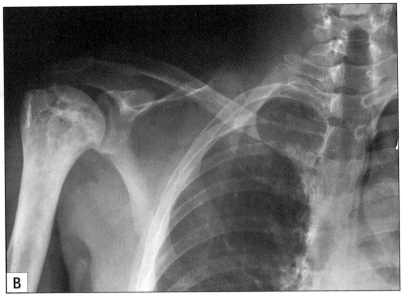

**FIGURE 8-44.** Gaucher's disease. **A,** This knee radiograph is from a 43-year-old man with Gaucher's disease who had experienced multiple episodes of joint pain, especially in the knees and shoulders. The left knee had become chronically painful and swollen. The radiograph shows widening of the medullary portion of the distal femur with a thin cortex.

Irregular areas of sclerosis are present, due to old bone infarcts with subsequent repair. **B,** Aseptic necrosis of the right humeral head is present. Irregular sclerosis of the proximal humeral shaft is also present, owing to bone infarcts with repair. (*Courtesy of* Thomas H. Berquist, MD.)

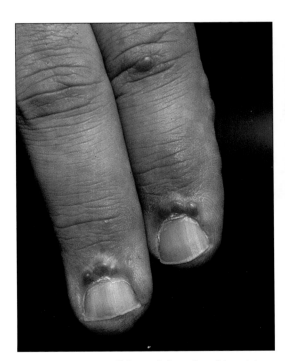

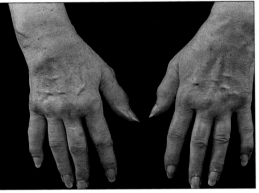

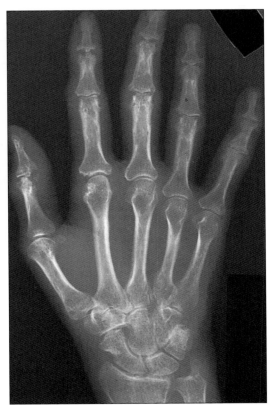

**FIGURE 8-46.** Multicentric reticulohistiocytosis. The patient presented with a symmetric seronegative polyarthritis and 2 years later developed the characteristic skin nodules on the fingers. The arthritis may be erosive and lead to "arthritis mutilans." Treatment with immunosuppressive agents may control the disease [21]. (Courtesy of William W. Ginsburg, MD.)

**FIGURE 8-45.** Skin nodules of multicentric reticulohistiocytosis. These characteristic nail-fold nodules have the appearance of "coral beads." Nodules may be numerous, grow to as large as 2 cm, and may involve mucosal surfaces [20]. (*Courtesy of* William W. Ginsburg, MD.)

**FIGURE 8-47.** Hand radiograph in multicentric reticulohistiocytosis. Erosive changes are present in multiple joints. Distal interphalangeal erosions are characteristic and may lead to pseudowidening of the joint spaces. (*Courtesy of* William W. Ginsburg, MD.)

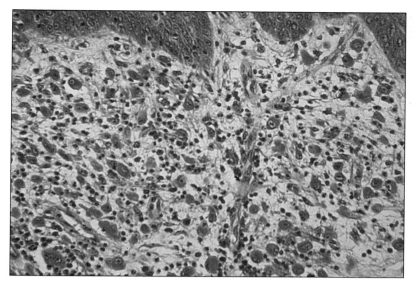

**FIGURE 8-48.** Multicentric reticulohistiocytosis, microscopic view of skin nodule. Dermal infiltrate of mononuclear histiocytes admixed with neutrophils and lymphocytes are characteristic of an early skin lesion (hematoxylin and eosin, X165). With time, more multinucleate histiocytes are evident with less neutrophilic and lymphocytic inflammation. The histologic appearance of the synovial infiltrates is the same as in the skin.

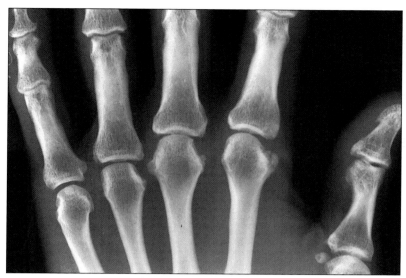

**FIGURE 8-49.** Wilson's disease. The radiograph is from a 39-year-old man with ataxia, tremor, and dysarthria. Kayser-Fleischer rings were present on ophthalmologic examination. Degenerative changes were present in multiple joints. Several joints, including the metacarpophalangeal joints, were surrounded by small ossicles, characteristic of Wilson's disease. (*Courtesy of* Thomas H. Berquist, MD.)

# References

1. Varga J, Wohlgethan JR: The clinical and biochemical spectrum of hereditary amyloidosis. *Semin Arthritis Rheum* 1988, 18:14.

2. WHO-IUIS Nomenclature Subcommittee: Nomenclature of amyloid and amyloidosis. *Bull World Health Organ* 1993, 71:105–108.

3. Lakhanpal S, Li CY, Gertz MA, Kyle RA, Hunder GG: Synovial fluid analysis for diagnosis of amyloid arthropathy. *Arthritis Rheum* 1987, 30:419–423.

4. David HG, Bridgman SA, Davies SC, *et al.*: The shoulder in sickle-cell disease. *J Bone Joint Surg Br* 1993, 75:538–545.

5. Reynolds J: The skull and spine. *Semin Roentgenol* 1987, 22:168–175.

6. Bassett ML, Halliday JW, Powell LW: Value of hepatic iron measurements in early hemochromatosis and determination of the critical iron level associated with fibrosis. *Hepatology* 1986, 6:24–29.

7. Ludwig J, Batts KP, Moyer TP, *et al.*: Liver biopsy diagnosis of homozygous hemochromatosis: a diagnostic algorithm. *Mayo Clin Proc* 1993, 68:263–267.

8. Feder JN, Gnirke A, Thomas W, *et al.*: A novel MHC class I-like gene is mutated in patients with hereditary haemochromatosis. *Nat Genet* 1996, 13:399–408.

9. Martinez-Lavin M: Hypertrophic osteoarthropathy. *Curr Opin Rheumatol* 1997, 9:83–86.

10. Bentley D, Moore A, Shwachman H: Finger clubbing: a quantitative survey by analysis of the shadowgraph. *Lancet* 1976, 2:164–167.

11. Bentley D, Cline J: Estimation of clubbing by analysis of shadowgraph. *Br Med J* 1970, 3:43.

12. Vazquez-Abad D, Pineda C, Martinez-Lavin M: Digital clubbing: a numerical assessment of the deformity. *J Rheumatol* 1989, 16:518–520.

13. Sly RM, Ghazanshahi S, Buranakul B, *et al.*: Objective assessment for digital clubbing in Caucasian, Negro, and Oriental subjects. *Chest* 1973, 64:687–689.

14. Cohen MD, Harrington TM, Ginsburg WW: Osteoid osteoma: 95 cases and a review of the literature. *Semin Arthritis Rheum* 1983, 12:265–281.

15. Snarr JW, Abell MR, Martel W: Lymphofollicular synovitis with osteoid osteoma. *Radiology* 1973, 106:557–560.

16. Jones BC, Sundaram M, Kransdorf MJ: Synovial sarcoma: MR imaging findings in 34 patients. *AJR Am J Roentgenol* 1993, 161:827–830.

17. Berquist TH, Ehman RL, King BF, *et al.*: Value of MR imaging in differentiating benign from malignant soft-tissue masses: Study of 95 lesions. *AJR Am J Roentgenol* 1990, 155:1251–1255.

18. Kyle V, Hazleman BL: The thyroid. *Clin Rheum Dis* 1981, 7:711–722.

19. Totemchokchyakarn K, Ball GV: Sarcoid arthropathy. *Bull Rheum Dis* 1997, 46:3–5.

20. Ginsburg WW, O'Duffy JD: Multicenter reticulohistocytosis. In: *Textbook of Rheumatology*. Edited by WN Kelly, ED Harris, S Ruddy, CB Sledge. Philadelphia: WB Saunders; 1997.

21. Ginsburg WW, Morris JL, Huston KA: Multicentric reticulohistiocytosis: response to alkylating agents in six patients. *Ann Intern Med* 1989, 111:384–388.

# A

Abdominal fat aspirate, 8.3f
Acetabular dysplasia, 2.12f
Acidosis, in osteomalacia, 6.8f
Acquired immunodeficiency syndrome, vasculitis-complicating, 4.29f
Acrolysis, 3.20f
Acromegaly, 8.1
  of hand, 8.16f
  in secondary osteoarthritis, 2.8f
  of shoulder, 8.16f
Acrosclerosis, in scleroderma, 3.20f
Adaptive devices, for osteoarthritis, 2.13f
Addison's disease, 3.16f
Adrenal hemorrhage, bilateral, 3.16f
Alendronate
  for osteoporosis, 6.6f
  for Paget's disease of bone, 6.13f
Alopecia, in systemic lupus erythematosus, 3.3f, 3.5f
Ambulatory assists, for osteoarthritis, 2.13f
American College of Rheumatology, criteria for remission of rheumatoid arthritis, 1.5f
American Rheumatism Association, revised diagnostic criteria for, 1.2f
Amyloid, classification of, 8.2f
Amyloidosis
  classification of, 8.2f
  clinical manifestations of, 8.1
  manifestations of, 8.3–8.5f
  secondary, 1.28f
    with shoulder pad sign, 1.27f
Analgesics, 2.2, 2.13f
Angiogenesis, in rheumatoid arthritis, 1.7f
Angiography
  for ocular vasculitis, 4.36f
  in Takayasu's arteritis, 4.20f, 4.21f
Angiitis, 4.1
Ankylosing spondylitis
  bamboo spine in, 5.14f
  bilateral sacroiliitis in, 5.11f
  clinical features of, 5.7–5.10f
  definition of, 5.1
  diagnostic criteria for, 5.6f
  early symptoms of, 5.7f
  hip and shoulder involvement in, 5.9–5.10f
  HLA-B27 testing in, 5.17f
  HLA-B27-positive and -negative patients with, 5.16f
  imaging evaluation of, 5.12–5.13f
  inflammation in, 5.13f
  sites of, 5.7f
  laboratory evaluation for, 5.16–5.17f
  management principles for, 5.18f
  prevalence studies of, 5.4f
  radiographic assessment of, 5.11–5.15f
  reactive bony sclerosis in, 5.15f
  recalcitrant enthesitis and synovitis in, 5.18f
  sacroiliac joint pain in, 5.9f
  spinal fracture in, 5.14f
  survival and familial aggregation of, 5.15–5.17f
  tenderness and decreased mobility in, 5.8–5.9f
  treatment of, 5.18f

undifferentiated spondyloarthropathies in, 5.23f
  uveitis in, 5.10f, 5.18f
Antibiotics, 5.21f
Anticentromere, 3.2
Anticoagulants, 3.19f
Anticonvulsants, 6.3f
Antigen presentation, major histocompatibility complex in, 1.6f
Anti-inflammatory agents, 2.2. *See also* Nonsteroidal anti-inflammatory drugs; *specific agents*
Anti-Jo1, 3.2
Antimalarials
  for ankylosing spondylitis, 5.18f
  for drug-induced lupus, 3.13f
  retinal lesions with, 3.14f
  for RS3PE syndrome, 1.45f
  for systemic lupus erythematosus, 3.1
Antimyeloperoxidase antineutrophil cytoplasmic antibodies, 4.12f
Antineutrophil cytoplasmic antibodies
  Churg-Strauss syndrome and, 4.12f
  pathogenetic mechanisms of, 4.5f
  in vasculitis, 4.4f
  in Wegener's granulomatosis, 4.14f
Antinuclear antibody testing, 3.10f
Antiphospholipid syndrome, 3.1
  clinical associations of, 3.15f
  clinical features of, 3.15–3.18f
  diagnostic criteria of, 3.15f
  treatment of, 3.19f
Antirheumatic drugs, 1.32f
Anti-ribonucleoprotein antibodies, 3.26f
Anti-ribonucleoprotein (RNP), 3.2
Anti-ribonucleoprotein (RNP) disease, 3.2
Anti-Ro, 3.2
Anti-Ro antibodies
  in lupus profundus, 3.6f
  in subacute cutaneous lupus erythematosus, 3.6f
  in systemic lupus erythematosus, 3.1
Anti-Scl 70, 3.2
AOSD. *See* Still's disease, adult-onset
Apatite crystal deposition, 2.9f
Arterial disease, sclerodermal, 3.22f
Arteritis. *See* Giant cell arteritis; Takayasu's arteritis
Arthralgia, in cryoglobulinemia, 4.25f
Arthritis. *See also* Osteoarthritis; Polyarthritis; Reactive arthritis; Rheumatoid arthritis; Septic arthritis
  chronic, muscle atrophy in, 1.19f
  Gaucher's disease with, 8.18f
  multicentric reticulohistiocytosis in, 8.18–8.19f
  osseous lesions in chronic sarcoidosis with, 8.17f
  psoriatic, 5.2
  in Sjögren's syndrome, 1.1
  skin nodules in, 8.18f
  systemic disease with, 8.1–8.19
  treatment of, 5.2
  Wilson's disease with, 8.19f
Arthritis mutilans, 8.2, 8.18f
  of hands, 1.15f
Arthrography, Baker's cyst, 1.20f

Arthropathy
  in amyloidosis, 8.5f
  with hemochromatosis, 8.8f
Arthroscopy
  of Baker's cyst, 1.20f
  of knee synovitis, 1.19f
Articular cartilage
  fibrous architecture of, 1.8f
  lack of in secondary osteoarthritis, 2.11f
Articular fracture, 2.8f
Articular synovial histology, 1.3f
Aspirin
  for antiphospholipid syndrome, 3.19f
  for juvenile rheumatoid arthritis, 1.37f
  for rheumatoid arthritis, 1.32f
Atlantoaxial subluxation, with basilar invagination, 1.21f
Autoantibody disease, with drug-induced lupus, 3.13f
Autoantibody testing, 3.2
Autoimmune myositis, 3.1
Avascular necrosis, 6.1
  of bone, with drug-induced lupus, 3.14f
  etiologies of, 6.13f
  osteomalacia simulating, 6.10f
  radiographic features of, 6.14f
  in sickle cell disease, 8.7f
  staging of, 6.13f
Azathioprine
  for reactive arthritis, 5.21f
  for Wegener's granulomatosis, 4.35f

# B

Bacterial arthritis
  changes in, 7.3f
  characteristic findings of, 7.4f
  differential diagnosis of, 7.2f
Bacterial infections, in HLA-B27-associated reactive arthritis, 5.21f
Baker's cyst
  arthrogram of, 1.20f
  arthroscopy of, 1.20f
  magnetic resonance image of, 1.20f
  in rheumatoid arthritis, 1.20f
Bamboo spine, 5.14f
Band keratopathy, 1.35f, 1.36f
Basilar invagination
  atlantoaxial subluxation with, 1.21f
  magnetic resonance image of, 1.22f
Behçet's disease
  anterior uveitis with hypopyon, 4.20f
  coil embolization in, 4.19f
  diagnostic criteria for, 4.18f
  magnetic resonance imaging in, 4.19f
  pulmonary aneurysms in, 4.18f
  vena cava thrombosis complicating, 4.19f
Bisphosphonates, 6.6f
Blue sclerae, 6.15f
Bone
  bowing deformity of, 6.12f
  diseases of, 6.1
  impaired resorption of, 6.1

Lymphadenopathy, in Sjögren's syndrome, 1.1
Lymphoma, grade IV diffuse large cell, 8.13f

# M

Maculopapular erythematous rash, 7.4f
Magnetic resonance imaging
  in amyloidosis, 8.4f
  of Baker's cyst, 1.20f
  in Behçet's disease, 4.19f
  for osteoarthritis, 2.4f
  of septic arthritis, 7.3f
  in Takayasu's arteritis, 4.21f
Malignancy
  myositis and dermatomyositis of, 3.1
  vasculitides associated with, 4.30–4.31f
Malignant lesions, 8.1
Marfan's syndrome, 6.16f
Marginal erosions, in rheumatoid arthritis of hands,
  1.12f
MCTD. See Connective tissue disease, mixed
Meningococcal infection, disseminated, 7.7f
Meniscectomy, 2.8f
Metabolic disorders, 1.2f
Metacarpophalangeal joints
  arthroplasty for rheumatoid arthritis, 1.14f
  hyperextension of, 6.15f
  replacement of in advanced rheumatoid arthritis,
    1.15f
  swelling of, 1.10f
  swelling of in early rheumatoid arthritis, 1.9f
  ulnar deviation at, 1.11f
  volar subluxation of in rheumatoid arthritis, 1.12f
Metatarsal resection, 1.16f
Metatarsophalangeal subluxation, 1.18f
Methotrexate
  for juvenile rheumatoid arthritis, 1.37f
  in osteoporosis, 6.3f
  for reactive arthritis, 5.21f
Methylprednisolone acetate, 2.13f
MHC. See Human major histocompatibility complex
Microaneurysms, in polyarteritis nodosa, 4.9f
Micrognathia, 1.34f
Microscopic polyangiitis, 4.3f
  differential diagnosis of, 4.10f
  fibrinoid crescent in, 4.11f
  glomerulonephritis in, 4.11f
  outcome of, 4.33f
  versus polyarteritis nodosa, 4.1
  prognostic factors in, 4.32f
  pulmonary infiltrates in, 4.11f
  treatment of, 4.34f
Microscopic polyarteritis. See Microscopic polyangiitis
Mineralization inhibitor, 6.8f
Morning stiffness, 5.1
Morphea, 3.1
  superficial, in scleroderma, 3.21f
Motor nerve palsy, 4.16f
Mouth ulcers
  in Behçet's disease, 4.18f
  in lupus, 3.4f
Multicentric reticulohistiocytosis
  hand radiograph of, 8.18f
  skin nodules of, 8.18–8.19f
  with symmetric seronegative polyarthritis, 8.18f
Multi-infarct dementia, 3.16f
Muscle atrophy, 1.19f
Muscle biopsy, for virus-associated vasculitis, 4.29f
Muscle-strengthening exercises, 2.13f
Myalgia, 4.25f

Mycobacterium leprae, 7.9f
Mycobacterium tuberculosis, 7.5–7.6f
Myelofibrosis, 8.8f
Myeloproliferative disorders, 8.8f
Myopathies, idiopathic inflammatory, 3.26–3.27f
  classification of, 3.23f
  clinical features of, 3.23f
  diagnostic criteria for, 3.23f
  types of, 3.24–3.27f
Myositis
  characteristic features of, 3.2
  classifications of, 3.1
  in rheumatoid arthritis, 1.26f

# N

Nail changes, 3.4f
Nail-fold capillaroscopy, 3.21f
Nail-fold capillary lesions, 3.25f
Nail-fold vasculitis, 3.4f
Naproxen, 1.32f
Naproxen sodium, 1.37f
Necrotizing angiitis, acute, 4.23f
Neisseria meningitidis infection, 7.7f
Neonatal lupus erythematosus syndrome
  fetal heart block in, 3.12f
  skin rash of, 3.11f
Neoplastic joint lesions, 8.13–816f
Nephritis, 3.7–3.9f
Nephrotic syndrome, 3.7f
Neuropathic joint, 7.8–7.9f
Nodular tenosynovitis, rheumatoid, 1.13f
Nodulosis, 1.22f
Nonsteroidal anti-inflammatory drugs (NSAIDs)
  for adult-onset Still's disease, 1.44f
  for ankylosing spondylitis, 5.18f
  for arthritis, 5.2
  for drug-induced lupus, 3.13f
  for juvenile rheumatoid arthritis, 1.37f
  for osteoarthritis, 2.13f
  for reactive arthritis, 5.21f
  for rheumatoid arthritis, 1.31f, 1.32f
  for RS3PE syndrome, 1.45f

# O

Obesity, in secondary osteoarthritis, 2.8f
Occupational therapy
  for juvenile rheumatoid arthritis, 1.37f
  for rheumatoid arthritis, 1.31f
Ochronosis, 2.8f
Ocular vasculitis, 4.36f
Olecranon bursa, aspirate from, 2.17f
Onycholysis, thumb nail, 5.20f
Oral ulcers. See Mouth ulcers
Orbital pseudotumor, 4.16f
Orcein staining, 4.23f
Osler-Weber-Rendu disease, 3.22f
Osteoarthritis
  adjuncts to pharmacologic therapy in, 2.13f
  classification of, 2.2f
  clinical features of, 2.1
  clinical management of, 2.1
  diagnostic methods for, 2.4–2.8f
  end-stage skeletal changes in, 2.12f
  epidemiology of, 2.1
  examination for, 2.2–2.4f
  joint inflammation with, 2.1
  management of, 2.2, 2.13f
  pathology of, 2.1

  premature, 6.10f
  primary, 2.2f
  secondary
    causes of, 2.1, 2.8–2.9f
    skeletal changes in, 2.9–2.12f
  symptoms of, 2.1, 2.2–2.4f
  therapy for, 2.13f
Osteoblasts, 6.3f
Osteoclasts
  giant, 6.10f
  in hyperparathyroidism, 6.7f
Osteoid osteoma, 8.14f
  sites of involvement of, 8.14f
Osteomalacia, 6.1
  causes of, 6.8f
  radiologic features of, 6.9–6.10f
Osteonecrosis, 6.1
  etiology of, 6.13f
  femoral head, 8.1
  radiographic features of, 6.14f
  in secondary osteoarthritis, 2.8f
  staging of, 6.13f
Osteopenia
  diffuse, 6.8f
  in untreated gout, 2.19f
Osteopetrosis, forms of, 6.1
Osteophytes, 2.1
  beak-type, 8.8f
Osteoporosis, 6.1
  bone mineral density measurement in, 6.5–6.6f
  bone remodeling unit in, 6.3f
  clinical and radiologic features of, 6.3–6.5f
  diagnostic criteria for, 6.5f
  drugs as secondary causes of, 6.3f
  epidemiology and pathogenesis of, 6.2–6.3f
  fractures in, 6.4–6.5f
  histopathology of, 6.4f
  risk factors for, 6.2f
  secondary causes of, 6.2f
  treatment of, 6.6
Osteosclerosis
  in fluorosis, 6.16
  of skull and pelvis, 6.17f

# P

Pachydermoperiostitis, 8.12f
Paget's disease of bone, 6.1
  clinical features and complications of, 6.11f
  histopathology of, 6.10–6.11f
  radiographic features of, 6.11–6.12f
  in secondary osteoarthritis, 2.8f
  treatment of, 6.13f
Pain, weight-bearing, 2.2f
Palpable purpura
  histopathologic appearance of, 4.7f
  in Sjögren's syndrome, 1.41f
Pamidronate, 6.13f
Pannus
  formation of with synovial hypertrophy, 1.30f
  invasive, 1.30f
Parathyroid gland, 6.7f
  adenoma of, 6.7f
Parotid gland enlargement, in Sjögren's syndrome,
  1.40f, 3.13f
Parvovirus, 7.4f
Patellar ballottement, 2.4f
Patellofemoral joint
  osteoarthritis of, 2.9f
  space of, 2.9f, 2.10f

Pathergy test, 4.18f
Pathologic fracture, 6.12f
Patient education, for osteoporosis, 6.6f
Pelvis
  osteosclerosis of, 6.17f
  radiograph of in Paget's disease of bone, 6.12f
D-Penicillamine, 5.18f
Pericarditis
  constrictive rheumatoid, 1.26f
  in juvenile rheumatoid arthritis, 1.36f
  in rheumatoid arthritis, 1.25f, 1.26f
Peripheral neuropathy, 4.25f
*Peromyscus leucopus*, 7.9f
Pes planus, 1.17f, 1.18f
Phospholipid-protein complexes, antibodies against,
  3.1
Photosensitivity, 3.6f
Physical therapy
  for ankylosing spondylitis, 5.18f
  for juvenile rheumatoid arthritis, 1.37f
  for osteoporosis, 6.6f
  for rheumatoid arthritis, 1.31f
Pigmented villonodular synovitis, 8.14f, 8.15f
Plasma exchange
  for cryoglobulinemia with hepatitis C virus, 4.35f
  for drug-induced lupus, 3.13f
Plasmapheresis, 3.19f
Pleural effusions, 1.24f
Pleural fluids, 1.25f
Pneumoconiosis, 1.25f
Pneumonitis, interstitial, 1.24f, 125.f
POEMS, 8.11f
Polyarteritis, 4.34f
Polyarteritis nodosa, 1.26f, 4.3f
  associated with hematologic malignancies, 4.30f
  classification criteria for, 4.2f
  clinical features of, 4.6–4.8f
  differential diagnosis of, 4.10f
  gastrointestinal manifestations of, 4.8–4.10f
  hepatitis B virus-related, 4.10f
  incidence of, 4.6f
  versus microscopic polyangiitis, 4.1
  outcome of, 4.33f
  prognostic factors in, 4.32f
  purpura in, 4.7f
  renal involvement in, 4.8f
  skin nodules in, 4.7f
  subcutaneous nodule and necrosis in, 4.32f
  vasculitis associated with, 4.31f
  viral infections with, 4.28f
Polyarthritis. *See also* Juvenile chronic polyarthritis
  adult-onset, 1.1
  of adult-onset Still's disease, 1.43f
  amyloidosis in, 8.1
  differential diagnosis of, 1.2f
  initial evaluation of patient with, 1.4f
  multicentric reticulohistiocytosis with, 8.18f
Polyarticular disease, 1.34f
Polychondritis, 3.27f
Polycyclic articular course, 1.1
Polycythemia vera, 8.8f
Polymyositis, 3.25f
Popliteal cyst, 2.8f
Port's disease, 7.5f
Prednisolone, 2.13f
Prednisone
  for RS3PE syndrome, 1.45f
  for vasculitis, 4.34f
Premature sex hormone deficiencies, 6.2f

Protrusio acetabuli, 6.10f
Pseudoarthrosis, 5.14f
Pseudogout, 2.1
  in hypothyroidism, 8.2
  in secondary osteoarthritis, 2.9f
  treatment of, 2.19–2.21f
Psoriasis
  clinical features of, 5.22f
  definition of, 5.2
  histology of, 5.21f
Psoriasis digit, 5.20f
Psoriatic arthritis, 5.22f
Psychologic support, 2.2
Pubic insufficiency fractures, 6.9f
Pulmonary arteries
  aneurysms of in Behçet's disease, 4.18f
  Takayasu's arteritis of, 4.21f
Pulmonary embolism, with antiphospholipid
  syndrome, 3.18f
Pulmonary fibrosis, 1.24f, 1.25f
  polymyositis with, 3.25f
  in scleroderma, 3.21f
Pulmonary infiltrates, 4.11f
Pulmonary metastatic osteogenic sarcoma,
  8.12f
Pulmonary nodules
  in rheumatoid arthritis, 1.25f
  in Wegener's granulomatosis, 4.15f
Pulmonary system, rheumatoid arthritis involving,
  1.24–1.25f
Pulmonary tuberculosis, with drug-induced lupus,
  3.14f
Pupil, irregular due to synechiae, 1.35f
Radiography, indications for, 2.8f

# R

Radius
  bowing of in Paget's disease of bone, 6.12f
  chondrocalcinosis of, 2.21f
Rash
  of adult-onset Still's disease, 1.44f
  butterfly, 3.2f
  in dermatomyositis, 3.24f
  facial, 7.5f
  in neonatal lupus erythematosus syndrome, 3.11f
  in systemic lupus erythematosus, 3.1
  in systemic-onset juvenile rheumatoid arthritis, 1.36f
Raynaud's esophageal dysmotility, 3.19f, 3.22f
Raynaud's phenomenon
  in cryoglobulinemia, 4.25f
  in scleroderma, 3.19f
  in Sjögren's syndrome, 1.1
Raynaud's syndrome, 3.1
Reactive arthritis
  definition of, 5.1–5.2
  diagnosis of, 5.20f
  extra-articular features of, 5.1–5.2
  infections in, 5.2
  postenteritic, 5.2
  presentation of, 5.19f
  treatment of, 5.21f
Reactive arthropathies, 2.9f
Reactive bony sclerosis, 5.15f
Rehabilitative interventions, for juvenile rheumatoid
  arthritis, 1.37f
Reiter's syndrome, 5.2, 5.19f
Remitting seronegative synovitis with pitting edema
  (RS3PE) syndrome
  clinical features of, 1.45f

hand and foot involvement in, 1.45f
  with Still's disease, 1.1
  treatment of, 1.45f
Renal biopsy
  in cryoglobulinemia, 4.27f
  for Henoch-Schönlein purpura, 4.24f, 4.25f
  immunofluorescence, 4.25f
  in scleroderma, 3.22f
Renal pathology
  in systemic lupus erythematosus, 3.8f
  World Health Organization classification of, 3.8f
Renal vasculitis, 4.8f
Reticulohistiocytosis, multicentric, 8.2
Retinal lesions, antimalarial-induced, 3.14f
Retinophotography, 4.36f
Rheumatic disease, with iritis, 5.23f
Rheumatoid arthritis. *See also* Juvenile rheumatoid
    arthritis
  aggressive, early, 1.10f
  American College of Rheumatology criteria for
    remission of, 1.5f
  American Rheumatism Association revised criteria
    for diagnosis of, 1.2f
  amyloidosis in, 8.1
  angiogenesis in, 1.7f
  Baker's cyst in, 1.20f
  bone scan of feet and hands in, 1.10f
  causes of, 1.1
  cervical spine involvement in, 1.22f
  clinical course of joint disease in, 1.5f
  clinical features of
    extra-articular, 1.22–1.28f
    in joints, 1.9–1.22f
  diagnostic criteria of, 1.2f–1.4f
  of elbow, 1.15f
  epidemiology of, 1.4f, 1.5f
  of foot, knee, hip, neck, and spine, 1.16–1.22f
  gender role in, 1.1
  genetic predisposition for, 1.1
  hip disease in, 1.21f
  homunculus for recording joint disease in,
    1.9f
  human major histocompatibility complex in,
    1.6f
  incidence of, 1.1
  laboratory features and synovial histology of,
    1.28–1.30f
  laboratory features of, 1.28f
  management of, 1.31f
  mortality in, 1.5f
  ocular involvement of, 1.24f
  onset of symptoms of, 1.1
  pathogenesis of, 1.6f–1.8f
  pathophysiologic stages of, 1.8f
  polycyclic articular course of, 1.1
  related conditions of, 1.38–1.45f
  remission criteria for, 1.5f
  in secondary amyloidosis, 1.27f, 1.28f
  in secondary osteoarthritis, 2.9f
  of shoulder, 1.16f
  Steinbrocker functional classification of, 1.5f
  synovial inflammation process in, 1.7f
  synovitis in, 1.30f
  systemic
    constitutional symptoms and signs of, 1.22f
    manifestations of, 1.1
  treatment of, 1.31–1.32
    principles of, 1.31f
  vasculitis associated with, 4.31–4.32f